NEUROGENIC
COMMUNICATION DISORDERS:
LIFE STORIES AND THE NARRATIVE SELF

NEUROGENIC COMMUNICATION DISORDERS:
LIFE STORIES AND THE NARRATIVE SELF

Barbara B. Shadden, Ph.D.
Fran Hagstrom, Ph.D.
Patricia R. Koski, Ph.D.

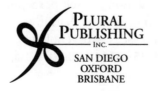

PLURAL
PUBLISHING
INC.

SAN DIEGO
OXFORD
BRISBANE

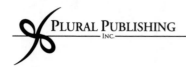
PLURAL PUBLISHING
INC.

5521 Ruffin Road
San Diego, CA 92123

e-mail: info@pluralpublishing.com
Web site: http://www.pluralpublishing.com

49 Bath Street
Abingdon, Oxfordshire OX14 1EA
United Kingdom

Typeset in 10½/13 Garamond by Flanagan's Publishing Services, Inc.
Printed in the United States of America by Bang Printing

Library of Congress Cataloging-in-Publication Data:
Shadden, Barbara B. (Barbara Bennett)
  Neurogenic communication disorders : life stories and the narrative self / Barbara B.
Shadden, Fran Hagstrom, and Patricia R. Koski.
      p. ; cm.
  Includes bibliographical references.
  ISBN-13: 978-1-59756-136-5 (alk. paper)
  ISBN-10: 1-59756-136-3 (alk. paper)
  1. Nervous system–Degeneration–Patients–Language. 2. Aphasic persons–Language.
3. Communicative disorders–Psychological aspects. 4. Autobiographical memory. 5.
Memory disorders. 6. Self-presentation. 7. Self perception. 8. Patients' writings–
History and criticism. 9. Discourse analysis, Narrative.
  [DNLM: 1. Neurodegenerative Diseases–psychology. 2. Aphasia–psychology. 3.
Narration. 4. Self Concept. WL 359 S524n 2007] I. Hagstrom, Fran. II. Koski, Patricia R.
III. Title.
  RC365.S43 2007
  616.8–dc22
                                                                    2007050050

Contents

Preface

Quality of life as an outcome has become prominent in health care and disability research in the past two decades. Similarly, life participation and daily functioning have become targets for interventions. Despite these facts, it is clear that the nature and severity of specific disorders rarely predict quality of life outcomes with accuracy. Nowhere is this more apparent than in considering outcomes for persons living with neurogenic communication disorders (such as those associated with stroke, dementia, amyotrophic lateral sclerosis [ALS], and Parkinson's disease).

As authors of this text, we began with a shared awareness of the profound impact of neurogenic communication disorders on those living with such disorders and with an interest in attempting to understand better those factors that might better predict broader quality of life outcomes. Our professional disciplines of speech-language pathology, sociology, and psychology each offered important theoretical constructs that could be applied to these efforts.

In our discussions and early writings, two concepts emerged as having explanatory power. The first was the idea of self or identity or personhood. Self and related concepts figure prominently in the theoretical literatures of many disciplines, and an exploration of self is characteristic of postmodern inquiries. We all maintain a belief in a sense of unvarying self, and challenges to this belief (internally or from the people and environments around us) may explain some of the variation in outcomes for persons with acquired neurological disorders.

Second, as we explored the impact of various disorders on a person's sense of self, it was apparent that we had to consider the way in which self is constantly being negotiated in different social contexts. As suggested by many theorists, self is socially mediated, and communication is a primary tool used to present and alter representations of who we are. Thus, self is a narrative construction in the broadest sense. While these concepts are not uniquely ours, what we realized was how profoundly an impairment of this communicative tool can and will alter self presentation and perception. It is not surprising that there is limited research on aspects of self in persons with neurogenic communication disorders. After all, researchers typically rely on narrative, on the written and spoken words of individuals, in order to study self and identity.

Sarbin (1986b) has stated that narrative is a root metaphor for human experience. At a basic level, narrative can be defined as telling stories. However, it is much more than that. Narrative is a critical cognitive tool for meaning-making in our lives. In fact, our everyday actions and utterances make sense only in the context of the various stories of our lives. Although Ricoeur (1992) suggests that lives are lived, and stories are told, he also notes that selves are constructed in interaction with others through behaviors and shared narratives. Indeed, in one sense, our stories become our identities. Thus we turned to the concept of narrative self as a guiding theoretical framework for our exploration of the profound and diverse life consequences of neurogenic communication disorders.

In addition to this concept of narrative self, we use the terms *life story* and *storying of self* throughout this text. However, we do not mean to suggest that self maintenance and renegotiation is dependent upon the actual telling of one's story (although that can be important in the sharing of illness narratives). Instead, we suggest that the storying of self also involves those multiple small moments of communication and interaction throughout each day that collectively impart a sense of who we are. It is these many small acts, as well as our shared stories, that are jeopardized by neurogenic communication disorders. If our premises are accurate, improving speech and language skills is an important but not sufficient target for interventions. Instead, we must find ways to understand better the impact of impaired communication skills on narrative self and those treatments that will allow us to address issues of narrative self more directly.

Once we adopted the concept of narrative self for our investigations of the impact of neurogenic communication disorders, we continued to grapple with the idea of self, as used and defined differently in our various disciplines. While there are many models of self in the current theoretical literature, we chose to focus on the specific populations we had targeted. As a result, we were able to settle on a four-domain framework for self that was conceptually rich enough to encompass our different perspectives. This framework allowed us to speak and write the same language with greater breadth and hopefully multidisciplinary insight than we had at the outset.

Our conceptual framework also evolved considerably as we explored the life stories and experiences of the key people who have informed our understanding of aspects of narrative self in the context of impaired communication and whose words are shared in this text. What began as an inquiry into aphasia was expanded fairly rapidly to considerations of other adult-onset neurogenic communication disorders, as each of us was drawn into the lives of individuals living with ALS, Parkinson's disease, and dementia. As we recognized the value of our perspectives when broadened in this manner, we were able to test our theoretical musings against the realities we were encountering, grounding our work qualitatively in a range of experiences and communications with individuals representing all of these domains of impairment.

We turned last to issues of clinical practice as informed by a focus on narrative self in multiple domains. We recognized a need to do some translational writing that allowed theory and life story to evolve into a meaningful, clinically useful process. Our intent was to make certain that the clinician—the person in the trenches with those living with neurogenic communication disorders—be provided with guidance as to how to proceed. Further, we always planned to return at the end to one of the nagging points of debate along the way—how to reconcile our multidimensioned model of self with the belief that an important and persistent sense of self carries us successfully through the life span, even when the communication critically needed for storying one's life is so compromised that it is no longer a functional tool.

Ironically, this plan did not acknowledge the fact that each of us had indeed engaged in an individual, as well as collective, meaning-making process in crafting this work. As we tried to provide an integrated perspective concerning what narrative self means in practice, we were failing to give voice to our unique insights as authors. Also, while we felt a need to validate our work by providing clinical guidance, we recognized that this need was rooted in the very impairment-based model we were trying to leave behind. Realistically, the conceptual framework we have developed is still in its infancy as applied to neurogenic communication disorders. As a result, the final section of the text is now enriched with three different perspectives on how we must move forward to support the ongoing storying of self for those living with these, and other, communication disorders.

Neurogenic Communication Disorders and the Narrative Self is organized around four sections, each of which has a targeted role in developing the ideas we present in this text. This sectional structure evolved over time as segments were written and modified to link theory to life stories and situations.

Section I establishes our framework for understanding the impact of neurogenic communication disorders on the narrative self. Chapter 1 introduces basic premises and a guiding theoretical framework. Chapter 2 presents a brief description of the specific neurogenic disorders that will be addressed in Section III. This description compares and contrasts specific dimensions of these disorders in order to establish a foundation for understanding the differential effects on self construction.

Section II explores in depth the interdisciplinary theoretical perspectives that inform this text. Each of the topics in Chapters 3 through 5 focuses on specific theoretical strands that collectively support the

model of narrative self we have developed: self, narrative processes (including life stories and illness narratives), and temporal/life span considerations.

In Section III, we describe challenges to narrative self associated with specific neurogenic communication disorders, focusing on impaired communication, impact on self, and narrative processes and consequences. We have made no attempt to address every conceivable neurogenic communication disorder. Instead, we have selected four disorders, amyotrophic lateral sclerosis, Parkinson's disease (PD), stroke-related aphasia, and dementia, based on the distinctive characteristics associated with speech production, language, and cognition outlined in Chapter 2. Our selection of disorders has also been influenced by our personal experiences with individuals living with these challenges. Therefore, aspects of the life stories of one or more individuals are presented in Chapters 6 through 9 to illustrate our core concepts related to narrative self when particular facets of communication are disrupted.

In Section III, we have chosen to frame our ideas in part through the words and experiences of real people. In some instances, the life story information emerged from semistructured interviews with persons with the disorder, their significant others, or both. In other instances, information was obtained from e-mail correspondence with one of the authors, from written responses to semistructured questions, from observations in personal interactions as well as treatment or support groups, and from diaries. At all times, the themes in each chapter emerged from the comments and behaviors of these individuals. Thus one chapter might give life span and other temporal considerations focus, while another only mentions them in passing. In addition to life span considerations, other recurring themes include the time line for the progression of or recovery from the disorder, issues of control, agency, and competence, and the social contexts and people who contribute to the ongoing storying of self. Challenges for significant others are examined in each chapter, although much more needs to be written about the narrative self needs of these individuals.

Finally, in Section IV, Chapters 10 through 12 address the implications of our exploration of narrative self. In each of the closing chapters, there is consensus that those who study and/or work clinically with persons with neurogenic communication disorders and with their significant others must constantly ground their work in the larger narrative perspective of an individual's need to continue the storying of self, the socially-situated narrative that is the essence of human existence. While these chapters are oriented towards speech-language pathologists, the information here is relevant for all disciplines working with persons living with adult-onset neurological disorders and suggests research domains of interest. Chapter 10 places the theoretical strands of this book within the larger context of postmodern theory. Chapter 11 explores the implications of theory from a sociocultural perspective. Chapter 12 revisits key themes developed throughout the text and suggests ways in which clinical activities can be shifted to respond more directly to the challenge of supporting the work of narrative self.

To summarize, in this text we suggest that the social role of communication in sustaining narrative self is fundamental to human existence. Undoubtedly, we need more treatment approaches that fit "outside the box" of specific deficit management when working with those who have lost or have disrupted communication. But it is essential for all of us who seek to be a part of the lives of these individuals to recognize that clinical engagement itself is a narrative event. When we interact with persons with neurogenic communication disorders, we become partners in the narrative processes that support the evolving sense of self or identity (Hinckley, 2007). It is our responsibility to understand these processes, as well as our role in and contribution to the communicative interaction that helps (or hinders) the person's moving on with life. We must learn to listen and provide narrative understanding for our clients and their significant others, avoiding the trap of focusing exclusively on speech-language deficits to the exclusion of their impact on narrative self.

We welcome readers from all disciplines and hope our preliminary theoretical work will provide the impetus for future research and interventions. Most of all, we hope that each reader will be able to use some part of this information to improve the quality of life of persons living with neurogenic communication disorders.

Acknowledgments

This text would not exist without the generous sharing of the many people whose lives have been touched by neurogenic communication disorders or who grapple daily with age-related changes in the life story. In fact, we probably would not have begun the journey to understanding narrative self without the experiences of two people in particular—*Harry Shadden* and *Steve Kressen*. In different ways, both men epitomize the fierce determination to retain a sense of self and to be recognized for who they are, despite impaired communication. Both also showed us the importance of considering self presentation in multiple domains—at the levels of personal biography, interactions and relationships with others, important life roles, and the broader social and cultural environment.

As our understanding of narrative self expanded, we expanded our work to other adult neurogenic disorders that affect communication, specifically Parkinson's disease and dementia. We are indebted to *Jerry Patnoe* and to *Flo Watkins* for guiding our work in this process.

Once committed to this project, we turned to clients, family, and friends to provide us with greater insight and to validate our theoretical perspectives or challenge our assumptions. The following list includes many who provided critical input and taught us the importance of maintaining a sense of narrative self despite unexpected disruptions in the life story. All three of us have learned and grown personally as well as professionally, thanks to the individuals named here. In addition to those named above, we offer many thanks to:

Wayne and Dottie Anderson

Penny and A. J. Ballard

Louisa Bennett

Linda and Jim Buckner

Sarah and Wade Burnside

Laura Cottern

Bruce and Emily Dippie

Jim Jackson and Barbara Taylor

Ruth Anne Kobleim

Sylvia Kressen

Judy and Buz Moxon

Dave and Jean Price

Jerry and Marie Putnam

Chris and Billie Simmons

Mike Smith

George and Sheryl White

Countless others also shaped our thinking and chose not to be recognized here.

We dedicate this book to
all of those whose voices guided us in this journey.

SECTION I

In this text, we suggest that the role of communication in supporting each individual's sense of self or identity must receive greater focus in research and in clinical practice. This is particularly true when a neurological disorder disrupts the well-established life stories of adults. We use Section I of this text to establish the foundation of or exploring the impact of such communication disorders on the process of sustaining a sense of self.

Chapter 1 introduces readers to the concept of narrative self and poses the question, "Why narrative self?" To answer this question, we first provide an overview of both the theoretical foundations for the concepts of narrative and self, as developed in the social sciences, as well as current clinical models that emphasize the social and functional context for understanding illness and disability. The chapter next presents the core constructs that will be used throughout the text, highlighting the ways in which self is dependent in part on narrative as a meaning making process and narrative as a social tool. We suggest that communication plays a pivotal role in the creation and revision of life narrative for all humans.

Essentially, we use Chapter 1 to build the case for using narrative self as a tool in our efforts to understand the impact of acquired neurogenic communication disorders. We believe that our collective perspectives from the disciplines of speech-language pathology, psychology, and sociology have allowed us to reshape current thinking about the interface between the storying of self and communication disorders that disrupt the act of storying. Thus, it is not that we have created a whole new theoretical base, but rather that we have merged disciplinary perspectives in a somewhat novel fashion.

In Chapter 2, we introduce the neurological conditions that create the communication disorders considered in this text. This is a cursory introduction at best, considering the wealth of material available on these topics. Our goal in this chapter is to provide the reader with an understanding of critical ways in which these disorders create similar challenges to narrative self, as well as important dimensions that distinguish each condition. To do so, we first elaborate on the importance of communication in self construction. Then two primary dimensions are considered in contrasting neurogenic communication disorders: (a) the onset and course of the disorder (disease progression) and (b) the communication aspects most affected. We suggest that the differences between these disorders can be understood, in part, by examining the degree to which each involves an underlying impairment of language, motor, or cognitive skills, as well as possible interface among these domains. We specifically explore connections between communication deficits and perceptions of self (internal or external) as well as the impact on health and illness narratives.

CHAPTER 1

Clinical Practices and the Narrative Self

What Is Narrative Self?

To begin this text, we ask, "What is narrative self?" To answer, we start with a brief vignette. On August 28, 2007, ABC News aired a Bob Woodruff special on "Senator's Road to Recovery," discussing the challenges faced by South Dakota senator Tim Johnson after a near fatal brain hemorrhage the year before. In an interview with Senator Johnson's wife, Woodruff asked, "Do you think he'll be able to walk perfectly again, do you think he'll be able to move his arm perfectly again?" His wife responded, "I don't really care, to be honest. I've got the Tim back that I fell in love with and that's all that matters to me." What Mrs. Johnson was saying was that the extent of her husband's physical recovery was not important as long as she knew she was sharing her life once again with the essential person, the core self of the man she originally knew and loved. Our goal in this text is to shed light on the impact of neurogenic communication disorders on this self.

Later in the same interview, Woodruff asked one of Johnson's physicians, "But you think, when people see him speak the way he does, a lot of people will think he can't

think?" And the physician acknowledged that might be true, even though Johnson's intelligence and competence remained unimpaired, along with his ability to carry on his job as a U.S. Senator. Why will some question Johnson's competence because of his altered communication, while his wife sees past these impairments to the person who is Tim Johnson?

So again we ask, what is *self*, and what is *narrative self*, which is the key concept addressed in this text? What is the self that embodies the Tim Johnson that his wife fell in love with? The concept should be relatively easy to define. Certainly, we use the term repeatedly throughout each day—myself, yourself, ourselves, herself. We refer to constructs such as self-concept, self-esteem, self-worth, self-indulgence, self-sustaining, and self-help, and seem to have no difficulty understanding the meaning of these words. A simple walk down the aisles of a bookstore will confirm the importance of self, as we see the hundreds and even thousands of self-help books on the shelves. Yet we stumble when we attempt to define the word self.

Reflect for a moment. We move through each day with a sense of who we are and with an intuitive belief that we have a relatively constant self or identity. Life would be extremely challenging if we did not have such a belief. We act and interact in ways that we feel are consistent with this inner self, even though most of us would be hard pressed to define that self if asked to do so. We know when we do things that are not consistent with our sense of self. Our perceived self is the product of an accumulation of life experiences and the meanings we have forged out of these experiences, the knowledge of our typical patterns of acting and reacting, our memories, the roles we play, our biographic realities, and our perceived status in the society.

Although we may feel that this self exists in a very private domain, it does not exist in a vacuum. The same words, actions, and interactions that confirm our persistent sense of a unified self are also received and responded to by others. On some level, we recognize that, when we communicate with others, we are making conscious or unconscious choices about which pieces of our self we will present, situated in the facts of our life, our interactions with others, our varied roles, and our place within society. In fact, these behaviors are what others use to identify us and to clarify how they should interact with us. This is self as socially situated or constructed. The responses of others are critical to our sense of ongoing self. They shape our sense of self by the responses they make to our behaviors and our words.

In our social interactions, others may comment on our behavior from the perspective of how consistent it is with the self they attribute to us. For example, with some surprise, a friend may say something like, "That is not like you to ask for help." A colleague may sarcastically state, "Well, you are the last person I thought would volunteer for this task." We also may be acknowledged and rewarded with positive recognition of acts that are consistent with whom we appear to be, as in "We knew we could count on you to step up and lead the group." If we are behaving in ways we believe to be consistent with our self or identity, and these behaviors are dismissed or devalued by others, we experience a threat to our sense of a continuous unified self. Sustained conflicts between our self perceptions and those of others can be deeply troubling, affecting quality of life in many ways.

What role does narrative play in this process of self creation and negotiation? We use the term narrative to capture the premise that humans make sense of their lives and experiences by creating stories that encapsulate our understanding. Thus, narrative is a cognitive process that reflects our selective understanding of our lives. Narrative also refers to the communicative exchanges through which we share aspects of our life stories. "The small and seemingly inconsequential, as well as the large and dramatic, pieces of life are woven together by the individual for self-understanding and for presentation to others" (Shadden & Hagstrom, 2007).

Thus, when we refer to narrative self throughout this text, we are targeting the role of narrative in self-creation, particularly the socially negotiated aspects of our sense of self. Narrative is thought-in-action, the acting out of pieces of our life story in communicative exchanges with others. Communication is critical in the sharing of narratives that validate and verify our sense of self, particularly when self is jeopardized by an event such as a neurological disorder. When we talk and interact, we are constantly communicating aspects of our self and life story. Others learn about us from the words we choose, the opinions we state, the snippets of our experiences we choose to share, even the responses we make to what others say and do.

When communication is disrupted in adult-onset neurological disorders, the life story is profoundly altered. It is human to wish to make sense of these alterations, to restore some kind of balance to the life story and to the sense of self. Typically, while we work through this process in our private reflections, we also rely on the responses of others as we share our modified stories and sense of self. This is where the concept of narrative self becomes so important. Ironically, the same neurological disorders disrupt the very communicative tools that we rely on for redefining who and what we are.

Our challenge is to explore how narrative self is jeopardized by neurogenic communication disorders and how individuals successfully and unsuccessfully attempt to maintain and/or renegotiate a sense of who we are. Our key premises are described in detail in Section II of this text. However, in the following sections of this chapter, we provide a brief overview of the theoretical foundations for these premises. We also define more explicitly the ways we will be using the terms self and narrative, how communication plays into the process of narrative self construction, and why neurogenic communication disorders pose such fundamental threats to narrative self. There will be some redundancy in our discussions, because we recognize some of these concepts may be unfamiliar.

Theoretical Foundations

Our path to a focus on narrative self draws heavily on current theory in the social sciences, theory that explores the nature and formulation of a sense of self and the narrative aspects of our lives, with emphasis on the role of social interactions in self construction. Our path is also grounded in evolving clinical perspectives on person

and function, the models that are being used today to expand our understanding of living with any of the disorders described in this text. Each of these theoretical foundations is discussed briefly in the following sections, before we frame the core concepts that will inform this text.

Perspectives on Self and Narrative

It is difficult to pinpoint where interest in narrative, self, and narrative self emerged historically, as the roots of these concepts are found in diverse disciplines. Exploration of self has its centuries old origins in philosophy and in religious studies. More recent perspectives on dimensions of *self* can be traced to the work of theorists such as James (1950) in the early 20th century. Self has emerged as a line of inquiry in various branches of psychology, sociology, linguistics, communication, and many other fields. Key constructs have been developed and debated in these arenas. Some of the debate results from different theoretical orientations. In this text, for example, there will be references to post modernism (see Chapter 10), as well as to sociocultural theory (see Chapter 11). Those interested in these theoretical frameworks will find citations for future reading in each chapter. However, because our work is an amalgam of theoretical approaches and ultimately has evolved out of our dialogues with persons living with neurogenic disorders, we wish to orient readers to core concepts without tagging those concepts with a particular theoretical label.

In recent decades, inquiries into the nature of self have focused increasingly on the individual as having agency, as participating actively in his or her life. Agency and empowerment figure prominently in today's attempts to understand narrative self for any individual. In addition, the idea of active participation in self-construction has led naturally to recognition of the highly social and interactive nature of these processes (Fivush, 1991; Fivush & Haden, 2003). Theoretical dialogues about the nature of self center around the degree to which the individual is seen as empowered in self construction, as contrasted with the premise that selves are so dependent on social construction and context that there can be little unity in one's identity.

There are multiple domains in which self operates. We all recognize that we appear to be different people, different selves, depending on our interaction partner, or the setting, or the role we are playing. In fact, there are many who assert that there is no single self, that as Holstein and Gubrium (2000, p. 24) suggest, a person "has as many social selves as there are individuals who recognize him and carry an image of him." Nevertheless, we continue to sustain a belief in a consistent self, an unchanging me. We can sustain that belief, in part, because our sense of self is linked to our knowledge of and ability to communicate our life narrative.

The theoretical construct *narrative* has also undergone considerable transformation over the past few decades (Hevern, 2004). In the 21st century, selves are seen as narrative constructions (Vollmer, 2005). For some, the concept of narrative is captured by the term story, giving rise to discussions of life as storied (Sarbin, 1986b), a concept whose roots extend back to Shakespeare's time and which was refined by Schapp (1976) to encompass the idea of living in a web or maze of stories that allow us to understand and provide meaning to our experiences.

Narrative figures prominently in today's attempts to understand human functioning.

Narrative intelligence and storying behavior, for example, have been linked to emotions, actions, decisions, identity, and experiences (Randall, 1999). What is important is that narrative refers to cognitive processes (Herman, 2000), the ways in which we attribute meaning to the events of our lives, weaving them together into a complex lifestory that allows us to function with some sense of unity of self. Indeed, a number of theorists suggest that the human mind is uniquely engineered for story construction and telling (McAdams, 1993).

An extensive literature in multiple disciplines attempts to explain development, adaptation, response to self- or life-threatening events, and lifespan changes through examination of narrative behavior. Of particular interest is the exploration of the illness experience in medical ethics. Illness is seen as threatening one's sense of self or identity (Frank, 1995). Illness narratives involve the telling and sharing of one's understanding of the life changes brought about by diseases or disorders, and these narratives are seen as providing the tools needed to redefine self and regain mastery.

This foregrounding of illness has, in turn, brought into focus the narrative processes that occur in clinical interactions. In different ways, recent works by Hinckley (2007) and Holland (2007) target the importance of the telling of one's life story in a variety of contexts. Hinckley's (2007) text, *Narrative-Based Practice in Speech-Language Pathology*, suggests that "stories are the way we conceptualize our own identities, the events of our lives, and share them with others . . . " (p. 4). She highlights the importance of sharing identities within the clinical process and sees narrative as " . . . a framework and a technique with which we can explore the difficult-to-define moments of interaction within the clinical process that have the power to become incorporated into our life stories" (p. 5). She also states that the more complex emotional and psychological elements of any clinical interaction are part of the frontier that needs to be explored in speech-language pathology, was well as other disciplines (Hinckley, 2007).

Based on these theoretical strands, we chose to focus this text on the construct of *narrative self*, loosely defined here as the story-framing processes we use to support our sense of self and which allow us to adapt to change. Wrigley (2001) has suggested that, "The continuing problem of narrative studies of the self involves constantly trying to grapple with the issue of how much the self is helping to construct the story (to author it) in an agential fashion, and how much of a person's story is a construction influenced by the social, cultural and historical environment of the narrator and the telling." The sociocultural construction of self is almost always dependent on communicative exchanges, and much of the theoretical work on narrative self assumes some ability to communicate one's narrative, to frame and adjust the communicative exchanges in which self is negotiated. Ironically, at the time when these skills are most needed, when faced with a neurological disorder, it is those communication skills that are impaired.

Later in this chapter, we will define more specifically our use of the terms narrative and self as they apply to our understanding of the life impact of neurogenic communication disorders. We will also build on current clinical perspectives that have encouraged practitioners and researchers to explore the way in which communication impairment disrupts the socially mediated life participation processes needed for a healthy sense of self.

Evolving Clinical Perspectives on Person and Function

In recent years, social models for understanding and treating communication disorders have gained greater prominence. Social models shift focus from impairment or deficit to explorations of the impact of a disorder on the person's daily functioning within a broader social and environmental context (Simmons-Mackie, 2000). One impetus for such a shift has been the worldwide acceptance of the International Classification of Functioning, Disability and Health (ICF) model for broadening perspectives on disease/disorder to a social understanding of disability, with quality of life and well-being as the goal for intervention (World Health Organization, 2001). In the context of this model, we now look beyond impairment of body structures and functions to a consideration of activity, participation, and function, particularly as influenced by environmental and personal factors. Environmental factors include aspects of the physical, social, and attitudinal world that can have an impact on the individual's performance. Personal factors address the background of an individual's life and living, including health condition or health state. These may include age, race, gender, educational background, experiences, personality and character style, aptitudes, other health conditions, fitness, lifestyle, habits, upbringing, coping styles, social background, profession and past and current experience (Simmons-Mackie, 2004; Threats, Shadden, & Vickers, 2003).

Virtually all the concepts of narrative self proposed in this text can be accommodated within the ICF and provide depth to the understanding and interpretation of major ICF model components. For example, one universal element in the literature on neurogenic disorders is the definition and measurement of quality of life, although quality of life may be more readily measured in some diseases (e.g., ALS, Parkinson's disease) than in others (e.g., aphasia, dementia). As a targeted outcome in the ICF model, quality of life can and should consider success in maintaining and reframing one's sense of narrative self.

The ICF model has been influential in shaping thinking about disability because disablement or functioning are defined as being determined by the interactions among these many variables. For example, in its report, *The Future of Disability in America* (2007), the Institute of Medicine highlights the fact that "Disability in the form of limited activities and restricted participation in social life is not an unavoidable result of injury and chronic disease," emphasizing instead the fact that the choices societies make also influence the experience of disability. The ICF model has spawned hundreds of articles addressing the functional and quality of life impact of specific disease processes.

The ICF impact can be seen in work with many different disorders. For example, a 2007 issue of *Seminars in Speech and Language* edited by Ma, Worrall, and Threats explores the ICF as applied to work with hearing impairment, TBI, aphasia, dementia, child articulation and phonology, child language, laryngectomy, swallowing disorders, motor speech disorders, and stuttering. A similar issue of the *International Journal of Speech-Language Pathology*, to be edited by Worrall, Ma, and Threats (in press) also explores the history and impact of the ICF.

There are other models of interest in examining the impact of neurogenic disorders. Kitwood's (1997) work on personhood and person-centered treatment has reframed dementia care for future generations. In Harre (1991) and Sabat's (2001, 2007) social

constructivist theory, many of Kitwood's premises have been elaborated to include three aspects of selfhood: personal identity, from the perspective of the individual; physical and mental attributes, beliefs, and beliefs about attributes; and multiple social persona. Clearly, a model with multiple representations of self as experienced personally and socially is consistent with the perspectives we discuss in this text.

In aphasia, various frameworks have been proposed to move from an impairment-based medical model to a social model that considers persons living with aphasia as situated in the broader social life context. The Life Participation Approach to Aphasia (LPAA Project Group, 2001) is an example of work that was influenced in part by the ICF and emerged in response to patient and provider demands for changes in the ways that individuals with aphasia receive treatments. Derived from an essentially social model for understanding the needs of persons with aphasia, as well as their significant others (Simmons-Mackie, 2000; Simmons-Mackie & Damico, 2007), intervention targets include both personal (internal) and environmental (external) factors. The LPAA is the subject of an issue of *Topics in Language Disorders* (Kimbarow, 2007).

Other models used in work with aphasia reflect this broader socially mediated understanding of life impact. For example, Parr (2001) created a Living with Aphasia model that situates the person with aphasia within immediate social contexts, communities, and society. This model targets these layers of involvement, specifying the outcomes of focused interventions at each level in terms of access to autonomy and choice of lifestyle, healthy psychological state, health promotion and illness prevention, enhancing communication, identifying barriers to social participation, and adaptation of identity (self-actualization). Shadden (2001) contends that the model is equally valid when applied to significant others.

Most recently, Kagan et al. (2007) have developed the A-FROM framework to facilitate discussion of issues related to social approaches to understanding and managing aphasia. At the heart of the A-FROM schematic is life with aphasia, which is influenced by and measured in terms of participation (community, conversation, activities, and roles/relationships and responsibilities), person (future, identity, feelings); environment (services, systems, policies, and attitudes), and aphasia (receptive and expressive impairment) (Kagan, 2005) The schematic allows snapshots of moments in time to be taken, with each part of the framework capable of being expanded as needed or desired. The value of this model is its breadth in encompassing functioning in so many different domains and roles and in its identification of "Who am I with aphasia?" as the central clinical question.

Brumfitt (1993, 1999) stated that language is powerfully linked to a sense of self or personhood, as mediated through social interaction, maintenance of core roles needing validation for consistency, and defining identity in relationship to others. In the following sections, we define broadly what we mean by *self* and how *narrative* processes play a role in sustaining a sense of viable self.

Establishing our Framework for Narrative Self

The Concept of Self

The concept of self is at the core of being human. Over the lifespan, we develop and modify representations of who and what we are that can be labeled, in the absence of a better term, *self*. Although we often view any concept of self as reflecting the unique aspects of being an individual, our selves typically are understood only through social interactions. In other words, current theoretical perspectives suggest that self is socially constructed (Guendouzi & Miller, 2006). Not surprisingly, the idea of self is not a unitary construct. Although we need and attempt to maintain some continuity and consistency in our understanding of self, the social presentation of that self varies with different interactions and contexts. Other terms used in the literature to capture the same essential construct are identity and personhood, although there is some controversy with respect to whether these represent equivalent constructs. Further, different taxonomies of self have been proposed and debated (Kitwood, 1997).

In this book, we suggest that the self can be fully understood only by taking several levels of analysis simultaneously into account. These levels are cultural (societal norms, values, beliefs, etc.), role-based (e.g., mother, college professor, pastor), interactional (specific interpersonal interactions), and biographical (a person's unique biology, physiology and previous life experiences). Consider for a moment the story of Senator Johnson presented earlier. His life narrative and sense of self were fundamentally disrupted at the cultural level (in a society where people generally devalue the competence of anyone who cannot communicate normally); at the level of roles (particularly given Mr. Johnson's high status role as U.S. Senator); in interactions (with wife, family and members of the public); and in terms of his biographical self (coming to terms with who he is now that stroke survivor has been added to the biographic particulars of his life). This concept of multiple domains of self will be discussed more fully in Chapter 3.

Selves are not just created and then accepted by others in all contexts. Instead, they are negotiated separately in every new situation. To negotiate a self, one must minimally use culturally acceptable symbols and appropriately present them for that situation. In other words, using Swidler's (1986, 2001) terminology, one must possess a cultural tool kit that contains the necessary tools and one must know how to manipulate that tool kit to preserve a sense of coherent self in moving from one context to the next. As part of this process, one must also have the power to compel others to take one's self definition seriously. In this text, we focus on speech, language, and communication as components of the cultural tool kit, and we explore what happens when individuals lose specific communication abilities or lose the ability to manipulate these skills within the tool kit. The work to be done with our tool kit is the narration of our life stories, and a major tool we use to do this work is communication. Our narrative communication allows us to present our selves and our life stories in terms of "the reasonably familiar identities" that Gubrium and Holstein (2001) say are essential to avoid "being seen as eccentric, if not outrageous. If we don't work with recognizable identities, our claims to selfhood will be treated as nonsense" (p. 13).

Human Narrative and Narrative Self

How does self get communicated to and negotiated with others in our lives? How does narrative function to position us in interaction with others (Wortham, 2000)? Most current theorists would suggest that the primary mechanism used to maintain one's sense of self is narrative, sometimes in the form of life stories. In fact, Charon (2002) and others suggest that " . . . self cannot be created, or even found, independent of narrative activities" (p. 61). It is hypothesized that we live by stories, and that from them, through them, we derive meaning in our lives (Bruner, 2002).

At a very basic level, narrative can be defined as telling stories. However, it is much more than that. Narrative is a critical cognitive tool for meaning making in our lives. Sarbin (1986) has stated that narrative is a root metaphor for human experience. In fact, our everyday actions and utterances make sense only in the context of the various stories of our lives. Ricoeur (1992) suggests that lives are lived, and stories are told, but selves are constructed in interaction with others through our actions and our shared narratives. Indeed, in one sense, our stories become our identities, and narrative identities are in a constant state of flux (Ricoeur, 1992). Narrative as communication is an interactive process that requires active work on the part of the narrator and listener (Shadden & Hagstrom, 2007).

The term "narrative" has multiple meanings in multiple contexts. While much of the literature defines narrative as story, or as a life story as told or written by each of us as authors, we expand the concept of narrative to include the idea of "thought in action" as Hagstrom suggests in Chapter 11. That is, people do not just talk about their self, they also enact a self, and those actions comprise our self as much or more so than the story we tell. In fact, many of our life stories are written after the fact, to take into account and make sense of our actions. Thus, the self is both language and action. Referring to a considerable philosophical and sociological literature, Holstein and Gubrium (2006) emphasize the importance of "talk-in-action" or "language-in-use" and these authors "tell the story of the self at the crossroads of narrative, social interaction, culture, and institutional life" (p. 96). The narrative we tell as a life story, as an explanation of what we do, as a story line with a plot and a rationale, is only part of the process of self creation. The narrative that we live in specific contexts, that we play out within social interactions—the narrative that we write by our actions, not our words—is the other part of the equation.

To construct the narrative that gives the scaffolding for our definition and presentation of self, we have a tool kit, as we mentioned earlier. Within this tool kit will be such things as speech, language, and communication, which receive focus in this text. We manipulate these tools to preserve a sense of coherent self in moving from one context to the next. We use our narratives to compel others to take our self-definition seriously. Thus, narrative is a story we compose, sometimes before the fact, sometimes after the fact, to create, explain, and present the self using (as we discussed in the previous section) cultural norms and values, roles, interactions with others, and our unique biographies as the raw material to be fashioned by our tools of speech, language, and communication.

Although humans are not necessarily aware of the purpose of the narratives we produce, we nonetheless live by stories that give meaning to life experiences. Our life narratives provide a kind of unity that is particularly critical at times when our biographical particulars are disrupted by major events, like a loss or a diagnosis of a serious illness. Ben Yishay (2000) defines these moments as situations in which a sense of identity is disrupted. Thus, an additional theoretical construct that informs this text is the growing body of literature about illness narratives. Through the work of Brody (2003), Charon and Montello (2002), Frank (1995, 2002), Kleinman (1988), and others, the medical community (and more broadly,

health care professions) has been asked to reframe its understanding of the patient/professional interaction to include and actively solicit illness narratives that will inform treatment. These narratives allow people to give meaning to the medical events that have altered their life paths and to continue a trajectory of self/identity across the lifespan.

The challenge to narrative self is particularly great when one considers how the ability to frame and share illness narrative is impaired because of loss of communication. Without full access to normal communicative tools, people cannot develop and share the illness experience as it alters their life story and requires new and different understandings of self without jeopardizing this sense of continuity in their life story. In recent years, a number of studies have addressed illness narrative experiences of those who have experienced a stroke. These stroke narratives provide important insights into the factors that affect the success or failure of the stroke survivor and significant others in moving on with life. In many of these studies, persons with significant communication disorders are excluded from the subject pool or choose not to participate. Clearly, there are exceptions, as can be seen in the work of researchers such as Armstrong and Ulatowska (2007a, 2207b). However, we are left with limited understanding of the impact of the loss of the communication tool on narrative self.

Although we will be using the terms life story and storying of self throughout this text, we do not mean to suggest that self maintenance and renegotiation is dependent on the actual telling of one's story (although that can be important in the sharing of illness narratives). Instead, we suggest that the storying of self also involves the multiple small moments of communication and interaction throughout each day that collectively impart a sense of who we are. It is these many small acts, as well as our shared stories, that are jeopardized by neurogenic communication disorders. In this text, therefore, we have turned to the concept of narrative self as a guiding theoretical framework for our exploration of the profound and diverse life consequences of neurogenic communication disorders. We will explore narratives associated with illness and health as well as the way in which adult-onset neurogenic communication disorders interact with other factors to jeopardize the process of ongoing storying of self. To do so, we must first examine more closely the communicative tools that play a role in this process.

Communicative Processes and Narrative Self

The critical role of language and communication is targeted over and over again in studies of self and narrative with some authors postulating explicitly that self emerges from and is shaped by language processes (Fischer, 1987; Kerby, 1993). Consistent with premises of life as storied, Kerby emphasizes that it is the selection, telling and interpreting of events from our past in the present that constitutes self construction. MacIntyre (1981) also states that the starting point for understanding identity and narrative is language.

What exactly does this mean? We know others and ourselves through daily social interactions, and the tool used to support these interactive processes is narrative communication in the broadest sense of the term narrative. Carey (1975) describes communication as a symbolic process that functions to produce, maintain, repair, and/or transform reality. As Holstein and Gubrium (2001) state, "interaction and communication are clearly the basis for the social *self*

. . . We 'talk our selves into being' in social interaction" (p.7). Thus they assert that communication is essential in the creation and presentation of self.

Communication is a complex phenomenon. To be successful, the person using communicative tools must posses: (a) the cognitive skills to frame the intention to communicate and to organize what is said; (b) the language skills needed to process and formulate messages; (c) the motor skills to turn these thoughts and language elements into movement of structures that create the actual sounds we hear as speech; (d) the ability to interpret and use various nonverbal behaviors to support comprehension or expression of meanings; and (e) the awareness of self and other that enables us to make appropriate choices in what we say to whom under what circumstances. Any of these elements, alone or in combination with others, can be the basis of the communication disorders discussed in this text. Given the multiple dimensions of self, and the complexity of the processes that must be managed to produce a successful communication, it is not surprising that those who experience adult-onset neurogenic communication disorders demonstrate unique profiles with respect to the impact of these disorders on narrative self.

The aspects of communication outlined above are pivotal to the actual event of telling one's story. *Storying* is a specific kind of communicative action that is associated with the development and maintenance of narrative self, as well as an aspect of narration that is particularly affected by neurogenic disruption (Hagstrom & Wertsch, 2004). What does this action involve? Storying involves an individual, whom we refer to as the speaking self, and others, those to whom the story is directed. These others may be physically present or may be individuals who at the moment are mental conversation partners. We have all had conversations in our minds with friends, family, teachers, and physicians. We establish our point of view telling them, giving them the story we want them to hear (or to have heard). Thus, one element of storying is that stories are constructed between the speaking self and others (Wertsch, 1991). A second element of storying is the relationship between "I" and "me." James (1963) used this relationship to analyze the role of the speaker (i.e., one who is producing the story) during storytelling. He stated that "I" references the story teller while "me" is the person about whom the story is being told. These positional words are essential to all personal stories as well as to the stories we tell about other people. An individual's perspective on herself in relationship with others is contained in the narrative.

In summary, although self construction is not totally dependent on communication, the storying of self that we describe in this text refers to individuals communicating through narratives to create or modify the self presented to others (Wertsch, Tulviste, & Hagstrom, 1993). The storying narratives, whether full-blown stories or brief communicative exchanges, may reflect multiple dimensions of self (as described earlier in this chapter and elaborated in Chapter 3). These narratives may be biographical; they may be about or have emerged from interactions with others; they may reflect roles taken or enacted by the storyteller or others, or they may be cultural stories.

Narrative Self and Neurogenic Communication Disorders

In the following chapters, we focus on aging, disease, and neurogenic communication disorders as more than just individual

biological facts. Instead, they are interpreted events in the lives of persons, families, and communities. Because we start with that assumption, our interest lies in how people create new selves under conditions in which they have lost essential tools, aspects of communication, from their tool kits. We believe that an essential process called *storying of the self* occurs, allowing people to move forward (or keeping them mired in the past) after they find themselves without these previously-used tools. Thus, we are not just interested in construction of the self, nor are we just interested in the narratives people construct; rather, we are interested in the crucial linkage between self and narrative that allows a person to create, with a story, a new self to face new challenges when old familiar tools for that construction have been lost.

We know little about how persons with communication disorders maintain and modulate their narrative self in response to life changes brought on by such illnesses or disease processes. In some instances, we understand better the narrative self consequences for the important social others in the lives of these individuals. Those in the social environment, whether significant other, paid caregiver, or virtual strangers, retain the communication skills needed to share their life stories and thus illuminate the impact of neurogenic communication disorder. However, our understanding of the roles of these social others, and the ways in which they can help persons with communicative disorders, remains limited.

Part of the challenge in understanding narrative self results from the multiple roles played by language and communication in human life. Impairments in language and communication create imbalances in exchanges between two or more people, actively disrupting the process of presenting and modifying the self. In this context

(Dowd, 1980), language might be conceptualized as a highly valued commodity that we use in social exchanges to establish our worth and, define the ways others react to us. In addition, loss of speech and/or language disrupts the individual's ability to use communication skills to respond to an illness and to forge a new life story. For those who have lost either the knowledge of the language system used in a given situation or their ability to manipulate that system, we need to understand better the impact of the loss of communication facility at a time when it is most needed to carry on the work of maintaining narrative self. Part of this work involves the creation of life stories that allow the past to be integrated into a present that acknowledges the communication impairment and other illness characteristics. Part of the work also requires addressing an altered future, and thus a major shift in understanding of the anticipated lifespan experiences. And all of the work requires recognition and validation by important social others.

We must examine the fact that these people have lost some of the tools needed or the ability to use some of their tool kit to effectively construct a narrative self. Persons with communication disorders do not stop having a narrative self when confronted with the loss of communication tools. And they do not cease having relationships with significant others, although the relationships are frequently altered in less than desirable ways. In this text, we want to return to the basic assumption that all of us strive to maintain a narrative self, an evolving life story, in order to make sense of life and to participate in and be validated by the surrounding social environment. If we start with that basic assumption and listen to those who have impaired communication abilities, we can learn much about the theoretical ways in which people not only con-

struct selves but also are able to negotiate and present those selves. We can explore the impact of losses of different aspects of communication and can develop a sense of the strategies that may be used to present oneself to others when feeling least privileged and most disadvantaged. We can learn about the way in which group membership and community enhance (or potentially detract from) a sense of acceptable valued self. We can identify at the individual level how and if critical relationships are reframed to accommodate changes in the narrative self, and whether specific interventions can be helpful in working to resolve illness narrative and reframe them into health narratives.

Summary and Caveats

In this text, we are focusing on the way in which neurogenic communication disorders create challenges to a sense of coherence and continuity in the constant storying of self. We probe the consequences of impaired communication when individuals have proceeded through their lives with "normal" communication skills prior to the onset of a specific disorder. We will use the words of such individuals and their significant others, as well as elements of their life stories, to explore the ways in which they can continue to construct a self, present that self to others, and resist or accept the imposition of a self by powerful others. By comparing and contrasting different diseases with their distinctive impact on communication behavior, we will highlight the role played by these unique characteristics on the ongoing storying of self. Our central premise is that any intervention with adults affected by neurogenic communication disorders should provide these individuals with ways to resume an active role in reconstruction or revision of the narrative self. Interventions that focus explicitly and solely on remediation of deficits leave critical voids in the lives of these individuals and their significant others.

In this chapter, we provided an overview of the major themes associated with a framework for conceptualizing narrative self. Each of these themes is elaborated further in Section II. One central premise is the notion of a cultural tool kit, with speech, language, and communication being specific tools for the construction and negotiation of narrative self.

Another premise is that an understanding of the life impact of adult-onset neurogenic communication disorders requires consideration of how impaired communication disrupts the ongoing storying of self. Acts of storying are the fundamental building blocks of narrative self. They become the foundation, scaffold the edifice, and continuously re-roof narrative self-structures. We are all place holders in these acts, all possible "others" in the stories being told by individuals and families living with neurogenic communication disorders.

This text makes no attempt to serve as a basic primer about the nature of all neurogenic communication disorders in adults or to provide a cookbook of assessment and intervention approaches. Instead, we attempt to provide exemplars of those dimensions of each disorder that provide powerful contrasts that allow us to understand better the ongoing challenge of maintaining and modulating one's narrative self in the face of such a disorder. In doing so, we have brought into focus seemingly disparate lines of research and clinical activity through use of a single unifying construct:

the *narrative self*. Our primary assertion is that an understanding of the ongoing storying of self must feature prominently in all that we do as clinicians, researchers and scholars of communication disorders.

In all probability, our work may raise as many questions as it answers. It is difficult to know how to shed light on the essential role of communication in creating, maintaining, and modifying our narrative self when the ability to communicate is radically changed. However, by targeting the issue of the impact of communication impairment on sense of self and/or identity, we hope that we will contribute to both the theoretical and clinical knowledge base. For the authors of this text, theory and practice have converged as we have talked with those experiencing adult-onset communication disorders, as well as their significant others. In particular, there has been a sense of "rightness" about the concept of narrative self as critical to understanding the lives of the people affected by communication disorders.

If narrative is indeed the most important tool used by humans to validate self, and to explain changes in life course, then disruption of the communication base of narrative behavior must be targeted in interventions. Further, our understanding of our roles as health care professionals must be broadened beyond targeting specific skills to address the use of improved skills in furthering the narrative self, in moving on with life. The following sections set the theoretical framework for our discussion of the impact of neurogenic communication disorders on narrative self. Our ultimate goal is to provide clinicians with perspectives that emphasize living with a neurogenic disorder, rather than curing the communication impairment.

CHAPTER 2

Neurogenic Communication Disorders

The term *neurogenic communication disorders* is a potentially awkward one that encompasses a broad range of illness or disease processes with an equally broad range of communication consequences. If this were a typical textbook about neurogenic communication disorders, there would be a need for a comprehensive overview of all such adult-onset disorders. From a communication disorders perspective, the list might include cognitive-communication disorders, aphasia, apraxia of speech, dysarthria, and right brain damage communication disorders. From an illness/disease perspective, some considerations would have to be given to stroke, Alzheimer's and other dementias, degenerative motor disorders (ALS, Parkinson's disease, pseudobulbar palsy, etc.), tumors, infectious disease processes, normal pressure hydrocephalus, and TBI, among others.

This is not such a typical textbook. Our focus is on the impact of communication disorders (and other associated disease characteristics) on one's ongoing sense of self or identity, particularly when the narrative tool is impaired due to an acquired neurological condition. Our premise is that understanding these processes will lead to interventions that are more truly person-centered and therefore more meaningful in

helping the person move forward with the life story. Thus we have selected exemplars of the process of communication breakdown and its impact on individuals with the disorder and their significant others. We have also chosen to frame this work in part through the words and experiences of real people.

The four medical conditions and associated communication disorders addressed in Section III of this text are: (a) amyotrophic lateral sclerosis (ALS), (b) Parkinson's disease (PD), (c) stroke-related aphasia, and (d) Alzheimer's disease (AD). Each of these conditions is described briefly in this chapter, with emphasis on the onset, course, and timeline characteristics that distinguish them, the nature of the communication impairment associated with each (with implications for narrative and life story), and issues of self. The overview in this chapter is designed to give the reader a basic understanding of the different challenges to narrative self that may be experienced by persons living with these disorders.

A literature review of existing research on topics related to narrative self in each disorder, and in normal aging, reveals an intriguing pattern. Using the disorder name (e.g., ALS) and keywords such as identity or self and narrative or life story, there were very different profiles in terms of the number and nature of articles returned in the search. For example, in looking at normal aging and life span changes related to aspects of narrative self, there were frequent references to the key words identity, self, narrative, and life story. A similar pattern was observed for research on Alzheimer's disease over the course of the past 10 to 15 years, despite the fact that this disorder historically has been viewed as one that robs people of their selfhood. In contrast, for aphasia, despite many years of discussion of loss of self or identity, most articles on narrative relate explicitly to narrative discourse as a linguistic behavior, specifically the ability to understand and frame story elements in the context of a compromised language system. While identity or self are frequently mentioned in abstracts or in the actual articles, these domains typically are not studied directly. Quality of life, however, does receive focus.

Why do different constructs (e.g., quality of life vs. self/identity) receive focus with different disorders? While there may be many factors influencing research focus, an important one is the nature of the communication impairment itself. For example, persons with aphasia, particularly those with severe expressive and/or receptive language impairments, cannot provide us with sufficient language for analysis of the narrative self being presented or cannot understand somewhat abstract questions of self or identity. Given these challenges, it is easier to study behaviors or perceptions that relate to domains such as life participation, revealing competence, conversational interactions, and psychosocial consequences (well-being, quality of life, depression), among many others. All of these domains can be linked to the concepts of self and identity, but the links must often be inferred. Narrative does not come easily to persons with aphasia. It can be extremely difficult for them to construct and share an illness narrative that captures their experiences, modulates the transition between past (pre-aphasia) and present self, and promotes a coherent image of future expectations.

Research on ALS and Parkinson's disease also focuses more on quality of life than on self, but the reasons for this focus are different. In the early stages of both disorders, there is no expectation that narrative self will be compromised in any significant fashion, and thus there is limited attention to the impact on narrative self. With ALS, the disease progression is relatively rapid, and new physical challenges are constantly emerging, challenges requiring the full attention and resources of both the person with ALS and significant others. For persons with Parkinson's disease, the course of the disorder is more variable and cognitive challenges may or may not develop. Thus issues of living with Parkinson's—of quality of life with PD—continue to be preeminent. In contrast, there is considerable attention to issues of self and identity for individuals with Alzheimer's disease, possibly because of the slow progression of language deficits, and their ability to construct narrative in the early stages. Given the perception that self is what is "lost" in dementia, it is not surprising that researchers and clinicians actively seek answers to the nature of self in this disorder.

In the following sections of this chapter, similar questions about research focus will be explored further. Each of our targeted illnesses and associated communicative disorders will be described briefly, with some of the most important contrasts among disorders outlined. This chapter is intended to set the stage for the theoretical examination of self and narrative in Section II and for the life stories presented in Section III.

The Illnesses and Associated Communication Impairment

Amyotrophic Lateral Sclerosis (ALS)

ALS is a progressive motor neuron disease whose exact cause is still not fully understood. The disease first received public attention when Lou Gehrig retired from baseball in 1939 after being diagnosed with the condition. ALS affects the upper and lower motor neurons that control voluntary muscles, with the first symptoms variable but typically associated with muscle weakness. At least two forms are distinguished. The bulbar form affects motor neurons in the cranial nerve system, with early symptoms typically associated with speech as well as eating and swallowing. The limb-onset or spinal form typically appears first in motor functions governed by spinal nerves—typically upper and lower extremity symptoms. Recent research suggests there may be a small subset of persons with ALS who demonstrate cognitive impairment towards the end of their lives, but this phenomenon is little understood. Between 90 and 95% of all persons diagnosed with ALS have the *sporadic* form of the disorder, one with no known genetic component. Over 5600 new cases of ALS are diagnosed yearly. While the typical age range for onset is between 40 and 70, cases have been identified in young adults in their 20s and 30s. ALS is more common in men than women in younger patients, with the gender difference disappearing in older adults. Average survival time is 3 to 5 years (ASHA, 2007a).

The speech disorder associated with ALS is *dysarthria*. Dysarthria is a motor speech disorder that has many variants. With dysarthria, muscles needed for intelligible speech (mouth, respiratory system, voice, and face) may become weak, slow, or uncoordinated. In ALS, the first speech symptoms may include weakness in oral or respiratory musculature, slurring of speech, loss of normal range of intonation, and reduced volume. Respiratory systems become increasingly compromised during the course of the disease (ASHA, 2007d).

Parkinson's Disease (PD)

PD is a motor disorder resulting from the loss of dopamine-producing cells in the brain. Primary symptoms include tremor, bradykinesia (slowness of movement), postural instability, and rigidity in limbs and trunk. Age of onset is usually over 50 years, although more early PD cases are being diagnosed. The disease is both chronic and progressive, but the course and severity of symptoms are highly variable. Prevalence in the United States is between 100 and 250 cases per 100,000. Although Parkinson's disease is thought of as a motor disorder, it can be associated with cognitive disturbances. These include slowed reaction time, executive dysfunction, memory loss, and dementia in 20 to 40% of all patients.

The speech disorder associated with PD, as with ALS, is dysarthria, although the characteristics of PD dysarthria are distinct from those found with ALS (ASHA, 2007d). In PD, symptoms include problems initiating speech, festinating speech (rapid rate with poor intelligibility), hypophonia (reduced vocal volume) as well as a hoarse or strained vocal quality, muffled resonance, and perceived stuttering. Intelligibility declines over the progression of the disorder associated with increased weakness in speech musculature. Communication can also be affected by the common loss of facial expression or "masking" seen in persons with PD. Because the motor system is involved, there is often a dysphagia, or swallowing disorder (National Parkinson's Foundation, n.d.; Parkinson's Disease Foundation, n.d.; Parkinson's Living, n.d.).

Stroke (Brain Attack) Aphasia, Dysarthria, and Apraxia of Speech

Stroke or cerebrovascular accident (CVA) occurs when the blood supply to the brain is disrupted, leading to death of brain cells. There are approximately 750,000 strokes each year, killing 160,000 persons. Stroke is the third leading cause of death in adults and the leading cause of adult disability. The symptoms and consequences of stroke are highly variable, depending on the part of the brain affected. There may be visual and other sensory problems, as well as cognitive deficits apart from any language impairment. Many individuals experience a one-sided hemiplegia or hemiparesis. Strokes typically occur in adults in the middle or late years.

Although not all stroke survivors experience communication problems, it is estimated that there are 80,000 new cases of *aphasia* each year, and one million living persons with aphasia (American Heart Association, n.d.; American Stroke Foundation, n.d.; Aphasia Now, n.d.; National Parkinson's Foundation, n.d.). Aphasia is a language impairment that results from damage to speech and language centers in the brain, typically in the left hemisphere that governs language in most adults. There are many different forms of aphasia, and it can affect the ability both to understand and to produce language. Some persons lose facility with the linguistic systems that govern production of grammatically complete utterances. Others have problems finding the word they want (anomia, word retrieval problems), despite knowing conceptually what they want to say. Language production may be either fluent or nonfluent.

Stroke may also cause the motor speech disorders *dysarthria* and *apraxia* of speech. Apraxia of speech is a motor speech disorder that results in an inability to target the positioning of speech structures and the sequencing of muscle movements for speech (ASHA, 2007b). It is caused by damage to the parts of the brain related to speaking. Other terms include acquired apraxia of speech, verbal apraxia, and dyspraxia. People with apraxia of speech have trouble sequencing the sounds in syllables and words. The severity depends on the nature of the brain damage. Dysarthria, as defined earlier, is a motor speech disorder resulting from weakness, paralysis, or uncoordination of the speech muscles (ASHA, 2007d). In stroke, the dysarthria typically results from weakness or paralysis of muscles on one side of the face, mouth, or vocal folds. Speech is slurred, monotonous, and associated with reduced intensity. Intelligibility is impaired; severity varies (American Stroke Association, n.d.; American Stroke Foundation, n.d.).

Alzheimer's Disease (AD) and Other Dementias

The term *dementia* refers to a group of disorders that are characterized by memory loss and other cognitive impairments that eventually result in an inability to care for oneself or relate appropriately to others. Most dementias worsen over time, although there are some reversible causes of dementia (e.g., infections, normal pressure hydrocephalus, metabolic disturbances). Disorders known to cause dementia include vascular (multi-infarct) dementia, Lewy body dementia, frontotemporal dementia, Parkinson's disease, Huntington's disease, and Creutzfeldt-Jakob disease. Alzheimer's disease (AD) is the most common form of dementia (between 50 and 70% of those diagnosed with dementia) and will receive focus in this text. Fifty percent of adults over 85 years of age are believed to be affected by AD. AD is a neurodegenerative disorder characterized by abnormal clusters of amyloid plaques and neurofibrillary tangles in the brain. At present, there are more than five million Americans with Alzheimer's disease, with the vast majority over the age of 65. The progression of the disorder is quite variable. Although death typically occurs within 4 to 6 years of diagnosis, individuals with AD can live as long as 20 years.

It is important to avoid confusion of early AD symptoms with some characteristics of normal aging. At least two major brain functions must be impaired if AD is considered as a diagnosis. Memory is typically one, while the others may be attention, calculation, language, visuospatial, praxis, or executive skills.

AD is accompanied by progressively worsening communication impairment. Both comprehension and production of language are impaired, typically because of underlying cognitive deficits, even though some persons with AD retain speech output (however meaningless) until the last stages. Given the underlying cognitive impairment, the communication disorder associated with AD is sometimes referred to as language of generalized intellectual impairment or as a cognitive-communicative disorder (Alzheimer's Association, n.d.; Alzheimer's Foundation of America, n.d.; ASHA, 2007c).

Similarities and Differences: What Dimensions Matter?

There are critical differences or similarities across disorders that can be projected to present unique challenges to the narrative

self and the experiences of persons living with the acquired neurogenic communication disorders described in the previous section. As noted in Chapter 1, the term "living with" a disorder is used when all those affected by the problem are being considered, not just a single individual. One major point for comparison is the onset and course of each disorder, the illness trajectory. The second major point concerns what underlying system is impaired in the communication disorder. Together, these two dimensions allow us to probe what impact a particular disorder can be expected to have on the narrative construction and reconstruction of self.

Onset and Course of Disorder

The disorders selected to highlight issues of narrative self differ considerably in terms of onset, progression or recovery, and timeline characteristics. Onset and timelines establish different kinds of identity or selfhood challenges and present unique obstacles to moving forward with one's life story.

For example, on the surface, it would appear that ALS and PD, the two degenerative neuromotor disorders selected for inclusion in this text, should present similar challenges to the narrative self. However, some of their differences in disease progression undoubtedly influence the work of presenting and modifying narrative self. A person with ALS is confronting an initially gradual onset degenerative neuromotor disease that will eventually rob her of motor control over any part of the body, resulting sooner or later in death. Frequently, diagnosis is delayed, particularly with ALS. Once the disease has been identified, the diagnosis carries with it an understanding of inevitable decline and the disease course tends to be relatively rapid. There is no threat to self here except insofar as a previously healthy, active person may begin to feel some sense of disconnection from the body that has served her well in the past. However, important life roles are altered and these may affect a sense of viable self. Because cognitive and linguistic functions are typically well preserved, the possibility of narrative discourse continues throughout the disease progression, although progressive loss of physical skills may impede this discourse. Typically, affected persons, as well as family members and friends, find themselves constantly reacting to new losses of physical function and new decisions to be made at such times of change. Further, the relatively rapid progression of ALS (typically 3 to 5 years from diagnosis to death) places high priority on physical body systems and demands energy and attention to survival processes.

In contrast, the progression in PD is much slower, and intelligible speech and language are retained longer, thus increasing the opportunity for doing the work of the narrative self. However, many persons with PD develop dementia towards the end of the illness trajectory. At this point, the burden of maintaining a sense of narrative self falls increasingly to the significant others.

Stroke-related aphasia and the cognitive communication impairments associated with Alzheimer's disease also provide unique onset and disease course contrasts. In Alzheimer's disease, the diagnosis is invariably preceded by dwindling cognitive functioning and associated fears, concerns, and attempts to hide deficits. The individual response varies, but the threat to narrative self, to competence and integrity of self, is felt at the outset because the probable diagnosis of Alzheimer's disease is associated with loss of self- or personhood. It is reported that, when Alois Alzheimer's first patient was confronted with her inability to write her name, she described this as a loss of self. In essence, Alzheimer's disease

(and other dementias) are typically seen as robbing the person of who she was, and, by extension, robbing loved ones of that person. The diagnosis is feared, particularly as we age. We almost hang on the words and interactions of persons with AD, looking for evidence that the person is still there.

The concept of "no one home" in the person with AD is already being challenged in health care. As the baby boomers age and the number of persons with AD in the population increases, there is escalating pressure to understand self and identity in this disorder. Is the person still there, and how is self manifested? What are the implications for care, and where does that leave the caregiver? We struggle to answer these questions, spurred on by the language and apparent communication that some persons produce until late in the disorder's progression.

In contrast, for persons living with stroke and associated aphasia (and other communication impairments), the transition from competent and normal occurs abruptly. One moment the individual is fine, the next moment, he or she is hospitalized and important physical and cognitive functions no longer work well, if at all. The threat to self is, in one sense, immediate and profound. Fear is dominant, often linked to concerns about medical survival. If a person has aphasia, he or she may not be able to discuss or to verbally frame this profound alteration of performance and the fears associated with it. That same communication impairment makes it impossible for the significant others in that person's life to anchor themselves in the social context of the relationship, to express themselves and their own fears. As the medical crisis abates, typically towards the end of any period of rehabilitation, family members suddenly find themselves facing what should be a celebration of going home, of moving on, but instead it may be a frightening feeling of disconnection.

The medical experience associated with diagnosis and early treatment also varies depending on the disorder. In stroke, the precipitating event is abrupt and disruptive. Exposure to hospitalization and the health care system in general tends to emphasize the relative incompetence and powerlessness of the person who is receiving treatment, robbing the patient of individuality and personal identity. The medical narrative is one in which disproportionate power is placed in the hands of the health care provider. The biographical disruption is profound. In contrast, for Alzheimer's disease, Parkinson's disease, and ALS, the gradual onset means initial and ongoing contacts with the medical system in order to diagnose a frequently evasive disorder. Because communication is not as impaired in the early stages of these disorders, particularly ALS and PD, individuals may still be able to project self as competent in initial health care interactions.

Communication Aspect Most Affected and Its Impact

The fundamental premise of this text is that adult onset neurogenic communication disorders create challenges to the ability to pursue ongoing presentation of self in social contexts. In addition to onset and disease trajectory, the four disorders selected for discussion are readily distinguished by examining the nature of the communication impairments and projected impact on framing of narrative self. What is of primary interest is the degree to which each disorder is the product of: (a) language impairment, (b) motor speech impairment, or (c) other cognitive deficits. Secondarily, deficits in both motor and cognitive domains may present complicating impairments affecting self presentation and construction. The schematic in Figure 2–1 conveys somewhat simplistically the overlapping influence of these three domains, with narrative self in the center, reflecting the fact not only that narrative facility itself is influenced by these

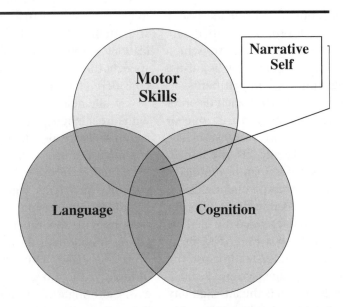

Figure 2–1. Motor, linguistic, and cognitive impairments of communication as they intersect in disrupting narrative self.

domains but also that self can only be expressed through the resources in language, motor, and cognitive functioning. The projected impact of different communication disorders on narrative self will be considered first. However, since those in the immediate social environment respond in different ways to these different deficits, particularly insofar as they allow others to recognize and accept integrity of self, it is important to comment on the larger picture of what society expects from "normally functioning" individuals.

In reading the following, it is important to remember that negotiation of self occurs through language in social interactions in culturally validated roles. Thus self requires more than language. It also requires the ability to remember and share one's life story, and the ability to make appropriate choices in self presentation. Self is linked to roles which are invariably compromised in the disorders discussed here.

Communication Effects on Self Presentation

The communication impairments associated with the four disorders described here differ in terms of the extent to which deficits are the product of motor, linguistic, or underlying cognitive impairments, as shown in Figure 2–1. Indeed, each disorder is also characterized by primarily one or some combination of two of these behavioral domains. For ALS and PD, the impairment domain is predominantly motor. As already noted, the primary communication impairment early on is dysarthria, a motor speech disorder characterized by deficits in speech output. With a pure dysarthria, a person's ability to understand or use the symbols of the language system is unaffected. What is impaired is the intelligibility of the language that is produced. Thus, in

theory, if a substitute for speech output can be found (e.g., augmentative and alternative communication, computers, writing), these individuals should retain the skills needed for ongoing construction and modification of the narrative self.

In practice, this distinction is not that clear. Part of one's presentation of narrative self involves the ability to efficiently and effectively manipulate language systems in ways that are appropriately fine-tuned to accommodate different social others and varied communication environments. The fine-tuning is problematic in both ALS and Parkinson's, partly because the communication begins to stray from the normal and accepted forms that validate the speaker. Further, deterioration of speech intelligibility is relatively rapid in ALS, particularly for those with bulbar onset. There are no specific speech therapy interventions that can alter the course of this deterioration, and the primary decisions to be made relate to whether to use some form of augmentative and alternative communication (AAC) or speech generating device (SGD). In contrast, with PD, the rate of loss of intelligibility is much slower than is found with ALS, and intelligibility can be improved by medications, surgical interventions, and specific speech therapy approaches. AAC may be considered later in the disease progression.

While neither ALS nor PD is associated with direct language impairment, communication skills are also dependent upon intact cognitive systems. As noted earlier, ALS and PD differ in terms of the likelihood that cognitive problems will emerge with the disorder's progression. For the most part, persons with ALS retain cognitive and linguistic functioning throughout the course of the disease. Thus the potential for thought, reflection, and communication exists, although the motor system impedes that expression more and more. The slower progression of PD means that the individual can communicate without support for a longer time with the potential for developing a credible illness narrative that supports coping with this disorder. Several aspects of PD limit this process. First, the subtle loss of speech intelligibility over extended time sometimes provokes increasing frustration with the communication process on the part of all parties. Frustration may reduce the likelihood of meaningful exchange of narrative. In addition, if cognitive problems emerge late in the illness progression, the person's ability to construct and present a viable self is diminished. We know little about how persons react to this loss of narrative skills, particularly if significant others become the primary tool in self expression, in speaking for the person with PD.

Alzheimer's disease and stroke-related aphasia affect very different components of the communication system. We have defined aphasia as an impairment in the ability to understand and/or use language symbols for communicative purposes, due to damage to specific areas of the brain that control language functions (see Figure 2–1). Regardless of type of aphasia or severity of impairment, it is clear that the narrative self is always challenged when confronted with aphasia. Typically, narrative requires use of language symbols, and presentation of narrative self to others requires considerable skill in adjusting the shared story to the communicative partner and context. Narrative is the meaning-making process that allows us to maintain and renegotiate our identity after a life altering event (such as a stroke). In most instances, aphasia is not a progressive disorder. If there is any defining trajectory, it is typically one of improvement in language skills for months and even longer post-stroke. However, the deficits in the language system associated with aphasia are not visible and therefore not understood well by the average person. Breakdown in social interactions due to language deficits may be wrongly attributed to a perceived loss of mental competence. Because the symbols of our narratives have been affected, it can be quite challenging for a person with aphasia to use AAC systems, since such systems also rely on symbolic forms.

In Alzheimer's disease, the language system is also affected, but the cause of language changes can be traced to underlying cognitive impairments, rather than damage to specific neurological language centers (see Figure 2–1). Unlike aphasia, the onset of Alzheimer's is gradual and early changes in language (and cognitive) behavior are subtle. Language performance deteriorates over time as cognitive functions become increasingly impaired. As Alzheimer's disease progresses, persons lose competence in multiple domains, while simultaneously losing memory for those biographical particulars that are part of what we rely on for storying of self. In essence, we expect Alzheimer's disease to be accompanied by loss of competence culminating in total loss of self. However, we often index this decline in competence and self by examining the language produced and the social interactions experienced with such individuals. What is particularly important here is the fact that many persons with Alzheimer's disease continue to produce language in an apparently interactive fashion even when cognitive decline is severe. Thus, unlike the language output of persons with a severe aphasia, the individual with dementia continues to provide us with linguistic behaviors that are open to interpretation and thus tantalizing with respect to what these behaviors seem to imply about the narrative self being shared. In AD, the impairment of presentation of narrative self is primarily the product of breakdown in cognitive functions, and the communication impairment is simply a byproduct of the cognitive dysfunction.

Issues of Self as Externally Perceived

To understand the concepts of recognition and acceptance of the integrity of self, it is important to acknowledge that humans are all somewhat programmed to look for and accept the "psychometric person" whom Sabat (2001) defines as the one we expect to meet and know in our lives. The psychometric person not only reflects average or typical behavior but also defines what may be considered acceptable deviations from these behaviors. Thus for adults with neurogenic communication disorders, their identities—their narrative selves—must be understood on at least two levels and exist on two or more continua. Sabat (2001) describes the self as representative mental and physical attributes which are socially presented. Kitwood (1997) addresses a similar concept in describing the neurological and social/psychological factors of personhood, and Guendouzi and Müller (2006) discuss three subsystems of self: (a) cognitive (which includes language); (b) sensorimotor; and (c) contextual (social). All of these taxonomies of self share an understanding that self consists of a person's characteristics (strengths, deficits, compensatory strategies) as well as the social presentation and validation of self. In the following section, emphasis is placed on the person's attributes, since the diseases discussed in this text call into question to varying degrees the integrity of a person's self. There are redundancies in this discussion, but they serve to underscore key constructs.

For both ALS and PD, although the physical decline is evident, we can clearly discern the person behind the disorders. Persons with ALS and the people with whom they interact have few doubts about the identity of the affected individual. In the earliest stages, these persons retain the ability to frame and reframe life stories, to formulate socially acceptable illness narratives, and to make some biographical accommodations to address the profound changes in their lives. Intact language systems can be used to maintain active life participation and to preserve some degree of agency and independence. In later stages, persons with ALS continue to have powerful advocates in their significant others who have faith in the unchanged narrative self of the person.

In Parkinson's disease, while the onset of symptoms is slower, the outcome is similar to ALS. There are opportunities for accepting the basic competence of the narrative self. Individuals have access for years to a relatively intact language system that can support framing of an appropriate illness narrative and creation of linkages from past through present into a foreseeable future. Late-stage losses in speech intelligibility, reduced facial expression, and cognitive impairments in some persons with PD can call into question the integrity of the narrative self.

In contrast, once a person with increasing cognitive difficulties is diagnosed with Alzheimer's disease, the label triggers a series of socioculturally determined expectations that the underlying disease process will impair and ultimately destroy the narrative self of the affected individual and, by extension, some part of the narrative self of significant others. Thus, at the outset, competence and integrity of self are the fundamental issues with AD. Many try to cling to the words and interactions (narratives) of persons with AD as evidence that the person is still there. Connelly (2002) notes that even those individuals who appear to lack the cognitive or communicative capacity to explain their lives and needs have a drive to connect. "Not only do the human qualities of the affected individual persist, the self persists . . . the intense longing for human connection" (p. 143).

Issues of selfhood and the integrity of identity become quite complex for stroke survivors with aphasia. Aphasia is not readily understood by the average person. Thus the inarticulateness evident in aphasic output, coupled with problems in comprehension and other neurological deficits, raise questions about whether this individual has indeed retained her prestroke narrative self. Ironically, the only way that persons with aphasia can confirm or validate the integrity of their narrative self is through communication, the very tool that has been impaired. The language impairment affects more than the expression of life stories and illness narratives that can help the person renegotiate a sense of self. The impairment also disrupts basic conversational interactions, the small talk or chit-chat that helps persons be recognized by social others (Pasupathi, 2006). At this level, changes in timing, in the flexibility of message formulation, of responses to cues signal that something is "off" about the person's presentation of self.

Further, most persons who have experienced stroke have been hospitalized for acute care followed by in-patient treatment in a rehabilitation facility. In these environments, many develop a sense of incompetence and loss of agency. Thus it is not surprising to hear spouses or adult children express concern about the loved in terms such as: "He's not the man he used to be," or "He used to be so smart, really," or "They really have changed, haven't they?" From the perspective of relative strangers outside of the immediate circle of family and friends, there is often a perception that the person with aphasia really is incompetent. Recent clinical research in aphasia has focused on the idea of helping the individual construct or reconstruct competence and on enhancing life participation.

Even graduate students in speech-language pathology have difficulty grasping the impact of aphasia on a person's life and self. Year after year at one university, when graduate students were asked what kind of aphasia they would prefer to have, about one third consistently expressed a preference for Wernicke's aphasia, reasoning that they liked to talk and "mean" things, even if they couldn't understand others and others did not understand them. What these students did not understand is the fact the communication, and beyond that, the expression of the narrative self, relies heavily on the recognition and validation of persons in our social environment. Communication without social connectedness is relatively useless.

In the preceding paragraphs, we have alluded to questions of whether individuals with different neurogenic communication disorders (and social others) view themselves as more or less marginalized and socially acceptable. The less acceptable the disorder appears, the more important it is to be able to express one's sense of narrative self in culturally and socially acceptable forms, whether linguistic or nonlinguistic (although linguistic behavior is particularly critical in the storying of self). The more marginalized the disorder, and the more impaired the communication behavior, the more likely we are to perceive the individual as displaying excess disability (Sabat, 2001, 2003). A perception of excess disability reduces the likelihood that the presented narrative self will be accepted and validated. This idea of excess disability is linked to the degree of stigma associated with a disorder.

An understanding of perceived stigma is crucial to working effectively with persons with a communication disorder and their significant others. The concept of stigma addresses one of Sabat's (2001) two defined aspects of self—the socially presented and validated identity. The question that needs to be explored is how we view the disorder, as something external to self versus an intrinsic impairment. Do those with specific kinds of diagnoses view themselves as marginalized or is the marginalization and stigmatizing due to the perceptions of others? Some of these questions will be explored in Section III of this text.

Stigma exists at the cultural level, in the playing out of our roles, in our interactions with others, and in our willingness to accept aspects of our biographical self. Thus stigma is linked to self in all its dimensions. For example, stigma influences the manner in which others interact (or avoid interaction) with the affected person. Stigma may also play a role in whether the communicatively impaired person and family members are willing to seek membership in the larger community of individuals with similar problems. By extension, stigma may determine whether individuals are willing to affiliate actively with this community through support group participation and related activities. Each of the disorders discussed in this text is associated with different types or degrees of stigma.

With ALS, it appears that the stigma of the condition is primarily the stigma that is associated with any severe disabling illnesses. The vast majority of the public find the condition horrifying and unfair, but there is little sense of being repulsed or frightened by the person, except insofar as most adults are uncomfortable with neurological problems. Indeed, there are relatively high levels of public sympathy for all persons touched by the disorder, because it is easy to imagine being mentally intact while one's body loses motor function each new day. Significant others often welcome opportunities to explain the disorder, further reducing the stigma. There appears to be little stigma attached to affiliating with an ALS support group. Instead, there is much to be gained in terms of mutual emotional support, infor-

mation updates, and strategies for coping on a daily basis, among others.

The stigma of Parkinson's is not as easy to characterize. The average person probably knows a bit more about Parkinson's than, for example, ALS. It is more common, and now has a powerful advocate in Michael J. Fox. As already noted, although the progression of PD is much slower than ALS, some aspects of the disease may make people uncomfortable. For example, the loss of facial expression makes it difficult to know how to interpret the person's intent or her engagement in the interaction. The same is true for the slowness of response that characterizes PD. Persons with PD live longer, and they and their significant others must learn to cope with evolving physical and often cognitive problems. Thus, the impact of PD on narrative self is highly individualized.

The stigma of Alzheimer's disease was acknowledged earlier in this chapter. There is probably no disease more feared that AD. In fact, early on, patients and family sometimes try to hide the impairment from others. It is interesting to note that families are much more comfortable sharing a diagnosis of mild cognitive impairment (MCI) than one of Alzheimer's, even though there is a high probability that MCI may evolve into full-blown dementia. As AD progresses, friends and family often find it difficult to continue to interact with the impaired person because of the perceived loss of self. There are many support groups for caregivers of persons with AD, along with an extensive research literature on the impact of the caregiving experience. It is only in recent years that diagnosed individuals are themselves seeking support, frequently through on-line support communities. Such individuals, often those diagnosed with early-onset AD, can now engage in dialogue on-line with caregivers, resulting in greater caregiver appreciation of the inner self of those afflicted with AD.

Finally, the stigma associated with aphasia appears to result primarily from a lack of public understanding of the invisible language disorder. This lack of understanding is verified repeatedly in research studies and is addressed through information materials and Web sites (cf. National Aphasia Association, Aphasia Hope Foundation, Aphasia Now). Family, friends, and strangers sometimes question the fundamental competence of the person with aphasia. In the medical model, the emphasis is on survival, and persons living with aphasia are expected simply to be grateful for being alive. As we move away from a medical, impairment-based model and toward a fully realized social model, we can begin to appreciate how even mild aphasia impairs the ability to negotiate successfully the social presentation of self. As discussed further in Chapter 8, it is not surprising that persons with aphasia and their significant others seek out membership in communities, such as support groups, where some level of acceptance and validation of self can be obtained (Shadden, 1994, 2006).

Illness Narrative

Implicit in the previous sections of this chapter is an assumption that the narrative self can only be maintained with some continuity if the individual is able to acknowledge the biographical disruption created by the disorder and formulate an account, an illness narrative, that bridges past self to present self, allows meaning to emerge, and promotes moving on of self toward some future point on the temporal continuum. What elements are necessary for the construction of an illness narrative that promotes a socially viable self in the context of

such profound alterations in life? Again, we return to the onset and course of the disorder and the central role of communication.

An illness narrative must be well crafted, using language that is appropriate, acceptably framed, and flexible (see Chapter 4). Thus, we would expect persons with ALS or Parkinson's to be more successful in creating such narratives than individuals with linguistic or cognitive-communicative impairments. Time is another critical issue. Disorders with gradual onsets theoretically would allow for development and fine-tuning of illness narratives more than those with abrupt onset. However, degenerative disease processes may provide greater challenges to sustaining a viable illness narrative, since the impact on narrative self is constantly evolving and since some deteriorating functions may be critical to the framing of the narrative. Finally, illness narratives require audiences, persons who are willing to listen and understand, who provide the needed recognition and affirmation of the evolving life story. These important social others may also have an important role to play in supporting or facilitating the communication of the illness narrative. At times, the life story cannot be communicated without the coconstruction and support provided by significant others. If a disorder is particularly stigmatizing, audience response will be affected by the stigma and associated stereotypical assumptions about competence.

Moving Forward

This chapter has provided the basic framework for understanding the communication disorders and disease processes selected for analysis in this text. In Section II of this text, many of the core constructs of Section

I are developed further from a theoretical perspective, including self, narrative and life story, and life span considerations in understanding narrative self. In Section III, theory is applied to the life stories of individuals living with acquired neurogenic communication disorders. Finally, in Section IV, each author highlights important thematic elements related to narrative self and suggests directions for moving forward. While the life stories and clinical implications chapters in Sections III and IV can be read without the material in Section II, the reader's appreciation of the issues will not be as full or complete.

SECTION II

In Section I, we situated clinical practices in a philosophy of function and introduced readers to our basic conceptual perspectives on narrative self, as well as the neurogenic disorders of interest in this text. In Section II, we examine more closely the underlying theoretical premises that provide a backdrop for exploring the life stories presented in Section III. Our focus is on the nature of self and its presentation and on the narrative processes, the "storying," that is the way we constantly negotiate and renegotiate self in social contexts.

Most people assume that they have a core self that travels with them through their life story, although it is subject to change. This perception of core self is associated with the idea of personhood. It would be difficult to operate effectively in life if we did not feel grounded in this sense of unique personhood. In Chapter 3, while acknowledging this perception, we introduce the idea that self is constantly being constructed, renegotiated in each new social situation. Four dimensions of everyday life are introduced as the primary elements out of which a self is constructed. These are described as culture, roles, interactions with other humans, and one's unique biography. All of these elements are part of a metaphorical tool kit that we regularly bring to each situation. Our ability to use our tools varies depending not only on personal communicative resources but also on the degree of personal agency and power one has in accessing them.

Language and communication are among the tools used to negotiate self construction, and it is these tools that are affected in neurogenic communication disorders. With such disorders, our ability to participate in self construction changes. It may be mildly impaired or become essentially unavailable. Chapter 4 in this section of the text lays out the narrative processes that can specifically be impaired.

In fact, it is damage to the essential storying of self, a communicative act, that constitutes the threat to narrative self that is the topic of this text. Chapter 4 provides basic definitions of narrative (personal and community) and identifies the close connections between narrative and self. In addition, narrative is described as a backdrop to illness. Within this context, theoretical perspectives on illness narratives are considered, along with discussions of the impact of communication impairment on illness narrative, perspectives of caregivers, the process of seeking biographical accommodation through the illness narrative, and tools supporting presentation of narrative, of life stories. Chapter 4 concludes with a brief discussion of narrative in the clinical context.

In writing this text, themes related broadly to time and temporality recurred frequently in the life stories we heard or read. By definition, narratives are framed in terms of time. Time is typically present in the presentation of the past, present, and possible future for narrative self. Time also implies stages in one's life trajectory, whether in the sense of Erikson's (1968) life stages or McAdam's (1993) presentation of premythic, mythic, and postmythic self. While life span considerations are touched on briefly in Chapter 4, temporal issues are given greater focus in Chapter 5. Much of Chapter 5 uses theoretical constructs of life span development from a gerontological perspective. Our intent is to emphasize the manner in which adult-onset communication disorders disrupt the lifetime trajectory of self. If the disruption occurs early in the adult life span, the challenge of renegotiation of narrative self is complicated by the perspective that this disorder has appeared at an inappropriate point in one's life course. If the disruption occurs in the lives of "older" individuals, the work of storying of self may be complicated by other age-related losses and society's devaluing of older persons in general. Chapter 5 sets the stage for the discussion of life stories and narrative self in Section III.

CHAPTER 3

The Self

In Chapter 1, we introduced our basic question, "How is the self constructed by those with neurological disorders that impair communication?" We offered the answer that, for anyone, the self is created using narratives or life stories. This answer is based on the assumption that the self is created in communication with other people. For people with neurogenic communication disorders, the ways in which the narratives can be written are fundamentally altered. In this chapter, we identify the raw materials that are available for people to create their selves. In the next chapter, we look at how those raw materials are put together into a coherent life narrative and, for those with serious illnesses, an illness narrative.

To be human is to have a self. The self is the person that we present to ourselves and others, that we use to understand and explain our actions. As humans, we are all continually engaged in the act of self creation. No matter how constrained our circumstances, how meager our resources, or how controlled our interactions, we are the ones who create our selves, but the self is never created in isolation. While individuals have unique biologies and biographies, what one comes to be is a social and cultural project. "[T]he self constructor is involved in something like an interpretive salvage oper-

ation, crafting selves from the vast array of available resources, making do with what he or she has to work with in the circumstances at hand, all the while constrained, but not completely controlled, by the working conditions of the moment" (Holstein & Gubrium, 2000, p. 153).

We often act as if we have enduring selves, because to do otherwise would be unbearably chaotic, but, in fact, the self is created situationally and in interaction with others. To argue that it is situated, though, is not to suggest that the self is eternally new. Rather, a person brings to each situation a self which has been created previously (Hewitt, 1989) and each situation itself is often scripted in predictable ways. Thus, "the reflexive project of the self, which consists in the sustaining of coherent, yet continuously revised, biographical narratives, takes place in the context of multiple choice as filtered through abstract systems" (Giddens, 1991, p. 5).

Giddens's statement is important because it points out several aspects of self construction. First, the self is biographical. Each individual is unique in his or her physiology, history, and life story. Second, the self is created in reflexive interaction with others, which makes it both "coherent and continuously revised." Third, the self is created in abstract systems, which are both structure and culture. Within structures there are patterned roles and role expectations; and culture provides us the symbols that we use to give meaning to the selves that we present. Finally, one has choices; one need never be exactly what is expected in a culture, in a structure, in a situation. While selves must be predictable, composed of parts that are culturally recognizable, we also have the freedom for individual expression, unlike any other.

What we are emphasizing is that people have agency—ultimately, they alone make choices about who they will be, but the choices they make will be based on their culture, in their roles, in a given situation interacting with others. What is important to understand is how they bring together the various resources of their biography, culture, and society to create a unique yet predictable self. However, to say that people have agency in the creation of the self does not mean that the self is always or necessarily created consciously. People can make choices about which values to believe, what goals to pursue, and so on without deciding that they therefore will be a given self. Sometimes, selves arise as a result of what we do, rather than being a conscious creation, as Swidler (1986) suggests.

Self, in the way that we are using the term, is a sociological construct and as such poses some terminological challenges for this interdisciplinary discussion. For example, the terms self and identity often seem to suggest that there is one single construct, but there are undoubtedly multiple senses of these terms, including social/collective, personal, and situational (Dowd, 2004; Mold, McKevitt, & Wolfe, 2003). There may also be important theoretical distinctions between self and identity (Gover & Gavelek, 1996), and between public and private aspects of self or identity (Shadden & Koski, 2007).

For us, identity, as typically described in the literature, is most closely incorporated in our discussion of roles. Self is a more global concept and also more personal—it incorporates the social/collective, the personal, and the situational (as we will discuss in the following), but it is also a creation of the individual. The self is a personal project.

Thus, in this text, when we talk about the self, we are recognizing the personhood of those with whom we interact. People operate on the basis of selves that they participate in creating, and to ignore that fundamental fact is to ignore the integrity—or personhood—of the individual. Self creation is fundamentally social and recognizing that can assist the clinician in her interactions with clients.

In the following, we have chosen to explore this fundamentally social nature of the self by examining four primary dimensions—the cultural aspect, roles, situational interactions, and biography. We then discuss the concepts of agency and power, which underlie all attempts at self creation. These theoretical constructs provide the foundation for discussion of the narrative self in neurogenic communication disorders.

The Dimensions of the Self

The Self and Culture

The human self is cultural. As we pointed out in Chapter 1, humans create themselves out of the parts that our society provides and we give those parts meaning. Geertz (1973, p. 5) defines culture as "webs of significance" that people spin, and argues that culture is basically semiotic, that is, a system of signs and symbols. We can also think of culture as composed of the ways that people live, work, and play together, using the things they have made to control or function in their environmental settings (Leeds-Hurwitz, 1993), as shared "cognitive schemas" (D'Andrade, 1987, p. 112), "publicly available symbolic forms" (Swidler, 1986, p. 273), or discourse (Hewitt, 1989). What each of these authors, and others, is emphasizing is that culture provides humans with the symbols—including language—that we use to "construct interpretations that create sensible, understandable, meaningful accounts" of whatever concerns us (Hewitt, 1989, p. 20) and to create selves. Symbols are meaningful only because humans give them meaning. The American flag is a piece of material, but it is also more than that, as we are so forcefully made aware when someone tries to burn it.

To be part of a culture is to use symbols that are meaningful not just to the individual but also to those with whom he interacts. "Individuals . . . actively invoke and formulate normal forms to provide meaning that all with a basic, assumed, shared cultural knowledge will grasp" (Faircloth, Boylstein, Rittman, & Gubrium, 2005, p. 931). Culturally adept people have and know how to use concepts that are culturally shared. Swidler (1986) and Wertsch (1991, 1998) use the term "tool" to capture this idea. Swidler (1986) talks about a "tool box," which contains "symbols, stories, rituals, and world-views which people may use" (p. 273). Examples are the rituals of "the pledge of allegiance" or "saying a prayer." One of the authors regularly attends a commencement ceremony at a military base in which she sits on the platform facing the audience. It is important that she understand that during the pledge of allegiance, one stands, looks at the flag, and places her right hand over her heart. It is also important that she know to bow her head during the prayer. If she did not do these things, it would be considered an insult, and perhaps worse, to all those in attendance.

A critical point that Swidler (1986) makes is that we tend to choose goals not because they are instrumentally more valuable, but because we have the (symbolic) tools to achieve them. For example, Willis (1977) provides a stunning example of working-class youth in Britain, who conspire in the creation of the very conditions that keep them trapped in poverty. Because they have come to define "mental work" as feminine, and because they view themselves as superior to women, they therefore see manual labor as the appropriate work for a man. These youths do not lack the ability to make reasoned, rational decisions about their future. Rather they choose behaviors that use the tools in their cultural tool kit—their beliefs about women and men, mental work and manual labor—in presenting a socially acceptable self to their own significant others. The boys are "the active, sometimes skilled users of culture" that Swidler (1986, p. 277) claims for all of us, but the culture that they use is that which is contained in their tool boxes, which ultimately ensures that they will remain working class.

So, at the level of culture, the self creator is given the symbols that provide meaning. If I am creating a self, for example, "mother," I understand that self initially through the symbols associated with that role and I will seek out those symbols. I will look on the Internet, read books, talk to others who have been mothers, talk to my mother. I will learn the language, the values, the emotion attached to being a mother.

Before moving on in our discussion, it is important to recognize that a challenge that arises in the construction of self for the person with a neurogenic communication disorder is the cultural perspective on illness and disability. Culture provides the symbols that give meaning to disability and these symbols tend to disadvantage individuals with impairments. In particular, cultural definitions of disability are often associated with perceptions of incompetence, lack of agency, and limited social desirability. This phenomenon is sometimes referred to in terms of stigma, and the stigma associated with any type of cognitive impairment tends to exclude individuals with disabilities from normal social intercourse (Beard, 2004; Stier & Hinshaw, 2007). In his *Toward a Model of Changing Disability Identities*, Darling (2003) suggests that there are a number of different "career paths" that may be followed by persons with disabilities, based on interactions and opportunities, which are considered in the next sections.

The Self and Roles

The reflexive self is created in interaction with others, within roles. Roles involve all of the self dimensions we have introduced— there are cultural prescriptions for how to play roles; roles are played out in interactions with others; and one's biography contributes a good deal to the playing of roles and vice versa. However, in this section, we focus specifically on what roles are and why they are important in the construction of the self.

Roles are expected patterns of behavior that give a person a social location. Hewitt (1989) argues that this social location is the "fundamental referent of identity" (p. 150). For people to create a self, they must be able to "objectify" themselves, see themselves from the perspective of another. Hewitt suggests that this objectification is based primarily on the person's roles. Prescriptions about how to play roles and how to interact with other roles are either shaped by culture or shaped by prior experience with people in those types of roles.

For example, we know how to interact with a doctor both because of our cultural experiences with that role (e.g., on television) and by prior experiences with doctors. We know how to behave as students in the classroom because we have all spent many early years in this environment.

Location in a social structure gives us authority and power to create certain types of selves and often requires specific characteristics for entry. For example, it is not possible to legally assume the role of doctor without lengthy training and certification about that training. Socialization for any role involves far more than imparting technical skills—one is also trained how to think about one's work, what values to hold ("thou shall do no harm"), what behaviors to engage in, what language to use. Professional jargon is used as much to separate the professional from the layperson as it is to efficiently communicate.

Playing roles is a continuous process of constraint and creation. As people enact their roles, they create structures (e.g., family, education, religion, government), but once created, these structures become institutionalized and constrain human roles. Giddens (1976, p. 121) says that "social structures are both constituted by human agency, and yet at the same time are the very medium of this constitution." Thus, we cannot explain self creation at the macrocultural or macrostructural level alone, nor at the interpersonal level alone. Roles are enacted by people in interaction with other people in specific situations but are affected by the patterns of interaction that have been created before they entered the situation. If a woman is anticipating the arrival of a child, she will begin to interact with others around the role of mother (e.g., baby showers, visits to the doctor) and in so doing will learn who she is expected to become.

While roles are critically important in the definition of the self, the role and the self must be kept analytically separate. If asked who they are, people will often respond with their most important role: "I am a college professor"; "I am a mother of three." However, regardless of this answer, the role that one plays is only part of the self.

The Self and Situational Interactions

Holstein and Gubrium (2000) argue that the self is constructed and presented in every social interaction and that every individual situation is the site of self construction. How we are able to use our cultural tool boxes to enact our roles will be dependent on our interactions with others. These are always specific to the situation in which we find ourselves.

When Giddens (1991) and others emphasize the reflexive nature of the self, they are pointing out that people must be able to stand back from themselves—objectify themselves, as we mentioned above—and be able to see themselves as others see them. That is, they must be aware of what others believe about them and reflect upon those beliefs, perhaps modifying their definition and presentation of self in response. This is sometimes a response to negative perceptions held by others. For example, as we have mentioned previously, when people with neurogenic communication disorders are viewed as disabled, their definition of self may be damaged.

People must also know how to take cultural expectations, values, beliefs, and norms and apply them appropriately in a given situation. In an elevator, it is appropriate to stand quietly and look at the floor numbers going by, but it would be considered a strange self indeed who did this in the middle of a sidewalk. If one is introduced to a friend's aging mother, it is appropriate to interact in a respectful and possibly defer-

ential manner. However, if the same woman is placed in a nursing home, interactions will occur rarely and when they do, the resident is treated verbally and nonverbally as incompetent.

One critical aspect of self creation is communication: "We 'talk ourselves into being' in social interaction" (Gubrium & Holstein, 2001, p. 7). As we pointed out previously, discourse, or more generally, semiotics, is critical for the give and take of self creation. While talk is not all of the matter, it is typically what others say to and about one that helps one objectify and therefore create and revise a self. One time, at a dinner party that one of the authors cohosted, she made a joke that was intended to present her self as witty. However, her guests (who had a different sense of humor) refused to accept that definition and, instead, interpreted her remarks as presenting a narrow and stingy self. That interaction was nearly 30 years ago, and she still remembers how this specific communication negated her proffered self and altered the self allowed in the interaction. With different people in a different setting, she may have been able to pull off the definition of witty.

Thus, it is only situationally that we see actual self construction, the actual use of cultural tools, and the actual enactment of social roles. And we see that those tools and roles are bent and shaped to our own interactions. Even in situations where all of the culture and all of the structure conspire to define people in certain ways, others can negate those views. For example, Bogdan and Taylor (1989) talk about people who refuse to accept official definitions of profoundly disabled loved ones as less than human, finding ways to interact with them in ways that create humanness.

And finally, we come to the individual actor, the set of physical, biological, and personality characteristics, one's abilities and appearance, the biographical self.

The Self and Biography

The self is the unique product of its own specific walk through life. No two people have the same combination of life experiences and it is out of these experiences that one draws on the raw resources to create a self. It is also here that one begins to create the "story" or "personal myth" of one's life (McAdams, 1993), which we will discuss in the next chapter, and it is here that we see the personal history or autobiography that so often determines our decisions about self.

People also, of course, have unique personality and biographical characteristics—one is male or female, relatively older or younger, abled or disabled in particular ways. One has been ill for most of one's life or one has "never been sick a day in my life." While these markers will be defined in cultural and social ways, they combine to provide a unique individual who cannot be ignored in our discussion of self. One may have power and refuse to use it. One may hold a role and be denied its benefits because of race and gender. One may have a characteristic that prevents admission to certain roles (e.g., if one has no talent for sports, one will not be playing in the finals at Wimbledon). And yet, if one has enough perseverance and determination, one may overcome many of these expectations. The biographical self, then, is one's unique combination of biology, physiology, personality, and life history as already written at a given point in time.

An Example

At this point, it might be useful to give an example of the ways in which a self is constructed. Let's take the case of Dr. X, a Caucasian female college professor from a blue-collar background. How does Ms. X come to be Professor X? We look first at culture.

From her culture (both U.S. culture and the culture of her profession), Professor X has gained assumptions, norms, values, and beliefs; that is, she has been given and has learned how to use a set of cultural tools that are now available for her use in constructing the self, "college professor." She is likely to be politically liberal, to believe that women are equal to men, to believe that humans can and should question received wisdom. She probably believes that knowledge can build on previous knowledge and this is good for society. She is likely to talk in professional jargon unknown to those outside her profession. It would be difficult to be a professor in the social sciences without at least some of these characteristics. Because she holds beliefs of the modern world, what Giddens (Personal communication, December 4, 1991) calls the project of the enlightenment, her postmodern students are likely to disagree with her belief that some sources of knowledge can be privileged. Because these are humanistic beliefs, her fundamentally religious parents are likely to disagree with her belief that received wisdom should be questioned; and because they are liberal beliefs, the layperson may argue that her knowledge does not make the world a better place. The use of these tools and not others is partly what distinguishes her as a college professor.

From culture, Professor X is given expectations for how to correctly play the role of college professor. She is likely to live in a particular part of town, drive a fuel efficient car, listen to classical music and NPR. She is expected to engage in research, publish professional papers in selected journals (or books, depending on her field). She is expected to refrain from cheating, plagiarism, and academic dishonesty in her own research, and she is expected to give grades because they are earned, not bought. She will use her cultural tool box to reinforce her presentation of a college professor self, emphasizing those tools that she knows how to use, while being affected by the lack where she does not have the necessary tool. For example, because Professor X has a Ph.D. from a state university, if she finds herself employed at an Ivy League university, she will not share the background of her peers and she will never have quite the same assumptions about the world as they. This will affect the ways in which she is able to play her role.

In her interactions with her peers, her superiors, and her students, if Professor X uses her cultural tool box to create the expected self and if she has the necessary tools in that tool box, then her self will be successfully created (for the moment). However, if she strays from the normative role performance, she will encounter resistance and if she strays far enough (e.g., engages in academic dishonesty), she may be expelled from the role altogether. Because there are a number of expectations for any role, she can choose which ones to privilege (such as emphasizing teaching over research), but if she works in a setting that resists those choices, she may again find herself subject to being expelled when she does not receive tenure. Thus, if at a research university, Professor X is likely to present herself to her peers in ways that emphasize her research record and the self that engages in that research.

This does not mean she has only one self. Our college professor will be one person in the classroom, another person at lunch with her peers, a third person at home with her spouse, and yet a fourth person at gatherings of her extended family. She will use jargon with her peers, explain the jargon to her students, and never use it with her families. She will present herself as a liberal with her peers, not discuss politics with her students, and avoid the topic altogether with her father.

Finally, Professor X will use her tool box in ways affected by her biography. Since our college professor is from a blue-collar background, there will be some tools that she never really learns how to use, but others that she possesses because of her background. She will never be completely easy with the privilege of her position, but she may find less of a division between herself and her working-class students. Interactions with others will as often be a source of unease as confirmation of her identity (Borkowski, 2004).

At every level of our analysis, if we change a characteristic of Professor X we will expect to see a different type of self. If Professor X lives in a different society (such as England), there will be different tools in her tool box. If she is educated in an Ivy League university, there will be different tools. If she is male rather than female, upper class rather than blue collar, employed in chemical engineering rather than the social sciences, she will have different tools. With different tools, there will be a different self. And ultimately, if she chooses to, she can present a different type of self even with the circumstances we have outlined. It may be harder for her to present a successful "college professor" self if she does not publish, but some have found a way; she may be pressured to be politically liberal, but she may choose to maintain the political and religious beliefs of her family; she may base her primary identity on her ethnic group rather than her profession. We must never forget that people have agency.

Agency

Agency is the ability to create the self that one wishes to have, to adeptly manipulate the tools in the cultural tool box, and to present an image of a coherent self (if one wishes to do so) across situations. Agency is mastery of the symbols used in a given situation. Agency is the ability to understand social interaction enough to be able to successfully negotiate it. Agency is knowledge of the cultural symbols, the ability to correctly predict which symbols will be privileged in an interaction, and the ability to use those symbols or substitute others.

The idea that selves are created situation by situation provides enormous opportunity for agency: "Since selves are socially constructed and situationally located, the social world is populated with more selves than people" (Hopper, 2001, p. 127). As Gubrium and Holstein (2001, p. 19) suggest: "Our ability to choose between options—to use some options in order to resist others, or to construct new ones—can be as liberating as it is overwhelming and debilitating."

Agency is not possible without power. Power is a resource that fills a cultural tool box with the appropriate tools and that animates those tools. We turn next to a discussion of power.

Power

For the purposes of this book, we define power as the ability to create a self that is accepted by others. Therefore, power is available (or not) at each of the levels of culture, role, situation/interaction, and biography discussed previously. As we discuss each of the levels of self construction, we will acknowledge briefly how power may play out in clinical interactions involving the speech-language pathologist (SLP).

Cultural Power

Bourdieu (1972/1991) reminds us that one may have power through symbolic resources as much as through economic or material resources. Bourdieu refers to this as cultural capital. It is not just the material usefulness of an object that determines its value, but also the meaning we bring to the object. We see this when a possession from, for example, Princess Diana, Jacqueline Kennedy, or Elvis Presley is made available for auction. In the clinical world, there are VIP clients, just as there are persons with limited cultural resources. In an equitable world, all clients would be treated equally. However, it is not uncommon for a clinician to be told, "You know, this is Mrs. X. The hospital wants us to make sure she gets the best treatment."

Cultural capital does not just refer to the possession of material items, however; it can also include the control of definitions, assumptions, values, and norms. In the clinical setting, the SLP controls the actual definition of the disorder being presented. This gives the clinicians considerably more power in defining their own self and in the negotiation of the client's self— the client will be at least partly defined by this diagnosis.

Power from Roles

The power that comes with role placement is critically important to the concept of self. This is two edged. On the one hand, with each role comes a set of preconceived notions of the self that will hold that position, and this gives power to the individual to act in accordance with that role. For example, an academic in a research university is expected to prefer independent research to teaching undergraduates. On the other hand, it may be difficult for the person occupying that role to bring into play alternate selves (for example, preferring to teach undergraduate students over engaging in research). An SLP occupies a number of roles within an organizational structure such as a hospital or rehabilitation facility. In addition to the obvious role of "professional providing services to the communicatively impaired," the clinician also occupies the role of "subordinate to his/her immediate supervisor." That supervisor may be responsible for monitoring and increasing productivity in terms of billable hours, and thus may view the clinician primarily as a source of potential revenue. In the eyes of other therapists in that setting (e.g., physical or occupational therapists), the clinician may play the role of "valued collaborator in team interventions." However, in the eyes of a physician who is not convinced of the efficacy of therapy, the clinician's role is less clear, except in its obvious subservience to the M.D.

Power in Interactions

At least in small task-oriented groups, such as those which involve the SLP, research has indicated that those with higher status characteristics typically have more power in interpersonal interactions (Kalkhoff & Thye, 2006). For example, the early literature on jury deliberations found that "proprietors" were more likely to sway the decision of the group than those in unskilled positions (Berger, Fisek, Norman, & Zelditch, 1977, p. 4). The power inherent in one's role also affects the power one has in interactions, and here the SLP typically has more power than the client. The client's power is dependent more on his ability to communicate. A highly verbal, socially interactive client has the power to compel the attention and interaction with a clinician in ways not available to those who are relatively speechless. It is important, therefore, not just to focus on the formal power held by a role's incumbent, but also the ability to negotiate an interaction.

Interactional power is also influenced strongly by the clinical perspective of the SLP. The movement toward socially-based person-centered therapy in communication disorders is an example of an attempt to change the definition of the self for both the clinician and client. A focus on the personhood of a client, not just the diagnosis, alters the clinical interaction by placing both parties on a more level playing field and empowering the client. What is altered in part is also the defined role of the professional, who must now focus on facilitating the client's search for a narrative self that includes a specific disorder. This has broadened the definition of self for the clinician but also certainly increased the ways that she may fail at successfully managing that role.

Power from Biography

Finally, power may come from one's biography. One's gender, race, and age; one's family name; one's experiences that comprise the life story completed to date; one's history of illnesses—all of these affect the power that one will have for creating a self. People who are abled find it possible to create and present a certain type of self more than those who are disabled, and those who are profoundly disabled may be stigmatized as less than human (Bogdan & Taylor, 1989). SLPs may choose to acknowledge biographical characteristics that empower the client, or may focus primarily on biography as defined by impairment. This is also true for the client.

Agency, Power, and the Self

Individuals have agency to create a self to the extent that they have the raw materials listed below. Each of these elements is predicated in part upon intact communication, which supports agency, provides power, and allows social definition of self. After the bulleted list of elements, we illustrate each with an example in which a speech pathologist is interacting with a client who has a communication disorder:

- *Cultural tools* that the person is capable of using. Example: The speech pathologist uses jargon unknown to the client, thus limiting the cultural tools available to the client for self creation, but enabling her own self creation as a professional with specialized and superior knowledge.
- *Roles* that enable or make harder a person's self creation. Example: The relative roles assigned to the speech pathologist versus the client again restrict the types of selves that the client may offer. The speech pathologist has a range of ways in which she may enact that role, but the client is required to operate (typically) under the medical model of relative incompetence.
- *Interactions* that provide ever-new sites for self construction, but which also have combined to form a history of self presentation. Interactions provide the locations where cultural tools may be used in accordance with role prescriptions and opportunities. Example: The person with a neurogenic communication disorder may be limited in interaction with a physician to the prescripts of the medical model but may find considerable opportunity for self creation in interaction with similar others in a self-help group.
- *Biography*, which includes biological and personality characteristics, life stories, and personal myths that allow an individual to create and present a certain self. Example: A woman is more likely to be a practicing speech pathologist than is a man; a client with aphasia who is younger is more likely to receive ongoing treatment than someone who is in his later years. A clinician who has personal experience with a particular disorder, such as with a parent's stroke and aphasia, may bring the understandings evolved from her own life story into the interaction with the client.
- *Power* to negotiate the acceptance of the self with given others in a specific setting. Example: In a clinical setting, the speech pathologist has greater power to set the parameters around possible self creation than does the client, for both the speech pathologist and the client. However, a high status client will have relatively more power relative to a lower status client. Relative to a medical setting, in a community center dedicated to the life participation of a person with aphasia, the clinician's power will be limited to supporting self acceptance and empowerment on the part of the person with aphasia.

The Social Construction of the Self

We have argued in this chapter that every aspect of self creation is a social project that is coauthored with nearly everyone

one encounters and that requires the complicity of others to pull off. At the level of culture, every object, every word, every value and belief is given meaning by that society. At the level of role, one's access to that position, the ways in which one may enact the role, appropriate and inappropriate actions within the role, and how long one is allowed to keep it are all dependent on others. Creating oneself in interaction with others means that one can only create a self if one is able to successfully present and negotiate the acceptance of that self, and if one has the power to resist definitions that others might wish to impose. And finally, although biography is sometimes physiological and personal, its meaning is always social. While one is biologically male or female, what it means to be male or female is determined by one's culture.

We turn now to an example that demonstrates how a self may be affected by a neurogenic communication disorder.

An Illustrative Clinical Scenario

Mr. Wilson suffered a CVA on August 2 and was admitted to acute care at the Medicine First Hospital. He was paralyzed on the right side and was unable to communicate at the time of admission or during the first full day of hospitalization. He burst into tears on several occasions when he could not say the words he wanted. The family asked about the communication problems and was told by the physician that these would probably improve over time. A neurologist is called in at the end of the first day and, observing fairly obvious aphasic deficits, requests a speech-language consult.

This scenario already illustrates some elements relevant to understanding challenges in creating or modifying self, particularly those associated with agency and power. Mr. Wilson and his family are relatively powerless in this situation, since both the fact of illness and placement in a medical setting define the person as powerless, having no role other than that of passive recipient of provided services. The family attempts to be active in seeking help for Mr. Wilson's communication, but their efforts are disregarded by the first physician, who knows that there is an SLP on staff but sees little value in the services she provides. Thus, the role of the SLP is defined in part by the physician who is, in this medical setting, at the top of the power hierarchy. However, the neurologist not only recognizes the communication disorder but also values the role of speech-language services, empowering the SLP by requesting a consult and indirectly empowering the family in their efforts to seek help.

The SLP sees Mr. Smith on the second day and performs an informal bedside evaluation, consisting of a few tests but no personal questions for either the patient or the wife. Fortunately, Mrs. Smith and one of the adult children are present, and the SLP provides them with a brief summary of her observations, as well as a diagnosis. The family is told that "Mr. Smith has global aphasia, which has very poor prognosis." Mrs. Smith bursts into tears and asks, "But will he be able to talk clearly again?" The SLP indicates that she doesn't know, then indicates that he will receive speech therapy while in the hospital, and possibly subsequently in a rehabilitation facility. Mr. Smith has begun to cry, seeing his wife so upset. His wife says she has never seen him do this before; it is like he is a different person. The SLP tells the family that this crying, called emotional lability, is common. She makes no eye contact with Mr. Smith while attempting to reassure the family.

So what has happened here? Again, issues of agency, power, and self are evident. The SLP has chosen to create her self based on the medical model. She uses unfamiliar jargon with the family, thus establishing her professionalism while simultaneously taking away the family's power to participate fully in the interaction. Mrs. Smith expresses concerns about what she sees as critical changes in "who" her husband is or was prestroke, particularly the crying behavior. Instead of addressing the wife's concerns about the fundamental integrity of her husband's self, the SLP simply labels the behavior with more jargon, thus reinforcing the family's sense of being powerless. By ignoring Mr. Smith during this discussion, the SLP also makes clear that he has no power in this situation and that who he is matters very little. The SLP defines Mr. Wilson as a patient and thus has very little interest in how either Mr. or Mrs. Smith has defined him previously. In this tension-charged setting, where the SLP has considerable power to impose a self definition, Mr. Smith has lost agency and is painfully subject to the definitions of others.

After 4 days, Mr. Wilson is discharged to the Better Living Rehabilitation Center in a nearby town. When admitted to that facility, a social worker takes an extensive case history from the wife and adult children, exploring everything from finances and employment history to personality style and family structure. Mrs. Wilson leaves this interview somewhat encouraged about the personal care her husband may receive while in treatment. The social worker shares much of this information at a staffing

held by the team treating Mr. Wilson. At the first meeting with him, a new SLP immediately begins making references to his life and family. While she knows that he does not yet understand everything she is saying, she recognizes the importance of connecting on the social, interactional level. Both Mr. Wilson and his family are given an opportunity to share their concerns and communication goals, and the SLP requests photos of family, home, pets—all of the personal things that are part of the biographical particulars of our lives. During the next three weeks, Mr. Wilson makes excellent progress in recovery of communication skills. As he improves, the SLP shifts her focus to more functional communication activities—the kinds of things Mr. Wilson will need to get through the day. He also begins attending a communication therapy group with others who have aphasia, and his immediate post-stroke depression seems to be lifting. At the staffing meeting held at the end of the 3rd week, it is the SLP who recommends to the physiatrist that Mr. Wilson receive inpatient treatment for one additional week, to further support his functional skills. The team supports her decision.

The situation has changed dramatically since Mr. Wilson was admitted to this particular inpatient rehabilitation facility. From the outset, family and patient are provided with opportunities to explain the biographic particulars of their lives, and the provided information is used by all team members to design a more individualized, personally relevant treatment program. All of this is very self-affirming, as is the SLP's continuing focus on those functional communication skills that will allow Mr. Wilson to play out his role as communication partner in everyday life activities. The more he is able to participate, the more likely he will be able to present a new self that can be validated by others. She is also providing him with action strategies for these situations, and with increasing control in the process of goal setting for his communication improvement and for his life post-stroke. Finally, in this facility, the SLP herself is allowed to play out more empowered structural roles. She is acknowledged as an expert, and her recommendations with respect to Mr. Wilson's care are validated and supported by the treatment team.

For this story to have the best possible ending, we might postulate that, upon discharge from the Better Living Rehabilitation Center, Mr. Wilson and his family began attending a stroke support group where they receive consistent support in their process of renegotiating who and what they are in life after aphasia. In finding this community, they begin to feel empowered. Other group members also provide them with interactions that allow them to move forward and with reinforcement for the difficult process of setting new life goals. Finally, if Mr. Wilson began outpatient treatment in a Life Stories Communication Group, he would learn to use a variety of tools to support his communication, and he would be able to share with others elements of his past, present, and hoped-for future in order to move past the biographical disruption of his stroke. He would also be able to experience success in presenting himself to others and in being recognized for the person he is today, a competent, empowered person who has aphasia.

One would hope that the early stages of Mr. Wilson's treatment in the previous case scenario would not be seen in health care today. Sadly, some version of this fam-ily's experience does play out in our hospitals all around the country. What is most important is an understanding of the complexity of the processes that occur and the ways in which the SLP may assist in the creation of new selves for the affected person and his significant others.

Conclusion

In this chapter, we have laid the foundation for this text's exploration of the impact of neurogenic communication disorders on self, emphasizing the fundamentally social nature of the creation of self. Humans are often inarticulate in the discussion of such abstract constructs as self. The ways that they actually construct and present a self to others is in the telling of life stories, their personal narratives.

We have considered the basic elements out of which a self is created—those elements provided by the culture, by roles, by interaction with other humans, and by one's unique biography. We have also suggested that power affects how one may access and use these tools, and we have emphasized that people have agency—within some boundaries—to create their selves. We have emphasized that all of these elements are packed within a tool box that may be more or less brimming with available resources for constructing the self.

In the next chapter, we move forward with our argument that the self is created through narrative. By taking each of the elements of the self we have discussed, using the tools in our tool box, and weaving them into a story, we create the self we offer in each situation. We turn to that theme next.

CHAPTER 4

Narrative Processes

One basic premise of this text is that life is essentially storied. As one of today's leading theorists, Jerome Bruner (2002), suggests, "There's some kind of underlying thing that gives a kind of unity and sympathy and possibility for the human condition continuing" (p. 3). This quote is particularly intriguing because it is remarkably inarticulate, a surprising observation given the usual eloquence of Bruner's writings. What the inarticulateness suggests is that narrative is not a simple construct. In the previous chapter, we introduced the raw materials that are available for self construction—cultural, roles, interactional, and biographical. In this chapter, we discuss how an individual's life story weaves together these raw materials to create a coherent narrative. Our goal is to understand the impact of neurogenic communication disorders on narrative self.

Exploring Narrative

The term narrative can be understood at many levels and in multiple theoretical contexts. On one level, typically addressed in speech-language pathology, linguistics, and developmental psychology, the term narrative refers explicitly to storytelling. The ability to understand and reproduce the key elements of what some call story grammar is a fundamental tool in formal education and informal learning about life. We study how children's narratives or stories develop, and we target narratives in speech-language treatment if children lag behind their peers in using the necessary narrative skills. We define those elements that must be present in a fully developed narrative structure, and we devise strategies to help children acquire and use those elements. The key elements of stories include setting, characters, initiating event, attempt to resolve, consequence, and reaction. Thus, narrative involves placing a series of events in some sort of order that implies chronological sequence and postulates causality. What is critical in this understanding of narrative is the fact that stories are creations, and the teller of stories can alter story elements to change the underlying coherence of the narrative. As Chambers and Montgomery (2002, p. 78) indicate, " . . . there are no unplotted stories."

Narrative can also be understood from a broader perspective of entertainment and socialization. As we mature, we begin to tell narratives to entertain and amuse others. On the surface, these stories may not seem to carry much weight in terms of sharing information about ourselves, but the choice of stories to tell often informs the listener about who and what we are and what we value. In has been suggested that much of our everyday conversation consists of some kind of storytelling. Some of these everyday stories are also told to communicate a message, based on sharing of a particular life experience.

Beyond this level of storytelling, we reach a more powerful understanding of narratives as life stories. McAdams and colleagues (McAdams, Josselson, & Lieblich, 2005, 2006a, b) point to the fact that humans are fundamentally storytellers, and Bruner (2004) notes that: "We seem to have no other way of describing 'lived time' save in the form of a narrative" (p. 692). At this level, narrative is viewed as an enculturated meaning-making process (Sarbin, 1986a, b). In other words, life is narrative and life stories are ongoing (Bruner, 2004). Common terms to describe this process include biographical work, framing of biographical particulars, meaning-making, and sense-making. As part of the meaning-making process, narrative can be viewed as a tool for expressing wants, needs, perspectives, and priorities.

McAdams (1988,1993) suggests there are two primary drives underlying our life stories: communion (relationships, intimacy), and agency (issues of power, mastery, and achievement). There is a dynamic tension between these two drives. People whose life stories are built around agency are those whose life activities are oriented toward the acquisition or display of power, autonomy, mastery, and achievement. They need to be strong, to have an impact on the world, to achieve success. In contrast, those whose life stories are framed around a desire for communion present life stories in which relationships with others play an important role. Such individuals are valued for their friendship and support. They belong to multiple social communities and act on communally held beliefs. Balance between the two drives is optimal.

When communication disorders disrupt the ongoing storying of self, it is important to understand the degree to which communion and agency figure in an individual's narrative self and the extent to which these processes are affected by impaired communication. Often, the stories that people attempt to share are designed to underscore the agentic or communal aspects of self that have been threatened by the illness. Those with a dominant drive to express and live agency will attempt to tell stories that support their view of narrative self as strong, independent, and accomplished (or express the loss of those elements). Those whose life stories are framed around strong needs for relationship and communion will try to share stories about people and relationships and caring (or about perceived losses of intimacy).

Bruner (1999) suggests that characterization of self or selfhood "rests upon a good story, a plot with Self as the agent that heads somewhere and gives continuity . . . we manage a certain autonomy while at the same time adhering to cultural forms" (p. 7). In this text, what is particularly important about this broader view of narrative is that it is inextricably linked with the process of development of self and identity. Damasio (1999) suggests that "consciousness begins when the brain acquires the power of telling a story" (p. 30). McAdams (1993) provides detailed accounts of how our personal self or myth evolves through stages from pre-mythic (childhood) through mythic (the realized and evolving self) and ultimately to postmythic (looking back from the perspective of advanced age).

The idea of a personal myth may be crucial in understanding the experiences of persons with communication disorders. One's personal myth is a self-created history of self, one that explains how and why events occurred and what they mean. The personal myth must be modifiable, because as our lives move on, different interpretations of life events must be constructed to be consistent with an evolving sense of self. Development of life stories and self results in greater focus on "I"—the self as storyteller, as contrasted with "me"—the self as the tale told (James, 1963). It is possible that one of the most destructive outcomes of an adult onset neurogenic communication disorder is people's inability to frame the "I," which leads to their dependence upon others and the environmental context for a definition of "me."

There is no question about the statement, "Stories matter" (Charon & Montello, 2002). The meanings we derive from our shared life stories become pivotal in informing the next stages of our lives (Singer, 2004). In discussing humans as meaning makers, Kitwood (1997) highlights that our social lives can be viewed as a series of narrative episodes, and the actions we take in new episodes are informed by the schema understood and the meanings assigned in previous life episodes. In one sense, our life stories are autobiographical, but autobiography is much more than the factual recounting of life events. More broadly, as Bruner (2004) suggests, the telling of a story is a truly challenging cognitive achievement. We must structure our experiences, organize relevant memories, segment and scaffold events. In doing so, we strive to empower ourselves in the present and in projected future circumstances.

Clearly, narrative, the telling of life stories, is a fundamentally social process. We create stories to meet the needs of our varied social roles (Singer, 2004), and we seek recognition and validation of our stories by those social others with whom we interact. Our stories are constantly being shaped and reshaped to meet the challenges of different listeners and different contexts as well

as alterations in the biographical particulars of our lives. In effect, as Beck (2005) suggests, "all narratives contain the voices of others, and require recognition of the identities of others" (p. 61). Not only do we require the recognition and validation of others, but they are also actively involved in the construction and reconstruction of our sense of self. In the context of illness, and even more specifically disease processes that affect our ability to communicate and render us metaphorically voiceless, it may be literally impossible to reconstruct a continuing life story and narrative self without the participation of others in this process.

Implicit in the preceding statement is the concept that social narrative requires the use of communication as the primary tool for conveying and modifying life stories. Narrative is a form of discourse, and narrative discourse typically occurs during the normal give and take of conversational interactions. These interactions can be viewed as negotiations. Each participant takes stock of what is known or presumed about the conversational partner, as well as the context for the conversation and the underlying purpose or need being met through the interaction. With familiar partners, little work is needed to make the necessary decisions about how the story is framed. With less familiar partners or in new environmental contexts, greater flexibility may be required, along with some trial-and-error negotiation of acceptable symbol sets and probes of shared experience.

The use of the term story should not be interpreted too narrowly. Story or narrative refers to any shared communication that provides the listener with a better understanding of the person who is communicating. Similarly, the concept of life story must be interpreted broadly. Although there are a number of approaches designed to elicit a life story or life history (cf.,

McAdams, 1988, 1993), it is not necessary to formally request the telling of the "chapters" of one's life to date. Bits and pieces of informal narrative can be interpreted in the context of life story and used to understand the self that is being presented in the interaction.

In fact, these bits and pieces, often called episodes (McAdams, 1993), are the primary elements that are shared in a natural communication interaction. Gubrium (2003) has attempted to define what constitutes a "good story" in the context of support groups for caregivers for persons with dementia. On the basis of his work with such groups, he concludes that the good story (a) rings true, (b) is engrossing, and (c) provides adequate but not excessive detail. By "good," he means successful in sharing of narrative self.

Our sense of self is being recreated and reordered constantly against the backdrop of daily experiences. At everyday crossroads in life, we create appropriate versions of self to maximize our success in interaction and managing small challenges. We do so through the narratives which are conveyed in conversation. Thus, communication in everyday conversations is a forum for self-narration. The success of these interactions depends on a number of factors, including the conversational partners' perception of the storyteller's competence and power and communication skills of the narrator.

In Chapter 1, it was suggested that presentation of self through narrative is only effective if the identities we project fall within some societal understanding of normal or acceptable. In part, the parameters that define normalcy or acceptability are being constantly negotiated. As Gubrium and Holstein (2001) state: "Broadly speaking, the self emanates from the interplay between circumstantial demands, restraints, and resources, on one hand, and self-constituting social actions on the other" (p. 9). Being different, however, does not totally disenfranchise the individual from participation within society. Being different may simply mean that one shares certain attributes or interests with others who form part of a larger community with which we affiliate. To understand this statement, it is necessary to understand the concept of community narrative.

Part of the cognitive challenge of narrative is creating and sharing life stories that mesh with the broader community (Rappaport, 1993). Thus the cognitive and linguistic processes that guide our narratives are shaped culturally. Community may be as narrowly defined as the group of colleagues with whom one eats lunch once a week or as broadly structured as the context of the community within which we live, the community with which one affiliates through religious preference, or the political party that defines one's beliefs. We can only participate effectively in these many communities if we understand the motives and characteristics of other community members, the reason the community exists, and the norms and practices for communicating what Holstein and Gubrium (2000, p. 12) refer to as discursive environments. However, our community affiliations influence our personal narratives.

If we reflect on people's responses to any disruption to their life story, to their expected life course, it is common to find statements like, "My friends have been there for me," or "The people I work with really stepped up to the plate," or "The church women's group reached out to me." All of these clusters of persons represent groups, or communities with which one is affiliated. Paul Rusesabagina (2006) movingly describes the power of groups in talking about his experiences living through Rwanda's darkest moments, stating:

We embrace the feeling of being dissolved into something bigger because at our cores we are lonely . . . we thirst for that unity, that lost wholeness. . . . That feeling of warm acceptance we get inside a group . . . is one of the most powerful human urges. (p. 73)

This concept of cultural group membership in one or more discursive environments is particularly important when the life story is disrupted by the diagnosis of a significant medical problem, such as those associated with the neurogenic disorders we discuss in this text. At these times, we are perhaps most needy of the understanding and validation of the larger social communities with which we affiliate—however we define those communities in connection with our unique narrative self. It is difficult to put into words exactly what it is we require from our narrative communities, because issues of self construction and the recognition of others are difficult to articulate. But the need exists and changes in community membership have a powerful impact on our sense of identity and self.

Ironically, as we experience the life changes that accompany a significant health crisis, when the comfort and familiarity of old ways of presenting narrative self are most needed, the communities that formerly recognized and supported a person's sense of self may become less accessible. These changes in social validation stem to a considerable degree from a breakdown in ability to communicate effectively who and what we are in the context of an unexpected shift in our life stories. Since communication remains a primary meaning-making tool, its impairment can be very

isolating. Thus coping with a neurogenic communication disorder may require definitions of the communities with which we choose to affiliate, as discussed later in this chapter.

Narrative and the Self

It should be obvious by now that it is almost impossible to discuss narrative and life story without considering the role of narrative in our creation and maintenance of self. Narrative clearly brings together the raw materials of self construction and weaves a whole story, one that will undoubtedly change as one moves through life or even from situation to situation. Since our focus in this book is on narrative self rather than either separately, it is important to combine these two concepts. Fundamentally, the cultural, role, interactional, and biographical elements of the self inform the plot one creates.

We exist within societies, within cultures that define appropriate and acceptable ways of functioning. Thus the term *cultural self* captures the many schema that govern how we are supposed to live together. While cultural symbols and knowledge are acquired gradually over time, they define expectations that govern one's understanding of one's self within the society. Culture also influences the expectations of others. Thus, we cannot really create a comprehensible narrative unless we start with the norms, values, beliefs, and ideologies of our culture. There are many cultural narrative processes that shape the cultural self. Examples may include laws and policies that govern behavior, cultural models conveyed through media and the Internet, and organizational procedures.

Our narratives also build on the culturally defined *roles* that we play now and have played in the past. The narrative of a college professor with Parkinson's disease, for example, is different from that of a carpenter with Parkinson's. A person who is a parent will create a different narrative when she is faced with ALS from someone who has never had children. A young adult acts and speaks and shares aspects of her self one way with a parent, another with a college instructor, and yet another way with friends. In effect, the narratives shared (including the way in which they are framed) allow people to present multiple selves defined structurally through roles. The success or failure of the self associated with each role depends largely upon the appropriateness and adequacy of the behaviors and the narrative processes that occur. For example, one type of vocabulary and set of topics is selected for use with one's peers, and another set is chosen for the employer.

Success in establishing a particular structural self depends on our understanding of the culturally defined roles *and* the communicative choices we make, as seen in the *interactional level of self creation*. At this level, language and communication are the primary tools in our cultural tool kit. Thus narrative processes—how and what we exchange communicatively with others —are the foundation for constructing and presenting the different selves we wish others to acknowledge and validate socially. When the communicative tool is damaged in the essential interaction between two or more humans (as with the neurological disorders discussed in this text), the cultural and role elements of self construction are also disrupted. Fundamentally, at this level, it is critical that others accept our narratives and reinforce them.

Finally, self is also authored by each individual who carries a unique cluster of *biog-*

raphical particulars that must be conveyed if the personhood of that individual is to be understood by others. Any of the disorders discussed in this text influence the biographical self in two ways. First, the disorder takes away skill in using the communicative tool needed to share one's uniqueness with another, in order to obtain validation. Second, the precipitating illness itself and the associated communication disorder actually change the person's life story in big or little ways. Those changes are perhaps best understood if we consider the role of illness narratives in the reconstruction of self.

Narrative as a Backdrop to Illness

As already suggested, the life story must be revised whenever we experience any kind of significant life change that creates a fork in one's lifeline, a point of disruption (Bury, 1982; Gregg, 2006). To be successful in allowing the individual to go on with life, these stories or narratives will essentially recreate the self to take the disruption into account. However, the successful creation of a new narrative, and thus a new self, requires the ability to communicate in social contexts about the narrative changes that are occurring. We are aided in our understanding of this process if we add two more theoretical concepts—the illness narrative and the health narrative.

As established earlier in this chapter, narratives provide a kind of unity to our sense of self, a unity that is particularly important when our biographical particulars are disrupted by major events, like a loss of a loved one or the diagnosis of a serious illness. When a person becomes ill, there are many life changes that must be addressed— challenges in terms of surrounding people, common environments, daily interactions, and required actions. The person's communication system and life story need to be particularly resilient to manage the challenges of these changes.

In effect, major life changes require reconstruction, renegotiation, and restorying of the self. The vehicle for effecting those changes is narrative communication. At such critical crossroads in one's life trajectory, at a time when we are most in need of communicative tools to negotiate these changes, those skills may be impaired as part of the presenting disease processes. Thus, the challenge is to find ways to use significantly altered sets of cultural tools after life-changing events when we are most dependent on known selves and familiar items in our cultural tool kits (Swidler, 2001).

In the past 20 years, there has been growing attention to the importance of illness (or more recently health) narratives in helping people cope with life changes associated with a major medical crisis. In medicine, the consideration of illness narratives has been linked to the study and practice of bioethics, with the implication that it is the responsibility of ethical medical practitioners to listen to and understand the narratives their patients try to share. This is particularly important given the fact that "the medical narrative trumps all others" (Frank, 1995, p. 5) and seeking medical care is often equivalent to narrative surrender. In other words, it is easy to lose one's individuality once one enters the medical system. One goal for clinicians should be to affirm and support the uniqueness of each individual seen for assessment and treatment.

The Illness Narrative

According to Frank (1995, p. 55), "illness is a call for stories." This quote will be repeated throughout this text because it is funda-mental to an understanding of what persons with neurogenic disorders need. As established previously, humans depend on narrative and communication in general to move on with their life stories in the context of an unexpected narrative disruption (Bury, 1982). The illness narrative provides a vehicle for healthy adjustment to threatening life events and for the search for meaning, mastery, and redefinition of self. These threatening life events create a kind of narrative wreckage (Frank, 1995, 2002), and one important role of the illness narrative is to tell the facts of this narrative wreckage in an immediate and literal way. However, "illness threatens not only the individual's physical integrity but also the individual's identity and sense of self in the world" (Stanley, 2004, p. 255), one's self-respect, and life plan (Brody, 2003). Thus, shared illness narratives allow one to repair the damage to one's sense of who she is and where she is going in life. The sharing allows others to witness, recognize, and validate the reconstruction of self that needs to occur (Caplan, Haslett, & Burleson, 2005; Haidet, Kroll, & Sharf, 2006).

This sharing is particularly needed to counteract the fact that most people navigate illness alone, isolated from the healthy, from loved ones, from the body, and even from one's self. In today's health care system, patients tend to become depersonalized. They lose autonomy, agency, control, and independence by virtue of being cast in the role of patient. In fact, Stanley (2004) suggests that the sick can "interiorize the sense that they ruin the otherwise 'normal' landscape" (p. 247). Ironically, while the burden typically falls upon ill persons to find a voice for themselves within the medical world, it should be the health professionals who take the initiative to elicit the stories that provide meaning to the illness experience. What is needed fundamentally is social validation. Without such validation, it is difficult if not impossible to make sense of one's suffering and to order one's life story (McKevitt, 2000). Thus patients need to feel that they are known as much for their humor as their cholesterol levels.

There are a number of important elements that characterize the creation and sharing of illness narratives (Hinckley, 2007). First, it is clear that there are different forms of illness narratives that reflect personal perspectives on the experience of living with sickness (Bruner, 2002; Frank, 1995). Understanding these perspectives is an essential part in helping people move forward. For example, some patients or their family members tell chaos narratives that capture the sense of profound biographical disruption they are experiencing but provide little direction for moving on. Three days after her husband's stroke, one spouse told the speech-language clinician, "I don't know what to do now. What happens when he comes home? I mean, he can't walk. I don't think I can lift him. And I don't know what he is trying to say." Clearly, the dominant motif in these statements is sense of chaos, of a world turned upside down. Physicians and other health care providers often attempt to communicate what are essentially restitution narratives, ones that emphasize the role of the medical professional in fixing or restoring the patient. To varying degrees, patients or family members may accept this version of the illness experience, but it is not one generated within the framework of the individual life story. The spouse described above was reassured by the doctor that her husband would be referred to "rehab" and that would help. For this woman, who had no understanding of what constituted rehab and no sense of the degree of potential recovery, the words were only minimally reassuring.

Many accounts of illness also take the form of quest narratives, in which the patient seeks to understand, to redefine self, to recast the life story. Such narratives have been described by others as healing narratives (McKevitt, 2000). These narratives take many forms, depending on the person's premorbid life experiences in general and her experience with illness specifically. For example, one man with aphasia told his physical therapist, "I know how. Therapy before. Now . . . how long, how much." His comments referred to the fact that he had experienced a small stroke several years prior to this one, had undergone physical therapy, and simply wanted to know how long therapy would take and how much he might recover. The husband of another stroke survivor told a support group, "We're not going to give up. We've tried the hyperbaric chambers and she got a little more movement in her right arm. Now we're looking at that new constraint therapy . . . checking out a place in Florida. That may be the ticket."

Another element that must be understood is the fact that most illness and healing narratives have common components (McKevitt, 2000). These include (a) a storylike form; (b) the retelling of events and experiences in an ordered fashion; (c) concern for the expression of meaning and coherence and for moving beyond the isolated personal experience to the collective one; and (d) an experience shaped for the listener. Note the importance of time in this framing of common elements. As discussed in Chapter 5, illnesses are time bound (Charon, 2002). In the narrative about illness, there are different kinds of times. For example, there is the real time playing out of the story, in all its particulars, through whatever part of the lifetime it occupies. There is also discourse time—the time required to tell the story, or retell over and over to as many listeners as needed to yield some sense of meaning.

In different versions of these narratives, it is particularly important to note the terms that are used to describe the illness, the person's current status, and the process needed to overcome illness. For example, some persons describe illness in relatively neutral terms, either labeling the problem with the correct medical diagnosis or referring to "my condition" or "my situation." Others focus on the process or their internal perception of the illness, such as one spouse of an ALS patient who described their medical journey as "fighting the monster."

Illness narratives also provide information that is important to the physical and emotional healing of the individual (Hinckley, 2007). To some degree, such narratives let us understand how the person conceptualizes the disease process, particularly whether it is seen as external or internal to the sick person. Stories also capture the patient's perception of her responsibility in healing and recovery. The language of these narratives indicates the degree to which the patient expects repair to occur, and in what time frame. Mold, McKevitt, and Wolfe (2003) discuss the fact that the biographical disruption of illness can be associated with a loss of sense of control, body, self, and life progression. Language also provides information about the patient's sense of perceived stigma associated with a specific disorder. Goffman (1963) suggests, for example, that simple loss of body control can be stigmatizing to some, resulting in a perception of an identity that is in some fashion spoiled.

This concept is consistent with the fact that most theorists see severe illness as having a profound effect on the identity of the individual and her significant others (Haidet et al., 2006; Stanley, 2004). Again, the medical system is partly to blame, since patients are not viewed as individuals but instead perceived as examples of particular disorders. For instance, it is not uncommon to find patients in the hospital literally labeled by their disease. Instead of referring to Mr. Jones, the retired mechanic with grown children, in Bed 2, Mr. Jones becomes the CVA in Bed 2. Patients and their significant others need to persist in refusing to be reduced to clinical material, using illness narratives to demand recognition for their unique experience of suffering. Recognition is central to an understanding of the illness experience of individuals and their loved ones. When people share their illness stories, they also hear the story simultaneously and absorb the reactions of others. The initial presentation of the story may be somewhat inarticulate and highly personalized (Frank, 1995, p. 3), but the sharing of the story makes the process one of social connection and allows the ill to regain their voice. In fact, expression of one's story of illness can open the door to other important narrative connections that allow people to renegotiate who and what they are (Caplan et al., 2005).

Community Narrative

At a time when the comfort and familiarity of old ways of presenting narrative self are most needed, the communities that formerly supported our sense of self may become less accessible or supportive, and new discursive communities may be needed. At such times, individuals may turn to alternate communities that have shared narratives that are more consistent with and accepting of the individual's newly defined self as person with ALS or stroke survivor or any other common denominator. Support or self-help groups are examples of such communities, as will be highlighted in subsequent chapters. Involvement with such groups can be particularly important to those whose life story disruption is characterized by the loss of communication. What is important about such groups is Rappaport's (1993) contention that they are best understood as "normative narrative communities where identity transformation takes place" (p. 239). The narrative emphasis reflects a focus on the individual within the social context, and the premise that " . . . the stories people tell and are told are powerful forms of communication to others and to self. Stories order experience, give coherence and meaning to events and provide a sense of history and of future" (Rappaport, 1993, p. 240).

Support groups serve many functions, some of which have been described elsewhere (Shadden, 1994, 2006; Shadden & Agan, 2004). In addition to support for the telling of life stories and illness narratives, and for keeping the story going, groups provide:

a. embracement (social validation and acceptance of life stories (Burle & Caan, 2004; Holstein & Gubrium, 2000);
b. information and resource sharing;
c. emotional release;
d. validation of old or new social identities;
e. empowerment (in dealing with others and in obtaining services);
f. a social context that acknowledges and validates the "unsettled lives" of participants struggling to come to terms with disruptions in their life stories (Swidler, 1986);
g. an extended timeline for social interaction that permits a more nuanced restorying of self.

What should be clear in this list is that community narrative can support all levels of self described in the previous chapter. Perhaps most powerful is the ability of support groups to transform stories from being accounts of *I* and *my* to *we* and *our*.

It is not surprising that the topic of illness narrative has begun to intersect with discussions of community and group membership (Davison, Pennebaker, & Dickerson, 2000; Rappaport, 1993, 2004; Roberts et al., 1999; Shotter, 2003, 2005). Personal illness narratives are more private, linked with identity development, maintenance, and change. By joining a group, individuals explore opportunities for a more public mechanism for identity development through exposure to the community narrative. The community narrative is the story told over and over and shared by most members. Such a story in a stroke support group might be the belief that "Everyone who has had a stroke can continue to improve over relatively long periods of time." To the extent that the community narrative is positive and empowering, individuals have the opportunity to transform their life stories to conform to the broader story of the group. In addition, repeated opportunities to tell one's story help us revise these stories, begin to eliminate or alter the negative aspects, and selectively remember those story elements that support identity reconstruction (Nelson, 2002; Rappaport, 1993).

Some version of the illness or health narrative is also an important tool in validating membership in new communities such as support groups. Barker (2002) refers to the formation of illness identities as a consequence of participation in self-help groups that are joined by a common medical or health narrative. In fact, the support group is one of the few places where having a particular illness or disability is a good thing. The support group is the context for Gubrium's (2003) discussion of defining the elements of a good story. For example, many support groups have developed an almost ritualized sharing of the common illness experience. In the sharing, the uniqueness of the individual is affirmed, but group membership is also acknowledged. The community narrative ritualizes what the community is like, how it came to be that way, and what is expected (Rappaport, 1993). Thus the story becomes *our* story, and a group narrative develops that affirms the narrative self of each member. In fact, the community narrative is neither more nor less than the story told over and over and shared by members. On-line support groups and discussion forums specific to particular illnesses also provide opportunities for developing a sense of belonging.

Alter (2006) has referred to the "magic of groups" when describing successful interventions at the Adler Center. Community membership can be a powerful tool for moving on with life. As noted earlier, however, support groups are not an option for everyone. Rappaport (1993) is quick to assert that, while there are healing properties associated with involvement with such groups, participation must always be voluntary. In other words, the community narrative must be developed spontaneously from within (rather than through professional management), allowing personal narrative to become intertwined with community narrative through the social interactions that occur within groups. Some individuals do not wish to adopt a new identity as a person with aphasia or a person with Parkinson's disease. They are working to overcome that part of their new identity, and the support group encourages them to do the opposite, to embrace this new part of their life story and this new identity. Others feel the need for community but find it elsewhere, such as church involvement.

Health Narrative

One concern in looking at illness narratives is the fact that the health care world tends to revert to classification and understanding of the illness experience in terms of a disease label. By relying excessively on the meanings generated by labels, it is possible to avoid confronting the human experience of the illness, focusing instead on narrow technical definitions of bodily function and dysfunction. More recently, from a biopsychosocial perspective, disease has come to represent intersections between the actual physical disease manifestation and the consequences in the interaction between bodily systems, psychological state, and environmental conditions (Kitwood, 1997; Kleinman, 1988). The term health narrative that has emerged in recent literature provides a broader framework for considering this biopsychosocial perspective. The idea of a health narrative allows consideration of the many narrative contexts in which an individual's health problem plays out: (a) with a variety of people, including health care providers, significant others; (b) with health organizations; and (c) more broadly, with the public domain. Harter, Japp, and Beck (2003b) state that:

> Health narratives emerge as complex performances in the midst of enveloping life and social narratives that can enable or constrain, stigmatize or empower, confuse or enlighten individuals as they attempt to restore continuity when faced with the disruption of illness, suffering, or trauma. (p. 29)

The Role of Life Stage in Illness Narrative

In the following chapter, the role of narrative processes across the life span will be considered, along with examples of clients for whom the disruption of life story was influenced powerfully by their stage in life's trajectory. As might be anticipated, age (or life stage) typically does affect the nature and content of the illness narrative (as noted in the description of Dennis's narrative in Chapter 5). Work by Faircloth and colleagues (Faircloth, Boylstein, Rittman, & Gubrium, 2005; Faircloth, Rittman, Boylstein, Young, & Van Puymbroeck, 2004) suggests that there is considerable discrepancy between expected outcomes in stroke narratives, as perceived by the medical community and by older stroke survivors. In this instance, old age was associated with narratives of decline and disability for medical practitioners as contrasted with narratives of hope and recovery provided by older patients. More and more, treatment options in health research literature on managing and coping with illness draws distinctions between younger and older patients, particularly in designing and providing interventions.

An understanding of the impact of neurogenic communication disorders on narrative self must involve consideration of chronological or biological age and life span. However, care must be taken to avoid any stereotypical assumptions about age and the construction of self in aging. This is particularly important when health care professionals attempt to provide opportunities for individuals to share their constructed illness narrative and to work through the process of reconnecting elements of the life story before and after the diagnosis of a neurological disorder. It is easy to slip into age-based assumptions about needs and interests, and about life goals. These assumptions tend to influence the questions asked and the topics pursued in conversation, and may limit expressions of self.

Communication Impairment and Illness Narratives

Monks (2000, p. 15) refers to "talk as social suffering," and Hurwitz (2000) acknowledges the importance of nonverbal as well as verbal communications in the stories offered as explanations of illness. Thus, the loss of communication *facility* undermines the illness narratives that can be used to respond to life change. The term facility is used here to imply a number of aspects of communication, including knowledge and use of the vocabulary and major rule systems of language, intelligibility of speech output, narrative conventions, and socially acceptable and familiar manners of expression (Beard, 2004; Becker, 1999; Guendouzi & Miller, 2006). For example, a marked delay before a person with aphasia processes and responds to a question is not familiar and acceptable. Abrupt unsignalled topic shifts on the part of the person with dementia lead to loss of the coherence that might be expected in typical communicative exchanges.

For some persons, there is an apparent total loss of communication. The person is unresponsive and nonparticipatory. In this context, the focus often shifts to others in the environment. One physician (Connelly, 2002) describes her experience of excluding a nonresponsive patient from a conversation with family members, effectively rendering that patient voiceless and abandoning any attempt to sustain narrative knowledge of the individual's needs. She focuses specifically on the importance of recognizing the patient's need for human connection, describing that as a persistence of self (p. 143).

The experience of illness is time bound in many respects, although the temporal aspects of different illnesses are highly variable (as discussed in Chapter 2). For illness, past, present, and future carry particular significance. These elements can be considered in the context of the course of the disease, the life story that is reframed to address the illness, and the point at which we may become bogged down in the reframing process. Exploration of past, present, and future is also needed to provide some sense of continuity to our lives and to the narrative selves we share with others. Life stage, including advanced age, influences the way in which individuals frame the illness narratives and others respond to these stories. All of these time-bound elements require communicative expression to be fully understood and dealt with as part of the life story.

Frank (1995) notes there are two kinds of emotional work involved in being ill. The first is the work associated with the emotions of being ill, and the second is keeping up appearances. Given the stigma associated with some illnesses, and the medical model of incompetence that still governs many health care interactions, the ability to communicate credibly and to present a narrative self of value and worth becomes critical. Impaired communication disrupts more than the sharing and shaping of life story as interrupted by illness. It also disrupts our ability to demonstrate that we are a worthwhile candidate for health care efforts.

Caregiver Perspectives

Frank (2002) suggests that caregivers who listen to another's story end up with narrative knowledge of that person because in listening, we are able to recognize the identity of others. He goes on to state: "I reserve the name 'caregivers' for people who are willing to listen to ill persons and to respond to their individual differences" (p. 48). The term caregiver is used rather loosely in this society. In the medical world, it can refer to a health care provider; however, Frank cautions us that treatment is not the same as providing care. Many health care providers lack the time, and some lack the inclination,

to truly listen and engage. Thus they fail to fulfill the recognition needed by a sick person, the need to be acknowledged as a person and as an "I" not an "it."

More typically, we identify as caregivers those family members and friends who have some degree of responsibility, shared or otherwise, for the person who is ill. Frank (2002, p. 6) says, "Caregivers are the other halves of the conversations I encourage the ill to engage in. They are also the other halves of illness experiences." In other words, caregivers have their own illness narrative to share and their own threat to narrative self as a result of the neurogenic disorders described in this text (Ganzer & England, 1994). Whether describing the care of medical professionals or the care of loved ones, Frank also notes:

> And as that person's life story becomes part of her own (caregiver-me), the caregiver's life is made meaningful as well. Care is inseparable from understanding, and like understanding, it must be symmetrical. Listening to another, we hear ourselves. Caring for another, we either care for ourselves as well, or we end in burnout and frustration. (p. 48)

Any illness of the body eventually moves outward to affect all those who relate to the ill individual. There are countless studies and texts addressing the needs and issues of caregivers, and many theoretical models of the factors that influence the health and well-being of these individuals (Lawton, Kleban, Moss, Ravine, & Glicksman, 1989; National Alliance for Caregiving and AARP, 2004; O'Rourke & Tuoko, 2000; Pearlin, Mullan, Semple, & Skaff, 1990; Schulz et al., 1997). None of the models is complete, however, without consideration of the degree of biographical disruption and the nature of biographical accommodation for the caregiver after the onset of illness of a loved one. Once again, communication is a critical tool in the process of renegotiating relationships and life stories, for the caregiver this time. If the illness experience cannot be shared, the burden of caregiving is immense. If the experience is shared, the renegotiation of life stories occurs within the framework of a sense of "we" or "us." No one's life returns to its previous state after a critical illness or terminal diagnosis. Caregivers, as well as the person with the illness, must deal with this reality. However, picking up the life story is much easier if one has been recognized as a person during the diagnostic and recovery process.

In Search of Biographical Accommodation

In many respects, this chapter's discussion of narrative, life story, and illness narrative depicts an essentially circular process. Schematically, it might be mapped out as shown in Figure 4-1. This figure does not adequately capture the temporal dimension

that defines these processes, but it does suggest that life story and narrative self are inextricably tied in with each other. When any disruptive medical event occurs (Bury, 1982), it must first be framed meaningfully in the sharing of an illness narrative. Part of this illness narrative may be recognition of the way in which the disorder creates challenges to the individual's sense of identity or self, challenges experienced through the filter of preexisting perceptions of narrative self, particularly those elements of one's life story associated with agency, control, and competence. However, the illness narrative is not enough. Eventually, there must be some form of biographical accommodation (Corbin & Strauss, 1991). As the illness story is told and retold, it becomes reconnected with the preexisting life story and self and clarifies the type and extent of biographical accommodation needed to move forward. It is at this stage in the cycle that finding alternate communities such as support groups may become particularly important in providing a mechanism for supporting both old and new selves. Biographical accommodation can take almost any form. For some, it is rediscovering ways to engage

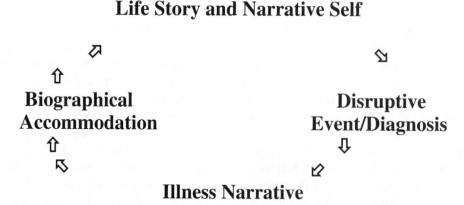

Figure 4–1. Maintaining and Modifying Life Story and Narrative Self.

in former hobbies with accommodations for the stroke-related challenges. For some, it is finding meaning in helping others, exemplified in Wayne's simple statement, "We are still here so . . . we do what we can . . . we give back . . . other someones need help." For yet others, it may be finding a way to return to work, perhaps in a different capacity.

Tools Supporting Narrative Communication

In the discussion of self in Chapter 3, the importance of one's cultural tool kit in negotiating self was underscored. In the present chapter, we have focused on one particular component in this tool kit—communication—and on the impact of impaired communication on the production of narrative needed to negotiate and renegotiate self. Faced with the reality of disordered verbal communication, there are many alternatives that potentially provide support for this process of negotiated self. While the meaning of tools varies depending on one's theoretical perspective, at least two constructs should be discussed here.

First, on a relatively concrete level, the concept of tools is linked in communication disorders with any device or aid, internal or external, that supports or improves communication. Certainly, it is appealing to consider the idea of "fixing" a communication deficit by substituting another vehicle for communication. In some of the disorders discussed in this text, communication devices figure prominently in the clinical perspective on treatment. Such tools will be discussed when appropriate, along with caveats about what they can and cannot do as part of the presentation of narrative self.

Second, other persons can function as tools in support of communication, or in coconstruction of communication, as is often described with aphasia. These others, typically key members of the person's intimate circle of friends and family, serve as animate tools, filling in some of the gaps left by the interactant's inability to communicate effectively through speech and language. The level of assistance of such animate tools varies. In one family, the daughter of a person with ALS interprets his broad gestures for a visitor, particularly those that serve the role of interactive questions and markers. In another family, the husband is so familiar with his wife's life that he is able to talk for her in social contexts, with nothing more than a look or small gesture to signal him to take this role. This idea of alternate tools in support of communication is an important consideration in clinical interactions with those with neurogenic communication disorders. The clinical process itself offers ample opportunities for use of tools in support of communications about self, if the clinician is sensitive to these opportunities.

Finally, tools may be a variety of beliefs, norms, values, and assumptions with which the clinician is less familiar. In this book, while we talk about the tools described in the previous paragraph, we are really focused on the tools of culture, role, and interaction that can be used in rewriting the biographical narrative of a person with a neurogenic communication disorder. This has broad implications for clinical work with those affected by these disorders.

Narrative in the Clinical Context

Clinicians spend their lives in the midst of narrative: listening to story fragments, interpreting word sequences, observing gesture, deciphering symptoms, ascribing causes, and suggesting treatments (Hurwitz, 2000). We have an ocean of words and offer ourselves to each other as links in ongoing stories. Clinical practice is predicated upon recognizing and responding to such links—whether symptom, sign, expression, mood, behavior pattern, or feeling. Clinicians project themselves in their daily interactions, just as they try to understand the selves of clients (Guendouzi & Müller, 2006). As already suggested, central to an understanding of narrative and narrative self is the recognition that our life stories take on particular significance in the light of a major illness or other disruption in the continuity of the story. In the past two decades, the evolving concepts of illness and health narratives have influenced medical interactions. Through the work of Brody (2003), Charon and Montello (2002), Frank (1995, 2002), Kleinman (1988), and others, the medical community has been asked to reframe the understanding of the patient-physician interaction to include and actively solicit illness narratives that will inform treatment.

The narrative processes discussed here are indistinguishable, at times, from issues of clinical discourse that have received focus in recent publications. In 2007, Hinckley addressed the topic of clinical discourse directly in a text that borrows from much of the same literature used in our work here. And in a 2007 issue of *Topics in Language Disorder*, Kovarsky brings together researcher/clinicians from multiple domains to explore the ways in which our clinical practices and core beliefs influence and are influenced by the discourse that occurs in the therapy dyad, in our writings about best practices, and in our studies of what makes efficacious treatment. Some of this work will be discussed further in Section IV of this text.

Hopefully, the following life stories chapters will help the reader identify challenges to narrative self experienced by those living with adult-onset neurogenic communication disorders. The four disorders selected for discussion in this text all disrupt a person's ability to renegotiate self through life stories. Each chapter will be framed around the communication problems experienced (and their life impact), the vulnerability of self, and the nature of life storying given communication impairment. Specific disorders, and indeed each of the individuals we introduce, differ with respect to the specific dimensions of self that are most vulnerable, the impact of loss of agency and control, the centrality of others in life storying, and the importance of community. Thus, no attempt has been made to follow a single fixed content outline in presenting these life stories. Prominence is given to those themes that emerged from the data as most dominant in each disorder.

In all chapters, however, temporal concerns are addressed. Time is a critical element in understanding narrative and life stories. In fact, Charon (2002) suggests that narrative does not exist outside of the context of time. The lifetime trajectory of self is carried in our many versions of our life stories, and the meaning we derive from sharing of life stories yields a kind of narrative intelligence (Randall, 1999). McAdams (1993) highlights this life span perspective in his discussion of the premythic, mythic, and postmythic states of storying of self. In life stories, there is a focus on past, present, and an implied future (in the sense of implications of the resolution of the story for subsequent action). Because meaning is inextricably linked to narratives, we constantly revise our life stories to reframe the causal connections and reshape our understanding of our selves. Thus, it is impossible to consider stories or narratives without the considerations of time, aging, and life span considerations found in the next chapter.

CHAPTER 5

Life Stories across the Life Span: Considering Time

"The body might have to bow to time, but what about the self?" (Charon, 2002, p. 60)

As noted in the previous chapter, it is impossible to consider stories or narratives without addressing time, aging, and life span considerations. While the term narrative itself implies the passage of time, it is also important to consider time from the framework of changes to life story across the life span. Concepts related to narrative self feature prominently in recent gerontological literature. Terms that have emerged in the past 10 years include narrative gerontology, biographical aging, narrative developmental intelligence, narrative identity as meaning-making, narratives or life stories of aging, and narrative temporality in the study of aging (Birren & Cochran, 2001; Birren, Kenyon, Ruth, Schroots, & Svensson, 1996; Bruner, 1999; Fivush & Haden, 2003; Kenyon, 2003; Kenyon & Randall, 1997; Randall, 1995, 1999; Randall & Kenyon, 2000; Randall, Prior, & Sarborn, 2006).

Randall (1999) states that gerontology lets us appreciate lives as self-authoring creations, with the desired outcome being meaning-making and self construction. One might also argue that the concept of narrative self is needed if humans are to understand the remarkable course we travel through a given life span. Certainly, aging plays a part in all four dimensions of self construction described in Chapter 3. In this chapter, we will consider temporality and aging as related to life span considerations and self, life storying, self, stereotype and the narrative of decline, and the social grounding of self in aging. We will close with a brief consideration of the boundaries of normal aging, using one man's story to demonstrate just how blurred the boundaries are between normal age-associated changes and impairment.

Aging as Temporality

Pick up any textbook that addresses aspects of gerontology and one of the first premises offered by the authors will invariably relate to the inadequacy of chronological time to explain life span development and aging. Indeed, as Baars (1997) suggests, chronological time is relative and the more important aspect of chronological time is the basic concept that humans live within a framework of past, present, and future. In the history of human development, the experience of time was first captured through storytelling. Ricoeur (1980) explicitly links narrativity and temporality, suggesting that narrative is the discourse form through which we express our temporal being or self. Narrative uses language to facilitate this process.

The two most important elements in our understanding of self are the past-present-future and the beginning-middle-end continua. Both are time based. Our biographical past illuminates the present or can shine a spotlight on current deficits and challenges. Similarly, our social past informs our present by providing a reference point for changing interactions and roles. Arguably, there is also a fundamental beginning, middle, and end structure to life (Baars, 1997), one that is captured through the biographical pieces that an individual determines to be important. In our perception of narrative self and sharing of life stories that express that perception, the "end" can be a true end to the life story, in the sense of the death of the individual, or it can be more loosely characterized as an endpoint, as in the moral of the life story we share (Becker, 1999). In either sense, we are constantly revising our autobiographical memories, based on individual needs and situational demands. Regardless of the endpoint, our life stories must lead us forward, in addition to reflecting and creating meaning for the past. Moving forward requires the ability to access the biographical particulars of our past.

From the temporal perspective, the idea of developmental stages is particularly appealing. The idea of stages allows us to minimize attention to chronological time, focusing instead on the other continua of past-present-future and beginning-middle-end. A life stages framework also allows us to consider changes in how others view our presented narrative self, as well as shifting priorities and evolving perspectives on self. A stages perspective allows us to focus more effectively on the fact that change is a constant across our life span, and our management of change depends in part on whether specific changes are consistent with a given life stage.

Life Span Considerations

In gerontology, it has been informative to consider life as a series of stages that capture the essential psychosocial challenges that dominate different chronological ages (Erikson, 1968; McAdams, 1988, 1993). While aging per se is not a disorder, any attempt to understand the changes to narrative self associated with neurogenic communication disorders must incorporate an awareness of the person's life stage. Indeed, if we consider narrative processes as acts of meaning-making, then it can be argued that we can understand an individual's development through the life stories they share. Bruner (1999, p. 7) postulates that life is indeed a work of art best understood in the telling. As humans age, life stories evolve, associated in part with life span changes to self as defined through culture, roles, interactions, and biographical particulars. These elements shape a person's evolving narrative self, and they are also elements disrupted by the neurogenic communication disorders considered in this text.

Chronological aging brings with it biological and cognitive changes and alterations in role demands, particularly in the later years. Just dealing with some of these normal processes requires a fluid sense of narrative self and the tools needed to reframe, in effect rewrite, the life stories that link our pasts to our present and the projected future. Singer (2004) suggests that learning and growing in the context of some of these changes and losses requires acknowledgement of what has been lost, or what may never be in our future (our lost possible selves). This process of acknowledgement and of moving on is frequently discussed in terms of stages such as those presented by Kubler-Ross (1997) and Livneh and Antonek (1997). In fact, in the communication disorders literature, there is frequent reference to such stages and to the need for clinicians to be sensitive to "where" the individual stands with respect to stages in acceptance and adaptation (Tanner, 1999; Tanner & Gerstenberger, 1988). These stages are important in understanding coping with specific disorders. In this text, however, we suggest that our understanding of these stages is acquired best through our listening to the life stories of those with whom we work. Further, we can be most effective in our interventions if we focus on recognizing and validating the individual's current life stories and presentations of narrative self.

Many theorists acknowledge that the most important and powerful life stories are those that are created around emotionally difficult moments, those involving loss, struggle, or personal crisis—what Bruner (1987) refers to as "trouble." In Chapter 4, these stories of trouble were discussed as illness narratives. Some of the losses associated with aging also evoke stories that address struggle and that end in some kind of resolution. In the context of normal aging, these times of trouble often constitute what McAdams (1993) refers to as developmental crises. While each person's experience of such crises is unique, their resolution paves the way for moving forward by modifying our narrative self in meaningful ways. If we cannot accommodate our life stories to aging changes, we find ourselves essentially stuck somewhere between past and present.

The idea of life span changes and life stages serves as a critical backdrop to our understanding of responses to neurogenic communication disorders. Such disorders are overlaid on the existing realities of one's specific life stage and any life span changes already being experienced. Thus the impact may be even more powerful and the biographical disruption may be greater. The concept of life stages lets us ask more appropriate questions in order to better facilitate the individual's moving forward in the context of such powerful changes. When the communicative crises that emerge violate life stage expectations, the challenge of restorying of self is greater.

One common life span consideration influencing responses to the neurogenic disorders described in Chapter 2 is typical age of onset. While chronological age per se is of limited interest, age indirectly marks the life stages of persons with communication disorders. As will be seen in subsequent chapters, the impact of impaired communication on narrative self can only be fully understood if we understand the developmental processes at stake. For example, Dennis is a comparatively young man (now 43) who experienced a massive hemorrhagic stroke before the age of 40. He is struggling to move forward from his past into a present and future that include aphasia and other neurological sequelae. However, he constantly "hits the wall" when he discusses the fact that he is young and was highly successful professionally before his stroke. Over and over, he alludes to the fact that he is not like other people. The primary way in which he is different is his comparative youth. On the one hand, he grieves for the loss of his professional identity, expressing a sense of hopelessness about the years left to him with no sense of purpose. On the other hand, he indicates that he cannot understand why others who are much older would want to spend any time with him. Thus chronological age is a huge barrier that blocks his continuing self narrative.

Dennis's age and life stage influence the narrative he creates. His story is clearly put together out of the tools he has collected at the cultural, role, interactional, and biographical levels of self. From the *cultural* perspective, he has learned that there are expectations about the way a man just entering his middle age in his world should act. He should be engaged in meaningful and lucrative employment. He should live comfortably and be in control of his life and actions. He should be valued and respected by others and should seek definition within a certain subgroup of the social community. Dennis's stroke has disrupted his ability to live in accordance with his beliefs, and thus he must rewrite his story, perhaps pulling from alternative cultural values and ideologies. Similarly, the *roles* that Dennis played prior to the onset of his illness were consistent with these cultural beliefs. He was an administrator at work, a primary breadwinner in a long-term relationship, a sought-out friend, a loyal son. These roles are all part of one's definition of self and all have been disrupted by the stroke, thus requiring a rewritten narrative.

At the *interactional* or *situational* level of understanding self, Dennis's communicative impairment and other alterations of nonverbal behaviors make it impossible for him to function as he did prior to his stroke, particularly within relationships and culturally defined contexts. His communicative challenges are apparent, disrupting the day-to-day interactions that might help him renegotiate his sense of self. He has not found acceptance in former interactional contexts, and cannot use the communicative cultural tools needed to redefine himself in

new roles. This has implications for writing a new narrative.

Finally, at the *biographical* level of self creation, Dennis must incorporate new physiological characteristics into his narrative. He suffers constant pain, he cannot walk naturally, his brain "shuts down" when presented with too many stimuli. Given that every level of self has been altered, Dennis is lost—he requires a new narrative to be able to go on. Later, in Chapter 8, his words will be used to share his sense of total disconnection from the particulars of who and what he was— physically, psychologically, socially—and to illustrate his struggles to rewrite his story.

Similarly, when we look at the life stories of persons with ALS, we often see young or middle-aged individuals whose narratives reflect their professional achievements and their families, particularly those with young children. Again, there is a sense of intrinsic unfairness about the developmental stage at which they are asked to address such life-altering changes. In contrast, when the 89-year-old neighbor begins to demonstrate signs of probable dementia, the reality is no less tragic but there is no sense of violation of the natural order of things.

There is one caveat in using life stages to understand the impact of neurogenic communication disorders on narrative self. Categories of life stages can mislead us into examining lives as discretely compartmentalized, despite the fact that personhood and self are continuous. Thus it is critical to remember that continuity of narrative self is maintained through life storying.

Life Storying in Aging

The preceding sections refer repeatedly to life stories and narratives. In recent years, a new genre of life story telling and age autobiography has emerged as a tool in understanding aging (Morganroth-Gullette, 2003). Fortunately, we seem to be moving past overly simplistic concepts of reminiscence as the most appropriate tool for dealing with the later stages of life span development. Gibson (2004) provides a more fully realized discussion of reminiscence in the context of sharing of life stories. In this text, she avoids the trap of suggesting that reminiscence or life story telling is just another clinical tool (McFadden, 2005) and instead acknowledges the constant revision of autobiographical memories and the fundamental grounding of sharing of life stories in the profoundly human quest for relationships. This constant revision is critical for the narrative processing that involves organization of life experiences and then filtering those experiences through the narrative experience (Singer, 2004). Revision and ongoing development are essential elements in an individual's experience of self and the responses of social others. In fact, it is argued that we create narrative to meet the demands of social roles. Randall (1999) suggests that life stories represent a kind of biographically accrued capital (as resource or power), and that the stories are texts that time has laid within us.

The centrality of narrative in human existence has already been established. In a seminal work on narrative and aging, Bruner (1999) offered four hypotheses for consideration of narratives of aging. First, and perhaps most important for this text, he suggests that "willingness or eagerness to 'story' one's life is tantamount to the desire to live" (p. 7) In working with persons with neurogenic communication disorders, that drive to continue to present an evolving self may be related to the more simplistic concept of motivation that is referred to repeatedly in the treatment literature. What Bruner's hypothesis suggests is that facilitation of ongoing storying of self should receive focus in our clinical work.

Bruner's second hypothesis is that the fullness and length of a life depends upon the self-credibility and "precedental" value of the running narrative that one keeps telling oneself "after the fact." What he suggests here is that process of maintaining and appropriately modifying the ongoing life narrative is a core human behavior, one that is particularly important to understanding aging, particularly successful aging. In his third hypothesis, Bruner takes on the concept of successful aging by suggesting that it is another way of referring to psychosomatic self. Of interest here is the suggestion that "the 'psycho' aspect of psychosomatic health may inhere in the sense of still-to-be-finished business that a life-story supplies" (p. 9).

Finally, Bruner highlights the importance of culture in defining one's choices for templates for framing the life story. In this text, we use the term culture very broadly, as does Bruner. Thus, culture may be as localized as the community found within one's church or as broad as expectations of one's employer about one's potential success in fulfilling job demands as one gets older. Culture also encompasses gender expectations as associated with age. For normally aging individuals, each society has different perspectives on what age group is valued and consequently empowered. The narrative self we choose to present in different contexts is dictated, in part, by our understanding of those unspoken age expectations. Indeed, life stories must mesh within the community of life stories if they are to be understood and accepted. McFadden (2005) suggests that creating a meaningful life story is a cultural imperative.

Our choice of narrative self to present also requires sorting through a lifetime of biographical particulars to select those most relevant to and valued in any given social context. Indeed, aging itself consists in part of the ongoing accumulation of those biographic particulars, with 80 years of life experience guaranteed to amass more personal details than 20 years of experience. Thus for storying of self, environments often play a critical role in sustaining a sense of continuity of self and in highlighting for others those artifacts that reflect valued aspects of self. Rosel (2003) describes the importance of familiar surroundings in maintaining knowledge of where and with whom one is aging in place. Krasner (2005) also writes about the need to study the complex relationships between self, space, and habit. He states that "longtime home residence represents a crucial imaginative structure through which elders define themselves and their life stories" (p. 210). Particularly for those who live alone, he suggests that there is a kind of creation of a self that is captured by the objects and environments of the home. Homes reflect time and life phases or stages. Homes and environments anchor our storying of self, particularly when we can bring social interactions into those familiar environments.

In addition to environments and biographic artifacts, both Bauer (2005) and McFadden (2005) emphasize the importance of dyadic factors in one's ability to create a narrative that is accepted by others. The importance of dyadic factors returns us once again to the fundamental social aspect of narrative (and thus, of coconstruction of narrative self). In fact, Blustein (1999) explores this concept of attempting to work clinically with an individual who cannot share a narrative self because he or she has lost narrative capacity. The issues raised in her discussion, particularly with respect to reciprocity and coconstruction, are similar to those raised in previous chapters.

Turning to a different aspect of self construction, roles, we see the importance of culture in defining acceptable templates for life stories in aging. In constructing and maintaining a sense of a viable, continuous narrative self, we are all influenced by societally governed role expectations. Role expectations with respect to family, work, health behaviors, and relationships (among many) play a critical part in determining how we shape the stories we tell and how we internally define ourselves. Further, these roles are consistently linked with different gendered expectations, and with fundamental age expectations. Basic roles, gender, and chronological age also influence with which community or subculture we choose to affiliate. For many aging individuals, at some level, there is a need to determine whether they accept or reject membership in the culture of the community of the aged.

In this context, Trethewey (2001) explored the experiences of midlife professional women as they confront growing older at work. Thus the concept of life span changes is linked here with key themes evolving from the master narrative of aging. The themes that emerged were those of loss, isolation, and diminished material resources. In this study, participants were not content to "buy into" the expectation of the narrative of decline. Their stories suggest that age themes are resisted in midlife narratives as an identity characteristic that is manageable. Trethewey's work leads logically to consideration of the broader impact of perceptions of aging on narrative self, discussed in the next section.

Self, Stereotype, and the Narrative of Decline

Clearly it is difficult to sort out themes of life story and narrative from broader considerations of self, identity, or personhood.

Further, issues of narrative self across the life span are inextricably intertwined with individual and societal perceptions of aging and the elderly and with narratives of decline. What is of particular interest in this section is how individuals address socially held perspectives on aging in framing a sense of narrative self. Given the breadth of this topic, only a few key points can be highlighted here.

Aging is not a disease or disability. However, chronological and biological aging are frequently associated with decline, loss, and risk of feared disorders such as Alzheimer's disease. Normal aging is associated eventually with decline in efficiency in most systems. Virtually every body system is at risk for some change or loss in functioning, although the individual differences in normal aging probably outweigh any generalities that can be provided. Change is gradual, almost unnoticed until some critical event highlights the fact of decline. For most aging individuals, the experience of chronological aging is often associated with loss of independence or control. This can be very disheartening in today's culture, which values personal autonomy and empowerment as themes defining perceptions of self and life expectations (Bruner, 2003, 2004; Dowd, 2004). For some, loss can be construed as defeat. Loss and decline are also markers of loss of control of one's life (Feldman, 1999). As one interviewee (Jessica) discussed in Chapter 9 said, "So that's another step when you get older, you lose your independence in a lot of things . . . and then that's another defeat for me."

Given the fact that many of these changes are normal, it is not appropriate to speak in terms of illness narrative. However, the concept of health narrative (Harter, Japp, & Beck, 2005a) or the idea of narrative of decline (Trethewey, 2001) may be helpful in framing core concepts. For at least some

of the neurogenic communication disorders discussed in the following chapters, individuals are already coping with preexisting challenges of normal aging prior to the onset of the communication disorder. Thus the threat to narrative self cannot be understood without understanding existing aging challenges, challenges to mental and physical systems and to interpersonal communication (Shadden, 1988b).

Further, there is stigma associated with aging, stigma usually understood best in terms of ageism and stereotyping of the elderly. Baars (1997) refers to the grand narrative of aging, usually communicated through the media. The two main markets for this grand narrative are (a) anti-aging products and (b) providing care for frail elders. Each market feeds stereotypes and stigmas of aging. A focus on anti-aging products and procedures highlights the desirability of youth and the unpleasantness of looking and feeling old. Targeting care for frail elders underscores the image of weakness and incompetence of older adults. It is not surprising that residents in environments such as long-term care often develop learned helplessness, a condition in which it is the person's perception of his incompetence, rather than any true physical or mental problem, that results in loss of independence.

Grenier (2006) has studied the concept of frailty—both *being* frail and *feeling* frail, focusing on how the concept captures social, economic, and biomedical practices that "collide as inscriptions on the bodies of older women" (Grenier & Hanley, 2007, p. 211). Grenier and Hanley suggest that "identity and self may serve as a protective mechanism from becoming frail" (2007, p. 225). Given societal stereotypes about aging and the elderly, it is not surprising that interactions between seniors and other adults can be compromised. Some of the common stereotypes about aging persons include dependent, incompetent, needy, weak, self-obsessed, and excessively talkative. These stereotypes prevail even among practitioners and preprofessionals in health care disciplines such as speech-language pathology (Shadden, 1988a, b). Over 3 years, in an undergraduate class in communication disorders, students were asked to use free association to respond quickly and without much reflection to the terms elderly and old. Over those 3 years, out of 96 responses, only 5 were in any way positive (e.g., wise, caring about family). Close to 95% of the students accessed negative stereotypes, even when most of those students said they "liked old people" or thought old people were "sweet." Thus it is not surprising that interactions with older adults may be disrupted by these dominant stereotypical perceptions.

If older adults are not viewed as viable or desirable partners in social exchanges, this may have powerful negative consequences on the social construction of narrative self for the older individual. Instead of being recognized for his individual strengths and unique self, the older person may end up being viewed as an exemplar of all elders, a class of individuals that are collectively viewed as less than competent and having little to contribute. Given the fact that our perceptions of self are highly dependent upon the views and responses of social others, aging individuals are at risk for narrative failure. At stake are considerations of self-worth and self-esteem and, more broadly, the issue of respect. These same issues of respect and self-esteem reappear in the life stories chapters of Section III of this text.

There is an extensive body of literature that explores the impact of age perceptions on interpersonal communication (cf. Giles & Reid, 2005; Shadden, 1997). More recently, attention has been focused on the degree to which aging is the dominant factor in altered communication, or whether the presence (or expectation) of a disabling condition such as hearing loss or dementia is the primary causal factor (Melton & Shadden, 2006). One implication of this interactive breakdown is the fact that a sense of stigma develops on both sides of the social exchange. Jessica notes, "It's a feeling that I'm not that interesting . . . I think of something and then I just say, you know, they're not interested . . . really . . . and they probably aren't. . . . " For older persons and their significant others, there is also acknowledgement of the fine line between normal aging and early dementia (Beard, 2004; Langdon, Eagle, & Warner, 2007) and considerable fear of the onset of cognitive decline. Given the centrality of communication in the process of storying of self, it is important to identify what can be considered normal changes in language and communication that accompany the chronological aging process (Shadden & Toner, 1997; Worrall & Hickson, 2003).

Whitbourne and colleagues have tackled identity issues in aging in a very direct manner, postulating multiple identity processes (particularly accommodation, assimilation, and balance), focusing on the challenges to a sense of self facing an aging society (Skultety & Whitbourne, 2004; Sneed & Whitbourne, 2001, 2003, 2005; Whitbourne, Sneed, & Skultety, 2002). They contend that the self is capable of remaining stable while changing over time. Further, at least for women, they note that identity processes are linked to self-esteem and must be studied from that perspective. From a different perspective, Miner-Rubino, Winter, and Stewart (2004) asked seniors to retrospectively assess their identity certainty in their 20s, 40s, and 60s. Identity certainty increased across the three age intervals, although women displayed less identity certainty than men.

Barrett (2005) also explores issues of situational identity, self-enhancement principles, role identities, and social identities focusing specifically on family and work roles and on health status. Of particular interest was the fact that family and work roles influenced identities through demands faced and perceived control.

As part of his discussion of narratives of aging, Bruner (1999) established what he perceives to be the critical element of life stories—the fact that something that he calls "trouble" disrupts the connections between agent, act, goal, means, and setting that are commonly found in narratives. His focus on trouble is consistent with others' framing an understanding of personal narratives, and more specifically illness narratives, around the concept of crisis, plight, transition, upset, chaos, and deregulation (Baars, 1997; McAdams, 1993; Randall, 1999; Singer, 2004). Much of the rest of this text will focus on illness narratives in the context of chronic illness. However, it is important to note that coping with specific communication disorders plays out against the backdrop of some other aging issues of chronic health problems or losses.

Gooberman-Hill, Ayis, and Ebrahim (2003) discuss the fact that stories matter most when dealing with such chronic illnesses, and Becker (1999) explores the role of storytelling in the management of pain in later life. Bruner's (1987) framing of personal narrative around the construct of trouble may also have implications for the role of narrative in successful adaptation to aging. Becker (1999) says that narrative can transfigure the experience of aging if appropriately formed and if presented to those who will really listen. The issue of framing the story appropriately is particularly important for those sharing narratives of advanced age. If any storytelling conventions are violated without justification, the narrator will be discredited (Beard, 2004; Becker, 1999; Guendouzi & Müller, 2006).

There is an extensive body of literature addressing the health care system and the medical treatment of aging adults. Similarly, much has been written about gerontological preparation in different health professions, as well as the degree of ageism found in such groups. Recent research has probed other aspects of the health care experience and self. In one study, Feldman (1999) reported that a group of older women in writing workshops identified factors important to their health and quality of life. The two major factors were their relationship to professional health care providers and the roles played by both service providers and these aging patients in maintaining health and well-being. In a separate work, Blustein (1999) explored loss of narrative self in the context of interpreting health care directives. While arguing that "interest in the integrity of one's life story does not disappear with the loss of cognitive function" (p. 21), she also discusses the idea of what constitutes treating a person like a person, ultimately suggesting that this means acknowledging the value of the individual. This process includes recognition that people have an interest in the future because identity is in part the product of the lived story, extending both forward and backward.

As part of the narrative of decline, illness and disability also occupy unique research niches within the larger literature on aging and narrative self. Montbriand (2004) interviewed a number of seniors in a Canadian city, eliciting life histories. All told of lives touched by chronic illness. The most pessimistic framed life stories in the context of present illnesses; in contrast, the most optimistic did not connect life experiences with illness. Harrison and Kahn (2004) studied the manner in which disability influences age perception and social integration for three aging women. They reported that women consistently expressed an age perception as younger than chronological age, despite disability circumstances. Social integration was linked to the ability to find an environment supporting chosen identities. What was important in this study was the finding that identity changed slowly as people aged if *expected* life events occur. Because these events are anticipated, they do not have the same impact as other less anticipated disease processes.

Social Grounding of Self in Aging

In this text, we have highlighted the premise that people's life stories evolve in social contexts. One's life stage clearly influences the expectations of others, as well as the level of biographical knowledge and experience we bring to the negotiation of self. Life stage may also negatively affect coping with a major life crisis (e.g., illness diagnosis) if such crises are unexpected in a life span perspective (such as ALS). But it is in the later stages of our lives that social expectations of and attitudes towards aging and the elderly may profoundly influence the maintenance of narrative self. The introduction of a diagnosis of Parkinson's, or stroke, or dementia must be managed on top of and filtered through the existing narrative challenges of aging in this society.

Several factors are at stake in considering this multilayered challenge to narrative identity. First, as we age, the groups to which we belong or with which we affiliate change. Group membership or affiliation should provide us with opportunities both for communion (relationships) and agency or empowerment (McAdams, 1993). For some, this change in affiliations associated

with aging is relatively comfortable. These are the persons who accept membership in the broad community of other older adults and even embrace this membership. For others, there is resistance to affiliating with other older individuals.

As is frequently described in gerontological research, chronological age is comparative. If Mrs. Burleson is 83, she will continue to talk about "those older people" and her definition is based primarily on who is older than she is. Age-based comparisons with others have been studied extensively. Heidrich has studied aging woman, noting that well-being is often gauged through social comparisons (Heidrich, 1999; Heidrich & Ryff, 1993a, b). Heidrich's work also explores older women's coping with physical symptoms and challenges over the course of 10 years. Despite physical changes and an increase in medical problems, a positive sense of autonomy was well preserved. However, there were changes in relationships with others and in aspects of psychological well-being. At the heart of these changes appeared to be increases in daily discomfort (pain, fatigue, weakness) that led to reductions in daily activities. Thus a sense of self in the context of aging can be influenced by many small life stressors in addition to other major life changes.

The Boundaries of Normal Aging

Later in this text, the impact of dementia on narrative self will be considered. One of the most distressing early challenges in dementia is an inability to determine with any certainty whether specific cognitive changes being observed in an aging individual are simply characteristic of normal aging processes or are instead harbingers of a more fully developed dementia to come (Shadden,

1988a). Indeed, the early warning signs of dementia are those that are also associated with typical changes in the aging body and mind. The implications of this distinction for narrative self are critical in any process of life storying, both for the aging individual and for significant others.

For the aging person and his loved ones, dementia is much feared. The stigma associated with Alzheimer's disease and other dementias is among the most powerful in our society. Part of the stigma, part of what is feared, is a loss of those biographic, interactional, and role aspects of self that the typical person anticipates with this condition. Dementia is associated with total loss of agency or control, as characterized by nursing home placement, which is the final residence of many with this disorder. While loss of self is feared, this same premise is used to console members of the families of those with dementia. Versions of the following comments are heard often: "Don't be upset. This really isn't your mother. Remember her as she was, because she's gone now."

As suggested earlier, the normal life span changes associated with aging are themselves often associated with stigma, particularly in a culture that values youth, independence, and agency. In the following chapters on life stories, it is important to keep in mind when in the life span these disorders are likely to occur. It is also important to recognize that those faced with challenges to narrative self as a result of chronological or biological aging will be even more challenged if confronted with a specific disorder resulting in communication impairment. To underscore the importance of these life span issues, this chapter closes with the story of Reggie. While it is impossible to capture the heterogeneity of the aging population with the words and experiences of a few, it is important to try to give a human face to the aging dilemmas described in this chapter.

A Lesson Learned through Reggie's Story

Reggie was the 89-year-old spouse of stroke survivor Lois, who had a mild receptive and moderate expressive fluent aphasia. Lois and Reggie were first brought to a stroke support group by an adult daughter who had moved thousands of miles to take care of her mother. In the initial two meetings, several things became apparent about Reggie. First, he had a severe hearing impairment, apparently age-related, and had considerable difficulty processing group discussions. Second, he frequently interjected seemingly inappropriate comments during the group, disrupting the focus of those who were sharing and taking a disproportionate share of the group's time. Most of his comments had little to do with stroke.

After the first two sessions, his daughter apparently spoke with him about these behaviors. At the outset of the next session, she took the group leader aside and indicated that her father occasionally became confused but had been asked by the daughter to wait his turn and plan a brief sharing. And indeed, that is what happened for many months. Reggie always waited for his turn and typically had notes to himself on a piece of paper. Sometimes he would tell a joke, other times he would share something from his past. The stories from his past seemed to be designed to validate his importance, but he always stopped talking after a brief time, indicating that it was someone else's turn. Even when spouses and family members split up into a smaller group discussion, he said little or nothing in that setting.

As is probably apparent, the group leader assumed that, in addition to presbycusis, Reggie was in the early stages of dementia. And so the pattern continued, even when other adult children of Reggie and Lois attended. The cues of the adult children suggested that they were not including him in the family discussions, so no one did. It was that simple—he was quite old, he couldn't hear, and he had dementia.

And then one day, in the family breakout session, Reggie appeared to be paying considerable attention to the discussion topic. The group leader turned to him and asked, "Have you experienced any of that with Lois?" And everyone was astounded when he answered, "Well, the only real conflict we have is when my hearing loss interferes with my hearing her, and she has actually said the right words, but I have to ask her to repeat it." And in one painful moment, the group leader knew that she had totally misread Reggie, assuming many things based on his age cues and his hearing impairment. It was a stunning realization. After the breakout session, the leader spoke with Reggie about her failure to include him adequately in the past and he generously indicated that it was understandable; the focus should be on his wife.

However, the story does not end there. Within the next week, Reggie had talked one of his children into coming by the office of the group leader and dropping off a copy of his autobiography, which he had been working on for some time. The autobiography was filled with lists and particulars of his professional achievement, and he had indeed been a very accomplished scientist. After that breakthrough session and the reading of the autobiography, the support group leader spoke with him about the autobiography and asked some additional question about his life. His responses were informative and appropriate. In future stroke group sessions, he seemed to have less need to have his time in the full group meeting but participated more actively in the family group, partly because everyone began to realize that he had something to add to our understanding.

The moral of this story is simple but extremely important for this text. First, one should never ever assume anything about a person simply because he or she is old. Second, everyone in the world of a person with a communication disorder is living the experience and has a need to share and reflect and be supported. And finally, we all need to share our life stories. While Reggie did so in a very direct fashion, through the literal sharing of his autobiography, others may need to do the same in less overt ways. Reggie needed validation, particularly in light of the time and attention that was being given to his wife. As a community, the group initially failed him because the group members collectively decided that he wasn't really able to participate fully. The lesson that should be learned from this is the need to recognize that it is not acceptable, on the professional or human levels, to respond to situational cues on the basis of stereotypes.

SECTION III

In the preceding section of this text, the reader was introduced to the theoretical base for understanding the impact of neurogenic communication disorders on narrative self. The following Section III explores the life stories and challenges to self experienced by those who no longer can use communication effectively as part of their cultural tool kit. For many readers, and indeed for the three of us as authors, these chapters are the heart and soul of this text. The people described within these chapters are known by us; our experiences with them served as the impetus for writing the text. We explore the life stories of those whose communication has been impaired because of ALS, Parkinson's disease (PD), stroke, and dementia in order to understand how and why narrative self may be jeopardized. At stake is the most important question we can ask: "How can we make a difference in the lives of these individuals?"

Section III consists of four life stories chapters. Chapters are sequenced loosely based on the communicative system affected. In Chapters 6 and 7, ALS and PD are discussed. Both are neuromotor disorders affecting primarily the speech motor system, although PD carries with it the possibility of some late stage impairment of cognition. Chapter 8 addresses language-based communication challenges in the form of stroke-related aphasia. Chapter 9 takes on the challenge of dementia, in which communication deficit is a byproduct of loss of cognitive function. This sequence of chapters allows us to consider escalating threats to narrative self, as we move through the underlying neurological systems that support storying of self.

Chapters 6 and 8 use the life stories of many to probe issues of narrative self in depth. ALS represents the extreme of severe degenerative motor impairment that leads ultimately to death, while the mind and self are relatively preserved.

On the other hand, aphasia associated with stroke and other medical conditions provides an opportunity to explore the potential for recovery in the context of impaired semiotic tools needed to negotiate the recovery trajectory. Unlike ALS, for persons who interact with those with aphasia, the intactness of self and of mental competence is often questioned because of the individual's inability to communicate in ways that validate self.

Chapters 7 and 9 address the challenges to narrative self experienced by persons living with Parkinson's disease and dementia (specifically, Alzheimer's disease). Each focuses primarily on one person to illustrate the way in which the theoretical constructs of this text can be applied to other communication disorders and can illuminate the unique experiences of individuals.

As we reviewed relevant literature for each chapter and began drafting content, it became apparent that a full-length book could be written on each topic. Choices had to be made in order to make the material more readable and focused. One of these choices has been to reduce the number of journal and text references on topics related to the life stories of those living with neurogenic communication disorders. For example, we have not cited much of the aphasia literature on quality of life, life participation, and social models for clinical practice. This decision in no way reflects on the importance of this literature. Instead, it allows us to elaborate the unique experiences of those living with aphasia, using their own words and life stories. The same is true for the other life stories chapters. We have also made no attempt in Section III to address the range of communication treatment options available to persons with such disorders.

Neither this section nor this text as a whole is meant to be a treatise about aphasia or ALS or Parkinson's disease or dementia. Instead, we have elected to build on the words and experiences of those whose lives inform this book. Adopting an essentially qualitative stance with respect to these data, we have identified themes or threads through the narratives available to us. The only common denominator across these chapters is the exploration of aspects of self and narrative, as they are affected by neurogenic communication disorders, and as they converge in our understanding of life storying and narrative self.

Beyond these themes, we have allowed the individual life stories to dictate other topics that will receive focus. Thus the reader will find considerable variety in the actual organizational structure of each chapter. For example, in Chapter 9 on dementia, the construct of self cannot be separated from other topics such as life story, illness narrative, and social others. Since dementia is fundamentally a progressive cognitive disorder, and since issues of self are at the heart of our understanding of this condition, Flo's story dominates the first portions of the chapter, and issues of self, life story, and illness narrative are highlighted as her dementia progression is documented. In contrast, in Chapter 7 on Parkinson's disease, Jerry Patnoe's story is laid out under headings that parallel the theory in this book, and the transition from illness narrative to new life story is emphasized. In Chapter 6, it is suggested that illness narrative is indeed the remaining life story for persons living with ALS. Thus in this chapter's organizational framework, many of the themes that emerged from interactions with persons with ALS are addressed under the heading of illness narrative.

Our goal is to guide clinicians and researchers to a better understanding of what it is about each communication disorder and each person living with such disorders that is important to our understanding of narrative self. For clinicians, our goal is to suggest what aspects of the individual's life story should receive focus in intervention, if we are to address the core issue of impact of communication impairment on narrative self. For researchers, our intent is to provide direction into different lines of inquiry that complement the existing literature on the life impact of neurogenic communication disorders. As will be seen, chapters of Section IV in this text provide each author's perspective on "what all this means."

CHAPTER 6

Life Stories in ALS

In exploring the life stories of those with amyotrophic lateral sclerosis (ALS), we may need to begin with the end—with the reality that ALS is the ultimate disruptor of life. The experience is one of clear, gradual motor decline, loss of speech, and death—often at an age when life should seem fullest and narrative self is evolving in all its complexity. So, how does one construct a new narrative—and negotiate a new self—when one is facing the end of one's life?

While many people living with ALS (PALS) undoubtedly experience a drive to find purpose and meaning in the present or past, there does not seem to be a consistent perception of narrative wreckage, in Frank's (1995) terms, despite the biographic disruption caused by the disorder. Certainly, the knowledge of imminent death flies in the face of most people's expectations, but it also seems that clear knowledge of the end allows some to focus more clearly on the present or to make choices to develop priorities for living. One factor that makes this possible is the relative preservation of mental capacities in ALS, including language and self-reflection. Even when speech intelligibility deteriorates, written language remains an option in some cases. In fact, for PALS whose speech is affected early on (bulbar onset), some limb motor skills for

writing or for computer-activated communication are available for a considerable time period.

Relatively spared mental abilities are also critical for the significant others who share the burden of ALS. There is something fundamentally secure about knowing that one's loved one can communicate if needed, even if the communication process is awkward and time-consuming. Unlike family members of persons with severe aphasia, who often have literally no sense of what their loved one is attempting to communicate, the families and friends of PALS learn that they can work together to understand communicative content and intent. The potential for coconstruction of the remaining life story empowers all those who are involved.

The existing literature on impact of ALS focuses primarily on quality of life (QOL) for the PALS and their friends and family members (Bremer, Simone, Walsh, Simmons, & Felgoise, 2004; Chia et al., 2004; Goldstein, Atkins, & Leigh, 2002; Jenkinson, Fitzpatrick, Brennan, & Swash, 1999; Mockford, Jenkinson, & Fitzpatrick, 2006; Nygren & Askmark, 2006; Smith, Crossley, Greenberg, Wilder, & Carroll, 2000, among others). Most of these studies use questionnaires to probe facets of quality of life.

We approach the task of understanding life with ALS somewhat differently. In this chapter, we explore the way persons with ALS pull from different dimensions of self—culture, roles, interactions, and biography—to rewrite their narratives or life stories, when ALS has fundamentally disrupted the previous story. The words of persons with ALS and their significant others have been gleaned from multiple sources, including written or spoken comments elicited in response to broad probes of the experience of living with ALS (with focus on communication), interviews with two spouses of PALS, the written "diaries" of one PALS who journaled his experience from diagnosis until shortly before his death and of another who began an autobiographical document shortly after diagnosis, and finally observations from interactions with PALS and their family members in the course of ALS support group meetings and delivery of clinical services. On-line support forums also yielded useful material. The existing literature on life impact of ALS is limited. Thus the reflections of those living with ALS become our most important vehicle for understanding these lives and how health care professionals can reach out and support the maintenance of narrative self.

Before going further, it is important to introduce those persons who have graciously shared their life stories in this chapter. The person whose legacy was a primary stimulus for the writing of this text is Steve Kressen, a man who held a high level administrative position in a large international retail company, and whose wife Sylvia and children from both first and second marriages brought real joy into his life. Steve's journals and e-mails inform much of this chapter. In the following brief quotes, it is easy to see why Steve's story is so inspirational. His words demonstrate the way in which the experience of loss of communication shifts over time with the physical changes associated with the disease and with the evolving understanding of the imminence of death. In the first quote, he is sharing his joy in finding a free shareware program called Click'it that would allow him to continue his work and his personal communications with friends and loved ones. In the second quote, Steve captures the heart of this exploration of communication and narrative self.

With my speech already a major source of frustration for both me and the listener, I had become increasingly reliant upon the written word. But as my arms and then my hands and in more recent weeks my fingers have weakened essentially to the point of paralysis, I had become more and more isolated, depressed, and not a whole lot of fun to be around. Vicious circle. Now I feel a sense of liberation, renewed energy and productivity, and general well-being. So get ready; I'm back. So little time, so much to say!

Barbara Taylor and Jim Jackson, married members of the University of Arkansas community, agreed to share their thoughts and feelings about the experience of living with ALS some months after Jim's diagnosis and perhaps 2 years after first symptoms. As caregiver, Barbara's explanation of the way Jim interacted prior to the disease onset is reflected in his current communication behavior. In turn, Jim describes the deterioration in his communication and intelligibility in rational, somewhat distanced terms in a manner consistent with Barbara's comments about his pre-ALS communication, highlighting the highly individualized experience of communication loss in ALS.

Barbara: Jim was never a talker, he's not one of those people who needs to have his mouth open to prove he's alive. I know there are some people who talk incessantly and who talk to remind themselves that they exist and he's never . . . he's always been fairly quiet, speaking when there is something to say and I don't expect chatter. I don't expect a kind of narrative going-on about how the day has been, so it may have not be as major a transition for us because of that . . . One of the things that I've always treasured about him is his ability to be silent and our ability to be together and not have to talk so that is the kind of broad context.

Jim: I had slurred speech for a long time before I had the ALS diagnosis; at least a year. Although it grew gradually worse, people still seemed to understand me. I just sounded hoarse, and many commented that my allergies must be acting up. As my speech continued to deteriorate, a few people began to have trouble understanding me, but most could. Over time that has changed and few can understand me now. What has surprised me most is how many could understand me for so long. Listening to myself, I thought the listener wouldn't understand but they did. That is my overall impression. As to how willing people have been to keep working to understand me, that has varied as one would expect from not very much to quite a bit. I can still write or type, although slowly, so I substitute that for the spoken word when needed.

The other couple who shared their experience of living with ALS is Wade and Sarah Burnside. Wade is a retired physician

who is much loved and respected in the community. His wife Sarah was also extremely active in the community, particularly in her church. Sarah's life and values had been deeply influenced by her earlier years living with missionary parents in Africa. In her adult years, in addition to raising three children, she gave to many—always quietly and behind the scenes—and also managed to pursue her passion for theater through acting, directing, obtaining a graduate degree, and supporting theater in the community. In the following quotes, we get a glimpse of what living with ALS means to them, particularly to their life stories.

Sarah (when asked about her priorities at the time of our meeting): I wrote a book about growing up in Africa—I'm doing the editorial notes now.
(When further probed about how she felt her identity had been affected by the diagnosis of ALS and her deteriorating physical condition, her written response was simple and to the point): There's a lot of me in the book.

Wade (When asked to reflect on the life changes he and Sarah were experiencing, he offered the following.): One other thought I have had in the past is . . . one of the things that happen in a situation like this is your priorities change. Like it used to be a priority to bake bread once a week or something. It's a priority to keep the flower beds weeded, keep the weeds out of the flowers. Things like that you just let it go.

Penny and A.J. struggled with coping with Penny's mother's ALS. This couple sought help early on in meeting the mother's changing needs. They did not live near her, and felt the helplessness that comes from an inability to see and assist in managing changes occurring on a daily basis. As Penny wrote:

> One thing that I feel is so lacking in the fight for ALS is any psychological help for both the patient/victim, and the caregivers/families/victims. There is no motivation, support, encouragement, or psych help at all. Everyone just fumbles around, trying to help, and getting very depressed.

Others in the ALS Support Group include Linda and David B. Linda's ALS has been slow moving, so she and David have had extended opportunities to reflect on their lives and their relationship and who share what they have gained from these reflections. Finally, Chris is a caring, affirming 71-year-old who has had many different jobs in his life, most recently owning a candle store in a nearby tourist town. His family is tight-knit; their love and mutual support are clear as he and his wife (Billie) and daughters join him at support group meetings. They often draw on their experiences with their hearing impaired child when dealing with the challenges of ALS. When Chris was asked to reflect on some questions about living with ALS, he volunteered the following in writing, showing his sensitivity to the plight of loved ones in addition to his own personal concerns.

> What is surprising to me is I have seen several cases where the ALS person is mad or griping or fussing at their caregiver for not understanding them. They are not thinking of the predicament their spouse is in. I know in certain cases it takes time to learn what their caregiver is going through. The ALS person did not bring this disease on themselves but I think they also must know

that their spouse did not bring the frustration on themselves either. So I think it is important for those with any problems that require the spouse's help to be thankful for what they have.

More than anything, these articulate quotes underscore the fundamental mental integrity of these individuals, along with their preserved capacity to reflect on life changes and give expression to the experience, sometimes with great eloquence. While recent research suggests that some PALS experience cognitive declines similar to frontotemporal dementia as the disease progresses, the majority remain cognitively intact. For the most part, those who contributed to this chapter are among the cognitively spared.

A central premise of this book is that impairment of communication potentially disrupts the process of storying of self that is necessary if one is to maintain some continuity in the life story. This discussion may be particularly important in dealing with ALS, given the fact that the rapidly changing physical/medical status of the patient tends to focus interventions on immediate physical challenges, with limited attention to the broader impact of the disease. It is appropriate to begin with communication, since speech intelligibility will always be impaired and our interests lie with the impact of that impairment.

Communication in ALS

The nature of the medical condition amyotrophic lateral sclerosis (ALS) was described in Chapter 2, along with a brief description of the dysarthria that is the primary speech consequence of this motor disorder. Communication impairment is a common theme in the narratives of persons with ALS. In a random selection of 20 entries on the Patients Like Me on-line forum, all 20 commented about communication loss, and 17 of the 20 discussed the powerful negative impact of this loss. It is not surprising that individuals who choose to participate in on-line ALS communities are those who value communication. However, in reviewing interview transcripts and clinical notes of interactions with PALS, it is apparent that the impact of loss of intelligibility is highly personalized, primarily due to premorbid communication styles, the role of communication in previous and current life activities, the responses of significant others, and the person's chosen ways of coping with the motor degeneration found in ALS.

One challenge in understanding the communication needs and experiences of persons with ALS is determining what people want to communicate about, and how they prefer to exchange this communication. Those whose stories lie at the heart of this chapter provide examples of how diverse and unique these needs and communication channels really are. For example, Chris began to write his autobiography shortly after being diagnosed with ALS. Sarah escalated her efforts to complete writing her early childhood autobiography, and Steve's priorities centered on continued work productivity, personal reflection, and connecting with important people in his life, primarily through writing. Jim continues to invest his energies in e-mail communications with a broad community of friends and acquaintances, and another support group member Dave devotes his time and communication effort to everyday interpersonal exchanges and activities such as playing card games and golfing.

As ALS progresses and communication becomes more difficult, both physically taxing and emotionally frustrating, people do begin to make unconscious or conscious choices concerning what to communicate about. These choices are highly variable but are always consistent with life priorities, and these priorities may not always be the same as those of caregivers. Communication impact is also very situation specific (Ball, Beukelman, & Pattee, 2004). Increasing communicative effort (whether verbal or using a communication device) along with varying degrees of adversity across social situations influence with whom PALS work to communicate and when or where.

All of the individuals described here have chosen to communicate in relatively complete and sometimes complex utterances, even as the physical challenges of communication escalate. For a long time, Jim persisted in spelling out complete words on his alphabet board even when the visitor had identified the target word. As it became increasingly difficult for him to use this alphabet board, his wife shared some reflections on Jim's desire to finish his message. One insight she offered seems particularly astute in the context of this chapter. She raised the question of whether the act of completing words might reflect a corresponding mental act of finishing a thought. If this is true for some, it might explain a variety of behaviors. While Jim needed to communicate about basic needs (suction, pain medication, etc.), it was also important to him to share the nuances of communication. Several months before his death, he could only communicate by responding nonverbally when others pointed to letters on an alphabet board. Remarkably, with his daughter's help, he wrote several beautiful poems during that time.

In addition, choice of words is particularly important to some. Just a week before his death, Steve was visiting with two speech-language pathologists (SLPs) in his home. At this time, he could only use one foot to activate a switch that operated his AAC device. Despite the effort required to communicate using scanning (moving systematically through letters and words and phrases to reach the desired target), he persisted in using complex sentences with elaborate vocabulary. When one of the SLPs figured out his intended message before the sentence was complete, Steve also persisted in spelling out the rest of the communication. The clinicians and Steve's wife joked with him about his love of words, and then one of the clinicians asked why he didn't take shortcuts such as just typing key words. Steve's response was, "That's not me." For Steve, his communication style was part of the self he presented to the world, and the decision to talk like he did pre-ALS was an affirmation of self.

Self and Life Stories

ALS is HOW I am, it will not rob me of WHO I am. (on-line discussion posting)

I have fought the good fight against the inevitable demise of the illness. I have prolonged my decline, I have maintained my dignity, I have continued to maintain an outward face. Now it is time to no longer do the things that promote my survival; rather it is time to do the things that will support my legacy. (Steve)

In these words, two persons with ALS characterize issues of selfhood and life story. Both quotes make clear that these individuals are determined to ensure that, regardless of the physical consequences of the disease, they retain the ability to create a self. In the second quote, Steve also presents a mini-life story, complete with elements of an illness narrative. This chapter section explores fur-

ther issues of self as intertwined with life narrative. The couples described here are engaged in construction of new narrative selves even as ALS takes its toll. Since the life stories carry the story of self, no attempt will be made to separate self and narrative.

Self and Culture

Some of the stories presented by PALS address the concept of stigma. Certainly, in Western societies, illness and disability are frequently stigmatized. Sabat (2001) speaks of the concept of excessive disability, noting that there is some point beyond which society's acceptance of disability does not extend. Perceived stigma limits our ability to use our cultural tools to construct a narrative self, and ALS typically exceeds the thresholds for normalcy and disability.

What, then, is the societal or cultural perception of ALS? For the most part, ALS is little understood, and the average person recognizes only the label *Lou Gehrig's Disease*. The behaviors that are visible are those related to physical decline, although loss of speech intelligibility may be perceived as an indicator of mental dysfunction and reduced cognitive competence. Sean Redmond (2003) uses the word *cripple* to attack the stigma associated with disability in general and ALS specifically:

I am one among some 30,000 patients of different ages, sizes and temperament who are under care for a disease, which has no known cause, treatment or cure. We're practically crippled. I say practically crippled because I've learned that being crippled doesn't necessarily mean we're emotional or mental cripples.

We live in a society where youth, appearance, and physical prowess are among the most desirable cultural commodities. For most persons, there is definitely a reluctance to "concede" that one has a disability. As Steve wrote 6 months before his death:

Recently I crossed one of few remaining bridges that, in this round at least, I am to traverse: I have left the workforce and accepted the federal descriptor "disabled." Ironic that now when my time is my own, when my acumen is crystal, and when my muse is a constant companion, my frailty is so devastatingly complete.

Steve's assertion of mental clarity is a reminder that even those who seem most reflective and most accepting of ALS continue to feel a need to remind others of their mental intactness. In interviews conducted for this chapter, respondents were asked to react to the question of which would be harder to deal with—physical or mental changes. Implicit in this question was an underlying probe about which would be harder to lose over time (personally) and which might be more stigmatizing (socially). Chris's comments reflect the complexity of this question and his sensitivity to the fact that everyone is affected by loss of functions.

At a certain point in time during this illness, I most likely will want to switch my opinion and prefer mental deficiency. I cannot help but think of what my wife and caregiver will have to do for me when I become physically unable to take care of myself. Most of my life, I have been mostly independent (except for Billie). To this day I do not depend on others to do the tasks I can do for myself. I am speaking of normal daily tasks. To one day be unable to do physical things would make me wish I were not able to know what was being done. It would bother me quite a bit to know what Billie had to do daily.

Jim also reflects on this question, stating:

As to the choice you present, I would prefer to have what I have (ALS) to stroke or Alzheimer's. The loss of physical functions is challenging, but compared to loss of mental ability, it's preferable. My father had a stroke and lingered several months following. I was one of several care givers he had. It was impossible to know whether I was dealing with him or the disease. I think probably always both, so when, e.g., on several occasions he thought I was his brother, and accused me of selling the farm, it could be stressful, and over time exhausting because rationality was not an option. I noticed similar effects on the other civilian care givers he had such as my stepmother. I don't know how the medical people deal with it. I never discovered any response that was very successful. In sum, I think having physical problems are better than having mental ones.

It is also important to note that acceptance is not an either-or phenomenon; some people are only willing or able to accept bits and pieces of the ALS reality at any point in time. This is evident in discussions of what the future may bring. For example, in an augmentative communication (AAC) evaluation with one couple who were being very proactive in recognizing a future need for communication technology, the wife said, "I guess I can see why someone might need scanning. *If* you lost control of your hands." And her husband stated later: "I'm just affected at the top. *If* it moves down, I may have to . . . do something" [emphasis added]. These statements demonstrate the remarkable power of the word if to stave off a complete acceptance of the implication of the ALS diagnosis.

For the people in this chapter, acceptance of diagnosis and of disability was often related to a single defining moment or event that brought home the reality of the ALS, its impact on each life, and its handicapping nature. In most instances, these defining moments were physical, and what mattered were the social and cultural implications of physical changes. In Sarah's case, Wade describes the following incident.

And then from there we went to Santa Fe for Elderhostel and that's when she fell and broke her arm and we piled in the car the next day and drove home and that was the point at which more fell on me rather suddenly and that from that point on I've been the chief cook and bottle washer. Because with the broken arm and plus some degree of weakness she really couldn't do much in the kitchen. But she was still eating so I was cooking for two at that point until January when she got the PEG tube. She was still eating a little bit but it was just a matter of weeks before she was eating nothing. Abrupt. Because she kept choking, that was one of the most frightening things because she would try to take . . . sometimes food and sometimes pills and there's nothing I can do when she was having one of those choking spells so in that sense in a way the PEG tube was a relief not have to swallow pills and to be able to get nourishment and pills without those awful spells of swallowing and choking. . . . That was the life-changing part.

Similarly, Barbara described an incident in which Jim fell while walking in their neighborhood, just prior to her leaving town for an important professional conference. The level of detail in this anecdote highlights its significance for her:

Interesting thing happened before I went to this big conference where I'm president, 60th anniversary celebration, huge thing—either a day or two days before —I'm in the office, get a phone call from Jim, well actually, my phone was doing something and I heard this funny little sound from it and I picked it up and I saw that I missed a bunch of phone . . . one of them was from Jim and then I had the phone out on my desk and it went (squeaky sound) and because it was out I saw that Jim had called me and he said I need help and I said, I'm there I'm on my way but he said I'm in the driveway and I thought Oh god. So I said I'm on my way and I raced down and got in my car and drove up and out of the corner of my eye I saw him sort of waving me down. He had been out walking by himself with a stick and was headed for home and he decided he wanted to sit down and have a rest and some of the neighbors have this retaining wall but the driveway was . . . so when he went to sit down he lost his footing. He pinned his right leg under him, his stick went clattering down the driveway and by the time I got there he'd untangled himself and he was sitting on the wall. I put him in the car got him home got the story from him. The only visible change was a scrape on his elbow so I cleaned that off, put a sesame street bandaid on it so it would be funny and thought oh my god . . .

You know, I worry about him still. So . . . on the one hand I'm continuing to work and carrying on as normal as Jim did through January before it became clear to him that he wasn't going to be able to work. Actually I think he's enjoyed not working at least that's what he says and I think it's probably right. . . . I guess I've had some practice in doing that and that feels fine and to know that whatever comes that that's when the correct response particularly will come to me . . . some sense that you will respond appropriately . . . that you'll do what needs to be done . . . and I know I'm sometimes pretty solicitous . . . we have a 2 year old granddaughter named Kylani and she's in the phase where she has to do everything herself, she has to put her shoes on herself . . . that's the way you are when you're two. You're learning to be yourself. There was some point when I was fussing over Jim and wanting to do something for him and offering to do something for him and he says no, I'm in my Kylani phase.

Clearly, Western society values independence. One cultural theme related to independence, dependence, and disability is that of "fighting" the disease. One spouse personalized ALS as the enemy, the "beast" or "the monster." In describing the battle, Steve says, " . . . we [he and his wife] struggle with the ravages of the disease, as if there is always someone else in the room. With ALS, we are never alone together." What a remarkable characterization of the experience. Terms such as "fight," "battle," "winning," or "losing" are common. Many on-line posts speak of not giving up, of holding on until a cure is found, of exploring every option, no matter how far-fetched. While the struggle is certainly personal, it is society that also is charged with finding the cure. The following excerpts exemplify the personal side of the battle.

I am just learning my ropes on my new career, fighting ALS. I believe, after all, it IS how you play the game (of living) that counts.

I enjoy life and refuse to give in to this disease.

Those who adopt an attitude of fighting the disease may see it as interiorized or exteriorized. For most, the fight is perceived as directed against some external threat. Some become impatient with the omnipresent external threat of ALS, as Steve notes: "Over the past year, as I've entered into this new phase of my life as an ALS PALS, I've noticed my disease can be (some days more than others) the center of my universe. I don't think that is totally healthy." Others feel the battle is interior and feel distaste and anger with the failing of their own bodies. Still others seem to feel a sense of integration with the disease, as Barbara suggests: "It's not something you have to reject or distance yourself from."

If disability, handicap, incompetence, and dependence fall at one end of a continuum, it is also necessary to explore the other end, representing agency, autonomy, independence, competence, and strength. At the cultural level, many whose lives have been affected become involved with national advocacy organizations such as the Amyotrophic Lateral Sclerosis Association (ALSA) or the Muscular Dystrophy Association (MDA) in local initiatives or national causes such as the development of a national registry for persons with ALS. Association with recognized organizations provides cultural validation for a new self that includes ALS.

At the personal level, issues of independence and competence in ALS tend to relate primarily to the physical domain (unlike aphasia and dementia). The gradual progression of the loss of motor skills can help some individuals adjust to changes more easily than, for example, the abrupt overnight loss of motor skills that can result from stroke. With guidance, PALS can find assistive devices and technology to sustain independence for a good portion of the disease timeline. Some resist these supports, as a way of resisting acknowledgement of disease progression. Others simply prefer to function independently as long as possible, without changing their daily activities. For example, Barbara indicates (with humor) that Jim:

> . . . really wants to do as much as he can for as long as he can do it. [I want to say] don't drive that car, that doesn't have power steering. I think you are out of your mind—of all the god damn things he does, driving is . . .

She also acknowledges, at the time of this interview, that they have found ways to continue enjoyed activities within only minor modifications, describing that:

> We are nowhere near crossing the line [of dependence]. And he probably supervises cooking more than he does cooking but he used to do a lot of it and Margot [his daughter] and I don't mind playing sous chef or following directions and making things he might have made in the past. . . . There's nothing that I will do that he doesn't want me to do. And I kind of have to monitor myself about being pushy. Because I can see for example that squeezing the key limes it's hard to do things that require squeezing and okay, I can do something else.

One issue of constructing competence or incompetence is the manner in which one has been treated by the health care system, the medical community. There are interesting contrasts between the experiences of persons living with ALS and persons living with aphasia, for example. Most of the PALS known to this author had no major issues with their medical experiences, although many were frustrated with delays in reaching a diagnosis and some expressed a desire for better listening on the part of physicians specifically. When Wade Burnside, himself a physician, was asked about medical experiences, he stated:

> I don't have any thing. I don't think I have a good answer to that.

Self and Roles

Structural tools for creating a new narrative include the roles previously played by the person with ALS and the roles that are now available to her. Communication is essential in most common roles. To the extent that one cannot assume new roles, creating a new narrative becomes more problematic. Not surprisingly, a recurring theme in ALS relates to the importance of communication in work/professional roles and activities. In an on-line discussion forum, a person with ALS writes: "I am a RN/BSN. Before I was disabled by bulbar-onset ALS I was a public health nurse. I miss my career desparately [*sic*]." This same person elaborated later in stating,

> All of this, including the consultation with other staff and contacts in various disciplines related to public health, all required clear speech. I was laid off two years ago, supposedly for budget reasons. I'm now on full disability. I miss my career more than I can say.

There is an extended on-line discussion of professions and disability, with one individual writing, "My job also entails significant public speaking and I am concerned I will get fired."

Chris writes about his earlier work as teacher, traveling salesman, and most recently store owner, and how critical communication was in all of these jobs. "So yes communication has been a very important factor in my life." For Steve, the ability to continue his work activities, which involved extensive written and spoken communication, was critical to his ability to cope with ALS. He comments on the issue of work productivity in many journal entries and e-mails.

> Despite the ALS, which has robbed me of my ability to speak intelligibly, has left me with only a couple of typing fingers, and forced me to become right-handed as the left wing is pretty well useless, I remain working, productive, engaged and somewhat naively optimistic about the future.
>
> Working is still important to my emotional and psychic well-being, and today was my usual day in the office. Happy to still participate meaningfully.

And in a public speech expressing his appreciation of his employer's support, he indicated that the company provided him with:

> . . . the specialized tools I need to remain productive. Because of them, I'm intellectually engaged and committed, and still able to add value. Because of them, ALS has not robbed me of my dignity.

Thus, for many persons with ALS, distress related to the loss of the job or the disruption of a productive career due to communication impairment continues to dominate their illness narratives and colors their quest to move forward with a modified narrative self in which profession is no longer central.

Roles figure prominently in on-line ALS forums where persons with ALS share their basic life stories. It is interesting to read these stories from the perspective of the biographic particulars people choose to share, and the focus of these stories on past, present, or future roles. For the most part, there is a sense of continuity in these stories, as people share bits and pieces of their past and present, along with determination to win out in the future. There is also a clear sense of what roles are valued and what roles are perceived as self-defining (whether in work settings or within the family, community, church, etc.).

> I am a quadriplegic and ventilator dependent. I am a fighter! I started writing poetry after I left work. You can read some of my poetry in the May/June issue of Neurology Now. Here is one. Resolved I refuse to die I choose to defy Prognosis (poor) I will see Daughters Graduate Marry Grandchildren I refuse to die I choose to defy Prognosis (guarded) I must Love Help Work Dream Eat chocolate every day I refuse to die I choose to survive Prognosis (good).

> I am married to a wonderful husband & caregiver with 4 beautiful children. I retired from the radiology field in 2003 (official diagnosis) after 24 years where I performed x-ray, cat scan & mammography. I was a member of the Woman's Professional Candlepin Bowling Association. I also enjoyed horseshoes, golf, softball & rollerblading. My decision to vent (3/06) was an easy one. I value & love my life. My hubby & children still need me. My computer is my link to the world as I can no longer speak. I still enjoy camping & boating. What I enjoy most is being with my family & friends. I love life!

> I am a 70 year old woman, married, with two sons and four grandchildren. I was an art teacher and public relations consultant and continued creating art projects after I retired. I am now writing

stories about my childhood and hope that these will be my legacy to my children and my grandchildren and beyond.

Former journalist, computer programmer until diagnosis. Was a runner and basketball player. Was always skinny.

These diverse stories share one common element—most are written by people who have the determination to continue writing their life story, changing some of the elements as earlier roles become lost to them. There is little dwelling on what these individuals can or cannot do. What is critical in working with persons living with ALS is an understanding of the importance of roles, even if those roles must be different from ones previously held. For Linda, her priority is her self-defined most important role, giving to her family, doing the things needed for their lives to go well. For Penny's mother, despite the fact that she was in her 70s, her most important role was found in her work for the parish in which she lives. Work is paramount to Steve in the time immediately post-diagnosis. Before ALS, one of Sarah's roles was reflected in her involvement with theater. She wrote about how people would describe her, "Love to act and direct. Loves theatre." She is quick to note, "But it does not have to be doing it," an apparent acknowledgement that some more active theater roles are now denied to her. And Wade describes many changes in how his time is used, including some losses in roles of regular church attendee and bread maker (literally). His new role of caregiver was not fully realized until Sarah broke her arm and required much more extensive physical assistance. Roles become inextricably tied in with priorities. It is as though ALS, with its clear reminder that time is limited, forces people to take stock of their different life roles and determine which will receive time and attention.

If the work of maintaining narrative self depends in part on the responses of others, it is not surprising to find that self is not challenged early on in ALS. The person can walk, talk, reflect on what is happening, and participate actively in daily decisions. At the same time, ALS brings with it dramatic changes in life roles and identities. In fact, a discussion of self is uncomfortable to some who show no hesitation when asked to speak about changes in life roles. Jim writes: "As to a sense of self, I don't know." And when Sarah was asked about how ALS had affected her perceptions of herself and others, particularly how her loss of communication might impair her narrative self, her response was, "I don't know. There's lots of me in the book" (referring to her autobiography of early years with missionary parents in Africa). She went on to explain that historically, she has always presented herself to others through writing.

Self and Interaction

While there are many differences between each person's experience of ALS as shared with a loved one, ALS seems to bring some couples together, and this is a critical factor in the interactional aspect of self creation. Barbara talks about the intimacy of shared knowledge and shared ways of being.

I think we share so much . . . so many approaches to things, opinions, preferences, what have you, and so many experiences, we have shared language, we have funny words we say, like oatmeal is not oatmeal but oakmeal things like that and that won't be there with anybody else I know. It really doesn't go away . . . He's part of who I am, Jim's part of me.

[The illness is now] incorporated into us . . . and I can go to this conference and dance . . . a couple nights in a row . . . and celebrate and relate to lots of people . . . and not feel guilty. Jim wouldn't want me to hold back.

And Steve reflects on the connectedness of selves, in writing to a dear friend and in describing his life with wife Sylvia.

To a friend: You have always been here inside me, and as you reach the half-century mark I want you to know that I would be honored to be counted among the many friends wishing you good luck, congratulations [*sic*], and Godspeed.

And about his wife: Sylvia is my soul-mate and my inspiration. We struggle with the ravages of the disease, as if there is always someone else in the room. With ALS, we are never alone together. But our love for each other remains strong and we feel blessed to have our days together.

The ability to express these feelings, with each other and with outsiders, is dependent in part upon the language skills of the person with ALS. It is not surprising that the sense of intact narrative self is more common in ALS than, for example, stroke-related aphasia, where words cannot be found to confirm these critical connections. However, as will be described later, there are some, such as Penny's mother, whose refusal to deal with any impingement of the disease on her sense of who she was essentially cut off important communications with family members about present and future needs. In effect, she chose not to use certain interactional tools in her tool kit.

Some PALS speak of concerns related to how their speech will be received and interpreted by others, as in the following on-line posting.

I have had slurred speech that has gradually worsened (with the fluctuations expected: significantly worse when I am tired or very stressed) for 17 months. So far this (along with choking) are the only symptoms I have. It is extremely frustrating! I am scared that I will get pulled over while driving and get taken in for "dui" (even if a breath-a-lyzer is negative they could suspect other drugs). I work in the medical field and I am afraid that my patients or other health-care providers will think I have been drinking. Unfortunately, I don't work with the same people every day (or even regularly) so I can't just issue a blanket "statement" about my speech. I HATE talking on the phone (because I never am easily understood) and I too feel very socially isolated.

Chris provides a similar story about customers in their store becoming concerned that he was coming to work drunk. In contrast, Jim indicates his surprise that others understood him for so long, sometimes attributing his altered speech quality to allergies.

For most, however, communication is simply the critical interactive tool for what McAdams (1993) calls communion, a means for staying connected with loved ones. Jim states rather simply: "Communication is very important since I live with other people." He makes no explicit distinctions between family communications and those with others, although he clearly interacts in different ways. And Chris elaborates on communication within the family, including evolving challenges with the ALS progression. He reports that early on, with some humor, he reasoned "the listener just was not paying enough attention to what I was saying." With considerable wisdom, he then highlights the fact that a breakdown in family communication can relate to more than simply the intelligibility of one's speech. "My wife, being more aware, knew that she was not just having a listening problem but also an emotional problem from the lack of communication. Communication with people is vital to life . . . " Chris also captures the daily impact of communication breakdown in the following description of profound alterations in the experience of traveling long distances when one person cannot speak:

> Here you are with your spouse who has been able to hear your voice since you have been together and now she can not understand what you are saying. Not only understand what you are trying to say to here but what you are trying to get across to her. Even with talking devices or paper and pencil, there is also a time element that is hard to overcome. Being in this spot I know. Just imagine going on a long trip like Eureka Springs to Houston with no words. Thank God for the radio. On any evening at home, again thank God for TV.

For others, there are specific family needs that need to be addressed, as Steve indicates in the following journal entry:

> I am bothered—no, troubled—by my inability to connect with my son Joey. With the girls, they intuitively seem to know how much communication lies in a gesture, a carefully timed glance, a change in posture. They are somehow able to downshift in order to match my excruciatingly slow top speed so that at least for a few daily moments we are clicking along stride for stride. Joey is

100% boy. He's charging forward, and you'd better keep up or get out of the way. He will need a man in his life to within an absolute sense of self while remaining selfless at the same time.

Penny and A.J. believed that communication with her mother was absolutely critical, and they have found ways to maintain this communication despite her resistance to using AAC:

> As we live in a different state than mom, we consider our selves very lucky that Mom, at her age, did have computer experience. Limited but she had some. So we bought her and us laptops, and taught her how to use the instant message program. We feel so very lucky that she can and does communicate with us, my daughter, my step sister, and even my brother and his daughters who are very local to her. This one program so far has been our saving grace as we could not at this point communicate with mom by phone. I only worry about when she loses her ability to communicate this way.

The issue of premorbid communication style emerged with most couples, as did hints of frustrations with current interactions. While Barbara's earlier comments about Jim's communication style underscore the importance of preferred premorbid communication strategies, Jim indicated nonverbally to the interviewer that Barbara sometimes didn't hear very well (communicated with a big smile). It was particularly informative to talk with Wade and Sarah about their interactive styles. Premorbidly, Sarah had been outgoing, very interactive verbally, the dominant communicator within the family. However, as Wade describes their interaction with each other:

We never have been real talkative. I mean like you know some couples you see them together they're constantly talking to each other and we can drive in the car for a long time and not I mean we don't have a problem with silence I see couples who just seem to be constantly in conversation and I wonder in the world they're talking about . . . I don't have that much to say.

Since the onset of ALS and the decreasing intelligibility of Sarah's speech, the interactive profile of this couple had changed. During a visit with Sarah and Wade, he noted that:

This is a problem that occurs right here with several people in the room. She gets left out of conversations. She listens but . . . it falls into talking to each other. There's a tendency for two people who are verbal to talk to each other and for the nonverbal person to be left out.

He described Sarah as somewhat on the outside, almost neglected, even in family conversations. Ironically, during this visit, when she was asked a question, if she didn't immediately move to her communication device to respond, others simply continued talking, often speculating about what her response might be. Finally one of the visitors pushed Sarah to explain why she didn't communicate more and asked for silence and attention from the others in the room. After a considerable delay, Sarah typed "When I listen, I learn." In a very deliberate manner, she got everyone's attention and activated the message. Immediately, both family and friends challenged this response, suggesting it was a "cop-out." She denied this vigorously, using gestures, head shakes, and facial expression. In a subsequent interview with Sarah, she indicated that she had been a talker for most of her life and now it was time for her to listen.

This apparent shift in previous communicative patterns might be rather challenging to family members, particularly since relationships are established and maintained in daily conversation. Wade described Sarah's new communicative behaviors as "inconvenient and frustrating" on occasion, particularly since she continued to use writing on a dry erase board as her primary means of communication and ignored the availability of the DynaWrite computerized device. However, Wade also noted that Sarah herself did not seem to be bothered by the slowness of her writing or her exclusion from group interactions.

The individuality of these experiences must be understood if we are to find ways for persons with ALS to tell their stories. What must also be understood are the communication priorities of persons with ALS and their significant others. In fact, health care professionals may need to guide the family through a discussion of such issues. Sarah clearly felt no pressing need to participate in the chit-chat give-and-take of social conversations. However, one major life priority for her was completing a book documenting her early life with missionary parents in Africa. An interesting example of communicative choices in support of interaction and relating to others occurred during a social visit when the completion of this book was discussed. Sarah indicated to Wade that she wanted him to explain how her daughter had given her a toy monkey named Pest to represent her pet monkey when she was growing up. One of the visiting friends said she had always wanted a pet monkey. Sarah became very animated and began gesturing to Wade that she wanted him to show the visitors the final draft of the autobiography.

After he got the manuscript, he and another visitor paged through the document for about 10 minutes. During that time, Sarah continued to try to communicate something nonverbally, but her intention was missed. Finally, when Wade stood up to put the manuscript away, Sarah managed to get his attention, letting him know that she wanted him to bring her the book. After additional time and considerable effort paging through the text, she found a photograph of herself as a child with her pet monkey and shared it with the friend who had originally expressed a childhood wish to have a pet monkey. In an evening of few communicative initiations, Sarah was willing to expend the time (almost 20 minutes) and effort to share this personal moment with a friend. It was truly a moment of expression of interactional self. For her, this communication was important and meaningful.

This rather lengthy story matters because it illustrates the challenge of understanding any person's priorities for communication. In a subsequent interview with Wade, he raised the question of Sarah's inconsistent responsiveness communicatively.

I guess . . . the one thing that has been a little puzzling is that sometimes when I ask her a question I don't feel like I'm getting a clear answer, like even a yes or no. She doesn't do a really clear yes or clear no, and then the tendency is to try to present choices, you know, you say something "do you want to do so-and-so or so-and-so?" Well how do you answer it if you can't speak? So recently I've come up with a method. I do it this way: do you want half of a hydrocodone or a whole hydrocodone (holds out hands), and she points at the appropriate fingers and that's been working. That's been a little bit of frustration to me— not getting a clear response . . . And it

may be that I'm impatient to have it sooner than she's ready to give it. She doesn't make a whole lot of effort to communicate other than something she wants or needs and then she can write it and then go from there.

Understandably for Wade, as primary caregiver, the communication that mattered most was the clear expression of her physical needs. Yet Sarah gave less attention and effort to these daily matters than to the personal sharing of a biographical moment with a friend.

At times, it appears that persons with ALS do not struggle as much as other groups with respect to changes in narrative self, at least as we have used that term in this text. Even though many PALS, particularly those with bulbar onset, experience communication loss early on, they seem to be relatively grounded with respect to who they are in relationship to people that matter. What is also evident, however, is the fact that the dreams of those with ALS revolve around a world in which they walk and talk effortlessly. Redmond (2003) refers to this in describing ALS as:

. . . a group of people who are dissimilar in many ways yet we're very much alike. In our dreams, we're able to walk, to run, to dance, to sing, to cry, to hold those we love and tell them how we love them. And *above* our infirmities, we can take to the heavens and fly unencumbered because our spirits are free.

Steve also captures similar dreams in the following journal entry:

But in my dreams there is no affliction. I am protection and safety for my family. I am wise in the ways of the world.

I am Sylvia's passionate, attentive life partner into the far distant end of our days. And even after I haven permanently separated from this malicious frame, as long as I am in the dreams of those I have loved, through them I will live.

While it is impossible to define simplistically the impact of ALS on self or identity, we can turn to representations of self in life stories, pursuing our fundamental premise that self presentation is indeed a socially grounded narrative process. Some life stories are shared interactionally, as described in this section. However, other persons with ALS have felt the need to chronicle their experiences beginning shortly after the diagnosis. Steve's writings begin with the diagnosis and move forward with the experience of living with ALS. Chris consciously chose an autobiographical approach as a legacy to his family, starting earlier in his life and following a clear chronological timeline. He also uses what he has written as an introduction of himself to others. For example, when first seen at a speech clinic, he brought his autobiographical text to share with clinicians. These stories serve many functions, but are particularly important in creating continuity for the biographical self discussed next.

Self and Biography

The quest to create a new narrative in the face of ALS must take into account that the progression of the disease seems to be defined outwardly by multiple losses. As one on-line ALS forum member writes,

Physical illness may shatter this illusion (of personal invincibility), and a patient may lose the feeling of safety inherent in a cohesive sense of self. This loss precip-

itates a panicky sensation that "my world is falling to pieces," and the patient feels a sense of personal fragmentation.

Certainly, from the outside looking in, most healthy individuals are struck by the extent and severity of the losses being experienced by PALS and may question how one maintains a sense of personhood in the context of these changes. Barbara describes an interesting situation in which a health care provider asked Jim, with great compassion, "What is it like to be you—in your body?" Jim's response—"It's okay." What is interesting here is the fact that this professional was clearly recognizing and validating Jim's narrative self, by asking such a personalized question in an effort to understand better what it is like to walk in those shoes. Instead of the expected outpouring of a sense of grief and loss, Jim's brief response captures his fundamental "okayness" with his life.

Although persons with ALS may be dying, it is still critical to privilege their biographical self. Ongoing storying of self cannot be facilitated unless one understands past biographical particulars and the extent of autobiographical drive present in persons with ALS and their significant others. We also need to understand the nature of the biographic disruption brought about by ALS and each person's unique needs to reframe the life story.

One final observation can be offered about life stories in the face of a life-threatening disease. When discussing Sarah's book about her early roots, Wade offered a remarkable story about growing up in a Louisiana town, split through the middle by race, and about the life parallels between him and a black child his age who grew up to be highly successful. The story in all its detail was truly fascinating, but what was more interesting was the fact that the sharing of this story was somewhat uncharacteristic of Wade. In a way, by sharing this story, he was also asserting his own sense of self through sharing of part of his life story.

Illness Narratives

As discussed earlier in this text, illness is a profoundly disruptive event in one's life story and thus is "a call for stories" (Frank, 1995, p. 55). Prior to the formal ALS diagnosis, previously healthy persons have already begun to feel a sense of disconnect from the bodies that had served them well in the past. The many individuals who contributed to this chapter all shared elements of their illness narrative, whether in separate writings or discussions with the author. As a result, a number of themes emerged from their words. The themes discussed here include response to diagnosis and management of change; considerations of time; and issues of control.

The Illness Narrative: Diagnosis and Change

The ALS illness narrative frequently starts with the story of the search for a diagnosis, the feelings of all involved when the diagnosis is actually made, and the losses in motor function that have occurred since then. There are additional landmarks, those defining moments when the reality of the disease sets in (a fall, a fracture). Steve describes the moment of diagnosis:

> Regardless of how many more I live to experience, it is a safe bet that I will never forget my 49th birthday . . . [visits to doctors, tests]. A few minutes later our lives changed forever. On Friday, January 12, 2001 with no preparation or forewarning, we were told that I had Amyotrophic Lateral Sclerosis, or Lou Gherig [sic] Disease. Not strong on bedside manner, the Doctor went on to inform us that most patients with the disease died within two to five years, and didn't we already suspect that this was probably what I was suffering from?

Wade also elaborates on the initial diagnosis and the way in which they told their children:

> So anyway that first appointment at the ALs clinic, their conclusion at the end of the day was a benign probably ALS a benign form. and I think they were saying a benign form because still her symptoms were limited to swallowing and speaking and she really didn't I mean she tested out pretty well on the muscles and everything.
>
> And so we proceeded on the thinking they said 'probably'. And we told all our children that, and they said they wouldn't accept that, they wanted another opinion. Well really this was a second opinion in KC, but anyway it was the first time that anybody had said ALS, but they said we want you to get another opinion. So then [our doctor] said . . . he had previously said maybe Mayo, so then he said let's do Mayo Clinic. It took a bunch of time so we ended up in April and the doctor said it was ALS.

What is relatively unique to ALS is the fact that the outcome—death—is known at the time of diagnosis (although not always fully absorbed). In contrast, with stroke, fears about the initial medical crisis give way to an unknown future that at least holds some hope for recovery. In effect, when the future is unknown, the illness story is constantly evolving. When the future is known, the focus may shift to present tense living and coping with the declines associated with ALS. Narratives of redemption and restitution typically only appear when a treatment trial is begun, or a new procedure is described in the ALS research literature. ALS support groups become forums for sharing and validation of stories of the search for diagnosis and for reporting of changes since the last session. Sometimes, extended time is devoted to narratives of the results from a recent medical evaluation, and there is an eagerness to learn from the experiences of others.

Many find ways to reflect on the physical and emotional experiences as the disease progresses. Early on Steve writes:

> I am struggling some emotionally, as I guess is to be expected. Letters arrived from Mom today which sent me reeling. A current one, affirming her love and indicating that she is pretty well focused on my disease . . . hourly! I hate being the center of attention . . . What a tearjerker, especially in my current condition, where every emotion is exposed like sunburned skin.

And Barbara reflects on change, and what remains:

> The mind is clear . . . and we could make a list of the things that are nice or not bad about ALS. I mean the fact that your digestive system continues to work and that you don't need a lot of help with toileting early on . . . cause I've seen how that's been for people with other illnesses. The fact that your skin still likes to be touched.
>
> Today is today and tomorrow, is something you deal with tomorrow when tomorrow comes. Now . . . now more than early on I can see progression of the disease. There was a while when it seemed to level out and then there'd be times when he'd seem to get worse and then that would level out for a while. Then there'd be another.

Jim responds to a request to describe onset and diagnosis in a very matter-of-fact manner:

> Initially, I was surprised with the diagnosis. I knew there was some kind of neurological disorder but I had not considered that it could be fatal. I anticipated it would be something for which there was a reliable treatment even if I were not able to be as physically active as before. However, the initial reaction did not last long, and within less than an hour—maybe even minutes, it's hard to remember—I had accepted the diagnosis as most likely accurate.

In each of these quotes, time is a critical player in the narrative experience.

The Illness Narrative: Time

> On some level, just beyond the line of sight or a quartertone above audible pitch, I sense that the endgame has begun. Subconsciously, everything seems to be speeding up.

Persons dealing with ALS cannot escape the inexorable specter of dwindling time, as stated so clearly by Steve in the above quote. By definition, the disorder is terminal. Thus, it is possible to project one's past, present, and future and to create a life story that gives meaning to that life trajectory. One of the challenges of this reality is that ALS can progress relatively rapidly, and each new month, or week, or day creates new physical/medical challenges, particularly with respect to loss of physical independence (what one son of a person with ALS described, with some irony, as a "very fluid situation"). Thus the question is, when and how do those affected by ALS find the time and energy to reflect on these changes and to recreate a life story and narrative self that includes the reality of an "endgame"?

Views of Time

Time can be viewed at many levels. For some persons living with ALS, time is viewed as a precious commodity that has allowed important interpersonal and professional work to be accomplished. For example, in a support group session, Linda shares the following:

> God has been real good to me—allowed me to be still walking when my daughter was dying in the hospital for three weeks.

She indicates that time also allowed her to help her dying mother and take care of the business of closing down the mother's house.

> God has allowed me to do what I needed to do for the family . . . I have been so blessed by all the hugs.

In the same support group session, Steve's wife Sylvia indicates that they were grateful for the time to get to know each other, to share the journey. Steve's determination to live life fully and his refusal to give in provided them with time for each other and for their children. The physical and communicative changes of ALS do alter the ways in which families spend time together. Wade, Sarah, and Chris comment on filling the hours of passing time when communica-

tion is no longer an option and physical constraints limit activities outside of the home. Wade and Sarah began watching hours of rental DVDs. When interviewed for this book, Chris was still able to do things many things around the home and indicated he did not look forward to the time when he could not do so. Unfortunately, he has begun to experience restrictions in home activities.

Another recurring temporal theme, particularly for significant others, is the concept of time allowing for a gradual acceptance of the deterioration of motor functions and independence. Most health professionals would assert that it is important to provide patients and their families with as much information about a disease as possible. However, for some caregivers, it appears that coping with crises as they arise—"one day at a time"—is much more manageable. For example, Barbara notes:

> I had looked up everything that that [sic] I could find that was connected with this. I went to the Internet and got a long list and I took it to the doctor and said okay is it this and if no why not and went down through that list and there were only a few that [sic] things that he couldn't rule out as possibilities and I think one of the ones I didn't want to talk about was ALS. It was there but I didn't bring it up and when he told him what he thought it was he [Jim] said "oh shit" because that we knew enough about it so that even without the detailed information we have now it was about the worst diagnosis you could get. It kind of is.
>
> I went down still hoping that they'd find it was Lyme disease or something like that. I was clinging to hope . . . and I thought that was a pretty human thing to do, I don't beat myself for that.

[In dealing with the progression of the disorder, and recent losses] So curiously . . . now it seems less awful than it did then which is really kind of interesting. The fear was in some ways worse than the experience.

And Wade asserts quite clearly that looking at the full implications of an ALS diagnosis at the outset might have been almost unbearable. As can be seen below, ALS changes may be manageable for some *only if* the endgame is not addressed too explicitly at the beginning.

Well, actually I guess when they gave us the diagnosis or what they thought was the diagnosis in KC by that time I was suspicious and it was almost a relief because [the doctor] said benign form and then he explained about bulbar onset and all that. I don't know if he was softening the blow by calling it benign because I don't see it as benign. . . . In one sense it was a relief even though the diagnosis was what I feared—benign made it more palatable.

I guess we said from day one, well we just take it one day at a time . . . don't try to be dealing with what's down the road just take it a day at a time. And I think we've been able to do that pretty well. . . . You know when you first get all the booklets with the information in it and you hear about BiPAP and PEG tubes and all the stuff suctioning—if you had to deal with all that right then it would just . . . you couldn't handle it. It's too much to think about all that stuff all those things going wrong and all that stuff being needed. And mercifully as symptoms progressed and progressed slowly and one more thing comes along, you think . . . I can do one more thing. I think it's overwhelming if you think

about it from the git go what you may have to be doing at the end. So we just haven't dealt with it that way, haven't tried to plan ahead. Just tried to deal with things as they arise. [All the ALSA videos] deal with the extreme, maybe they don't deal just with the extreme, but they certainly include the extreme and that's sort of a downer . . . looking at those videos and once was enough.

Clearly, for some, information is often best received in bits and pieces that are relevant to living today. Health care providers must attempt to develop a sense of the degree to which persons with ALS and their significant others can cope with some of the harsher realities of the disease as it progresses over time. There are subtle cues about the person's ability to cope with specific outcomes. For example, in the last quote, Wade notes that the videos include what he perceived to be the "extreme"—an indicator that he may not be comfortable with acknowledging these extremes. And Barbara's current philosophy is captured best in the following:

And I don't have any preconceived notions. I don't know what's going to happen I don't and I'm okay with that. And again that's our—the founding Zen master for our school—his most famous phrase was "only don't know" "only don't know" not knowing that place before thinking, not assuming but just dealing with what is when it comes.

The burden is upon the health care provider to be vigilant with respect to verbal and nonverbal cues about comfort zones. What is the person willing to accept and willing to project into the future? What really matters—to the person with ALS and significant others? These issues often emerge in the context of making decisions about AAC. The SLP recognizes that the individual may very well need to use scanning in the future to access a communication device. However, that may not be a part of the ALS story that the client or a family member is willing to accept at that point in time, as discussed in subsequent sections.

As noted earlier, the comparatively gradual nature of the decline in ALS allows everyone affected to adjust, accommodate, and accept changes as they occur. Time is simultaneously the villain of the story, and the single most important tool that allows for reframing of the life story, or renegotiating one's sense of self or identity. In other words, time allows all concerned parties to do the narrative work necessary for moving forward. Whether they choose to do so is a different question.

Life Span Issues

In ALS, the theme of life span issues often merges with considerations of time. Certainly, ALS strikes at a broad spectrum of chronological ages across the life span; the particular life stage of involved individuals must be considered in framing interventions and in providing opportunities for narrative. In one ALS support group, the ages of PALS range from 37 to 79. Needless to say, the challenges for the 37-year-old with young children are vastly different from the challenges for the 79-year-old, although the impact is equally devastating. Life span issues are also critical for the families of persons with ALS. One young man in his 30s had to decide whether to move his wife and children to a different state in order to be with his father who had ALS. He was in the midst of building his career, and his wife and children had strong roots in the community and needs of their own. For Penny and A.J., who live hundreds of miles from her mother with ALS, those family members living closer geographically were not willing or able initially to project the future needs of the mother, because they were experiencing their own forms of denial. The distant daughter bore the burden of being the realist while simultaneously being the one "creating problems" for the mother.

Aging, particularly physical aging, also plays a role in how an individual's body responds to ALS. As Jim writes,

I'm older now and with time I have changed and I would change whether I had ALS or not. Compared to before ALS symptoms, my body is much weaker, there is more fatigue, weight loss, impaired speech, inability to continue in my job, everything physical takes longer—everything! Lung capacity has decreased drastically. Motor skills are less, e.g., using buttons, removing jar lids—in general, whatever I used my hands for, I either can't do that now or have limited ability to do it now.

But the good news is . . . However, now I can read whenever I want, watch TV if I want to, sit outside and watch the birds, enjoy the day, go for walks even if they are short and the terrain must be taken into account, see many more visitors than I could before. I can take an afternoon nap, sleep past 5:00 A.M. when I used to get up. Have a beer for lunch during the week if I want one. Not be concerned about work, whether I'm there or on time. Dress however I choose. Listen to music whenever I want. Since I can't talk, I don't answer the phone. Overall there is a balance. There are limitations as in the first part of this paragraph but there are positives as in the latter.

Jim's statement of balance may reflect his own personal philosophical and spiritual beliefs. However, his perceptions of the positive aspects of this process are probably influenced by the fact that chronologically, he is closer to the age at which many begin to think of retirement and reflect on personal priorities in life.

Time for Reframing the Life Story

From a broader perspective, the temporal progression of ALS can be viewed as a process of constant reframing of life story and understanding of self. McAdams (1993) discusses in considerable detail the evolution of our personal myth, our life story, as we progress from early childhood into adulthood and finally old age. He particularly notes that in midlife, we begin anticipating the end of the story, and later, we look back to generate a sense of meaningful continuity across the life span. For persons with ALS, there is some certainty about when the end of the story is going to occur, even if it is not linked to old age chronologically. Thus, there is a need to identify life priorities, to make certain that there is some logic and meaning to their lives when viewed in perspective. As Judy said in a recent support group meeting, "I told my son that he had a wonderful opportunity to make choices for the rest of his life."

The following series of quotes from Steve's writings captures the sense of his perception of quality of life and evolving narrative self as time moves on. Some of these quotes are used elsewhere in this chapter, but it is the sequence of the narrative that requires their repetition here.

April 2001—At the outset, Steve is strong. He refuses to give in to the disorder, and he refuses to stop living his life fully. He is philosophical about how he needs to approach that challenge.

I am living with this disease, not dying with it. I am convinced that what makes the difference at the end of the day is

attitude in approaching the problem. I refuse to engage in pointless arguments. I will not be dragged down by people who thrive on negative energy. Living is not about acquiring at someone else's expense: rather, it is about sharing what one has to the mutual benefit of all. By not descending to the level some people chose to live in, but by rising above it, I will be around for years and years to come. And a positive sense of humor, a firm religious faith, and wonderful friends and family . . . don't hurt either.

By September of 2001, Steve's journal bears witness to the many strategies he is using to remain in the game. Records chronicle constant manipulation of medications and supplements, with less and less attention to these details as time goes on. Certain patterns emerge—he reaches out with increasing frequency to loved ones, making peace, and he also seeks information and inspirational stories from the Internet. By the end of this first year, Steve is relying more and more on the poems and writings of others—works that explore the endgame, the ending, and the way of ending. He writes:

Despite the ALS, which has robbed me of my ability to speak intelligibly, has left me with only a couple of typing fingers, and forced me to become right-handed as the left wing is pretty well useless, I remain working, productive, engaged and somewhat naively optimistic about the future.

Closing in on the end of the second year, he clearly seeks to understand the nature of his struggle to enjoy life. In October of 2002 he writes:

My battle for continued participation in and enjoyment of my own life and the lives that surround me make it abundantly clear that our time here is short, and that we must never lose sight of the blessing and gifts each of us are given daily. . . . The sublime essence of life is in the living of it.

And more than 2 years from diagnosis, when he is being honored by his employer, he acknowledges that the time has come to shift his life focus.

But insufficient energy and changing priorities on how to expend what is left are forcing a new plan to unfold. With a progressive disease like ALS one comes to a point where the focus shifts. I have fought the good fight against the inevitable demise of the illness. I have prolonged my decline, I have maintained my dignity, I have continued to maintain an outward face. Now it is time to no longer do the things that promote my survival; rather it is time to do the things that will support my legacy. Put another way, I know that self-will has kept me figuratively putting one foot in front of the other for the last two and one half years. I realize that as I mark my 3rd anniversary with ALS it is now time to turn my fate over to my God, and to spend whatever time remains helping to make my passing as easy as possible for my family.

And about a year before his death, Steve wondered in writing whether he would have done things in his life differently if he had known he would die early. In answering this question, he asserts:

I keep coming back to the realization that in order to have today's full measure of blessing, I had to live exactly this life. There is no hesitation . . . I would do it all the same way.

Only days before his death, he reflects once again on the process he has gone through, and on the fact that he is indeed writing his life story—and is uncertain whether this is the story he wants to leave as his legacy.

Upon reading my last entry, it quickly becomes obvious why I have so few of my notes generating replies. Even when I am not writing about dying, it appears that I am writing about writing about it! Who among the living would fixate so completely on this ultimate demise? I know that the writing has thus far been aimed at keeping my head and heart from exploding under the sheer mass of mental anguish and emotional torment that ALS delivers each morning. Do I really want this to be a /the record I put on the final chapters of my life?

Steve's writings are a clear testament to his sense of narrative self, and his active framing and reframing of his life story. While most PALS cannot be as articulate as Steve, or as consciously reflective, his words should guide us in our thinking about the impact of this disease on narrative self. To be effective in interventions with PALS and their significant others, we must see the uniqueness of each individual, hear their live stories, acknowledge their many selves, and validate their existence.

The Illness Narrative: What Do Persons with ALS Seek?

ALS is an equal opportunity disease, robbing both young and old of life and of loved ones. It is also a disease that engages people passionately in the "good fight" against the disease. In the construction of the self and the writing of the life narrative, it is important for the ALS patient to maintain some type of control over her life. In the following, we look at several themes of the life story that pertain directly or indirectly to the issue of control, including dignity, acceptance, and closure.

Earlier in this chapter, it was suggested that persons with ALS wish to be treated with dignity and accorded self-respect as they cope with this disease. This appears to be true of all of the ALS patients whose stories inform this chapter. However, different issues may be at stake in defining dignity for each individual. Steve was particularly concerned with preserving dignity in his professional life. Thus he worked for much longer than would have been deemed possible, because he chose to use every available piece of assistive technology to maintain the productivity that he equated with dignity. He also sought dignity in his personal relationships, reaching out to those in his present and past to ensure that these relationships were connected and valued. He registered his disgust with his physical appearance.

Sarah also valued personal dignity highly all her life. Between her missionary upbringing and her southern background, her life was lived graciously and she lived with ALS's changes with similar grace. Until shortly before she died, she continued writing thank you notes and appreciation letters to friends and family. Sarah had a great love of theater and appreciation of the spoken word. Once her speech became difficult to understand, she relied primarily on handwriting to communicate, eschewing the communication device that would "speak for her." In all probability, some of her reluctance to use the device came from the way it sounded and the way it disrupted the normal rhythms of conversation. Sarah would not have found that dignified. In planning her funeral, she made clear that her death would also be one celebrated in scripture and music . . . with dignity.

There are others who prefer to ignore or deny the disease's presence, taking no steps to plan for the end or even to control their current health. Many of these individuals are also seeking a kind of dignity. Penny's mother has resisted any planning for her future, despite Penny's efforts to help with anticipating needs (such as a communication device, walker, etc.). Most recently, she sent a message to Penny indicating that she wanted no interference, no heroic measures, no communication devices. In a sense, it appears that ALS seems undignified to her, and she can only maintain her dignity by denying it. As Penny and A.J. state:

Mom, at 74 years old and what I consider to be a very proud woman, upon receiving her diagnosis of ALS, thought she could remain in denial and then keep her kids in denial. Unfortunately for Mom, I am a rebel and choose to not be in denial. . . . As AJ says, mom has not acknowledged the monster, so she fights the care givers and doctors.

Acceptance and closure also appeared frequently in conversations with those living with ALS. Later in this text, persons with aphasia will be described as needing acceptance from others. For those living with ALS, however, the acceptance that is needed is often internal. The one overriding reality is that PALS will die from this disease, unless a cure is found quickly. One can cling to the hope of a cure, and by doing so sometimes extend one's life span by the choices that are made. Ultimately, though, the life story is one with an ending in the relatively near future. Most of Steve's words throughout this chapter reflect his active process of coming to terms with this reality. Sarah defined closure as the completion of her autobiography, and once that was done, she truly felt she had closure on her life.

The Illness Narrative: Social Situatedness and Social Others

In the illness narrative, there must be social others. As in all life stories, interactions with a variety of others help to create our plot. Clearly family plays a major role in the social world of those with ALS, particularly because family members understand the narrative self of the PALS better than most others. Moreover, as the disease progresses, the social world of the person with ALS becomes increasingly constricted, often confined to contacts primarily or exclusively with family. Sometimes, the spouse speaks for and coconstructs the life story that the PALS wishes to share. In an on-line post, one wife wrote:

> XXX is a wildlife biologist and wildland firefighter, retiring from the U.S. Fish and Wildlife Service upon ALS diagnosis in Aug 2004. He lives in a small prairie town with his wife of 7 years and an indulged golden retriever. His woodworking shop was the envy of all who laid eyes on it. Initial reaction to ALS diagnosis involved buying a 53-foot sailboat and sailing it from San Diego to mainland Mexico on a 2-month voyage. He now spends an inordinate amount of time reading political blogs on the internet.

There is affirmation in this story, but there is also humor. For example, the comment about "an inordinate amount of time" is a loving "dig" at the husband's preoccupation with these blogs.

In this section, the social others of greatest interest are family (and close friends), caregivers, and larger communities such as support groups. They are central to the narrative self of those with ALS, but they also must find ways to renegotiate the life story.

Family and Friends

Receiving the diagnosis of ALS disrupts the equilibrium that is maintained in most functional families. Thus, while people living with ALS are struggling to contend with the physical changes of the disease, they are also engaged in a process of trying to reestablish that critical equilibrium (Norlin, 1986). It is not possible to understand the illness narrative of the PALS without understanding some of the family dynamics and relational challenges that are also being experienced.

For many who have shared their lives in this chapter, their relationships with a spouse or significant other are indeed love stories. Steve writes of Sylvia:

> Sylvia is my soulmate and my inspiration . . . .In some strange and intangible way, our love for each other has been reinforced and strengthened through these last few weeks since the diagnosis. We are closer and more connected than ever before. Perhaps it is the uncertainty of how long I will be around, or the fear of not being together in our old age, as we had planned. Or maybe it is just the need to confirm to each other continually that together we can beat this thing. We are decidedly in love.

And Jim says about his wife, Linda, "It's brought Linda and I closer. Sometimes I love her like a teenager." Most PALS are also aware of the feelings of significant others, although it can be difficult to discuss. When asked about Wade, Sarah wrote: "He's very reticent but sometimes will cry." And Wade did indeed seem to be able to express sadness through tears without any apparent embarrassment.

In some instances, the family world remains somewhat mysterious to outsiders. One woman with ALS was always accompanied to support group meetings by one of her children, usually a daughter and son-in-law who brought their new baby as well. During these meetings and in clinical contexts outside of the group, no mention was made of the husband or the husband's caregiving efforts, even though he lived with his wife. Efforts to probe further in this situation were deflected by either the person with ALS or the children. There are also couples whose relationship was already somewhat dysfunctional prior to the ALS diagnosis. Some may respond by drawing closer, others by pulling apart.

Children of PALS often struggle with accepting the diagnosis; for many, this is the first direct confrontation with the mortality of a parent, and the pain is very real. The early life stories of any of us begin with a world in which the parent is central. Even in adulthood, part of the biographic particulars of the former child's life story is the existence of the parent(s). Not surprisingly, there appears to be great sensitivity to their needs on the part of the parents. Sarah has clearly reflected on the needs and individual differences of her children. She explains:

> Kirk and Lorie who live in Farmington do stuff for us. Allen was feeling a little despondent because he can't. But I wrote him a letter that helped. Had part of a poem "To an Adopted Child." Helped him. I wrote the same letter to Kirk. Carol was feeling so far away. So Wade has her coming once a month. That helps, too! She helps Wade with dish washing and odd jobs.

Two of Wade and Sarah's children were able to attend support group meetings and share their emotions in an honest and caring way. Dave and Jean's adult son and daughter-in-law also attend support group meetings with their parents, indicating

that they learn a great deal by listening to others.

If each family presents a unique pattern of relationships, those with friends and acquaintances are even more diverse. About friends, Sarah comments:

> Friends and family keep coming to see us—never boring! And bringing food for Wade and flowers for me.

And in an on-line posting, one PALS writes:

> I try to live my life to the fullest each day, but it is getting more difficult as the ALS progresses. I do have wonderful friends that give me a lot of support.

For many friends and acquaintances, it is extremely difficult to visit with the person with ALS, primarily because of the motor deterioration and the barriers to communication. After struggling with making the decision to visit Jim, a friend commented, "It wasn't so bad. I don't know what I'm afraid of . . . it's just so hard to see and I don't know how to act." Those living with ALS often understand these difficulties, and some are very accepting. Barbara writes:

> I mean I don't have any negative feelings toward those who aren't able to do it. Cause I know that some people can and some people can't and it's okay and I've got good friends who I know just can't handle it and . . .

Barbara is particularly insightful on the topic of friends and acquaintances.

> People who come and who enhance . . . one of his friends from college came . . . she had a high school reunion in Tulsa . . . and she came to see him on her way back home. Lot of people like

that who are part of Jim's life and my life . . . friends . . . his friends, my friends, our friends . . . people who are just treasures for both of us . . . and those people we love and love having around and in those instances, absolutely the more the merrier. There are friends who are life enhancing and there are friends who are life-disruptive. . . . But people who are friends . . . even some people who I think we though of as more acquaintances than friends who have been so wonderful at coming, visiting and checking in.

Barbara also acknowledges the topic of boundaries with others.

It's boundaries. It really is. And you've got to have some boundaries in order to . . . you've got enough to be taking care of your partner and of your situation and those who are around you and who are life enhancing...and why be around those others with bad energy.

It's not as if it's going to make any difference to them. . . . In a funny way it doesn't matter if you are not welcoming to those people . . . it's been a good exercise. . . . To say, okay, there are certain people that are not part of this and that's okay.

Each person living with ALS, indeed each human, has a different set of boundaries with respect to social others. In order for those others to reach out, to make a difference, these boundaries must be understood. And boundaries often evolve as the physical progression of the disease limits access to social contexts outside of the home. In the early stages of ALS, it is important to help the patient and her family continue to participate in social activities that matter to them. One common example is eating out, an activity enjoyed by many, one

that is fundamentally social in nature. As physical changes make the eating of food more challenging, some PALS become reluctant to be seen publicly while they are eating. An important social context is removed from that person's life. Wade also noted that Sarah's ALS progressively restricted their ability to attend church, another important social context for both of them. As opportunities for social interaction become more and more limited, the social world becomes constricted to the home. Without visits from friends and family, all members of the family will lose some of the necessary validation that comes from the recognition of others.

Caregivers

We now consider caregivers. Who are the caregivers of persons with ALS? They are adult men and women of virtually any age and a variety of relationships with the patient, including younger children. Often they are the same family and friends described above. They express as broad a range of hopes, dreams, and fears as is imaginable. Linda's husband Jim offered the following in a support group meeting: "It is a privilege to be Linda's caregiver." The following are examples of statements about caregiving from an on-line Web site. The themes are varied, but many express a desire to find a way to help, to deal with the daily struggles, to learn from others' courage, and to affirm the value of the good fight.

My 42-year-old brother was recently diagnosed with ALS. I've been a professional journalist for more than 20 years at a national newspaper and I can't believe I can't do something to make my little brother better. I've registered at this site to lend solidarity to my brother and the extended ALS community. Beyond that, I'd like to become better informed about the disease itself, promising treatments and clinical trials, and the daily struggles and courage that you all exhibit in battling this cruel affliction. Above all, I am here to find hope.

My name is Don and I am the caregiver for my wife Linda. She was diagnosed in November of 2003 with Bulbar ALS. I retired early in order to be at home with her. We enjoy traveling and antiquing. We live in Tennessee and I would like to hear from you about how you deal with all of this.

I have been a healthcare professional as Director of Recreational Services at a rehab hospital as well as working as a leisure consultant for nursing home activity departments for the past 25 years. My husband was diagnosed with ALS in 2002 and now I am a caregiver at home as well. We will eventually conquer this disease!

From the outside looking in, many would see the task of the ALS caregiver as almost unbearably difficult, watching as a loved one deteriorates physically in front of one's eyes, shouldering more and more of the burden of simply getting through the daily challenges of eating and toileting and moving from chair to bed. Certainly, the physical and psychological burdens are real, and there are constant, often escalating concerns about finances and other family needs. Caregivers themselves may feel that they are living a chaos illness narrative with no sense of who and what they are in this ALS new world. Fatigue is common, as Wade notes:

That's been one of the major changes for me. I used to read in bed every night, I didn't read long but I've always had a book I'm reading and I would just get in bed and start reading and maybe not read two pages but eventually I'd finish the book. Now when I go to bed I'm too tired to read. I still have a book at the side of the bed, haven't read it in weeks. Sit here and read part of the newspaper and go to sleep reading it. So I'm not doing any reading really except the newspaper . . . and that's somewhat of a change. . . . But now I'm too tired . . .

And Chris indicates:

What I am about to talk about now is something that I have had on my mind for quite some time. The longer I meet with people with ALS there is something that goes unspoken in the ways I have seen it. "Caregivers." Caregivers can be a spouse, children, family members or some one hired or supplied by a health organization. The caregiver has a job that is, in many cases, not appreciated in many ways. I can only speak from the position, of having bulbar ALS. The caregiver position has to be the one the most frustrating jobs in the world. Here you are with your spouse who has been able to hear your voice since you have been together and now she can not understand what you are saying. Not only understand what you are trying to say to here but what you are trying to get across to her. Even with talking devices or paper and pencil, there is also a time element that is hard to overcome. Being in this spot I know.

However, many caregivers, particularly family, find some comfort in the fact that the spirit, the narrative self, of the person with ALS is untouched by the disease. When asked what they feel would be most difficult to deal with—the physical challenges they confront daily or a loss of mental capacity (as in Alzheimer's disease), the responses are complex but share many elements. Barbara makes reference to her aging mother in explaining:

> In some instances it's something that really creates major major [*sic*] impairments . . . the cognitive stuff . . . and that's the blessing of ALS I mean that it doesn't. [I would choose] Physical in a moment. That's actually a question that I had thought about long before because my mother was a physical mess and was mentally fine until really a few days before she died. She spent her last five years in a nursing home, and the staff loved her because she could talk to them she was clear she was bright, she was interested, she was interactive and this for a very shy person . . . in any case at least she wasn't gaga and I often thought if she could have had one of those machines from Dr. Strangelove that could be her body . . . it would be great. It would have been fine.

She reasserts how important it is that "the mind is clear." Earlier, Barbara's husband Jim responded to a similar question by asserting his preference for physical over mental impairment.

Persons with ALS often reflect on these issues without external prompting, as noted earlier. For example, Steve suggested, "But now I'm facing an illness where the body will eventually fail, but the mind will be strong and facile as ever." He describes his death in terms of "being permanently separated from this malicious frame." In a subsequent entry he adds:

> I love a good turn of phrase, a clever conversation. I have a knack for a well-written letter or memo. Hugging my children, raking the yard, shaking hands, kissing my wife . . . . Today I need help taking a drink of water or brushing my teeth. As the body melts, the mind remains alert. I have complete clarity that I am witnessing my demise.

Earlier, Chris described his own preferences, but he acknowledges the complexity of the question, for himself and his wife, in the following.

> This must be the most unanswerable question I know. The answer is something I have a hard time determining which is best and which is worst. I have come to the conclusion that it depends on the individual. I believe the mental loss would be worse for me. As much as I enjoy working in the yard and being outdoors, I think I am better off if I still know what is going on. There is a downside however. Being aware of the fact that the end is coming and the results are already determined weighs on a conscious mind. My wife not only knows the consequences but will have to all the physical day to day obligations that are required. Mental deterioration must be hardest on loved ones who wish to communicate with you. Everything can be discussed if you are lucid. Physical disabilities create problems also. Moving a person who has lost use of their physical body can be worked out with our modern machines, and knowledge.
>
> Maybe it would be a blessing if the ill person was not aware.

Ironically, at a recent ALS support group meeting, Chris's wife Billie unexpectedly began to talk emotionally about the fact that "no one tells you that the mind may be affected." Chris was present, although it was hard to determine his reaction. Other caregivers in the room were clearly taken aback. The facilitator acknowledged that this was not a comfortable topic for anyone, noting that cognitive changes, if any, in ALS are not yet well understood.

Significant others also experience the biographic disruption caused by ALS, and their life stories are also altered. During the battle with ALS, disrupted communication affects the caregiver's narrative self, taking away or altering those interactive moments that are self-defining. A working wife of a man with ALS may find that formerly important life roles (e.g., employee, part-time aerobics instructor) disappear or become strained, while new roles (e.g., nurse, physical therapist) are added to her repertoire. For many, the task of managing the physical demands of ALS escalates rapidly in the later stages of the disorder. There is little time to reflect on needs and feelings, to explore how one's sense of self has been altered by these life transformations. Sometimes it is only after the death of the loved one that the full impact of the experience is felt. While living with ALS, caregivers have neither the time nor the emotional resources to confront the life transforming experiences they are undergoing. Support groups can be important to all persons living with ALS.

Support Groups and Communities

Within the study of social psychology of illness, research has established that support groups (also called self-help or mutual help groups) are used more by individuals who are experiencing what are considered to be stigmatizing disorders (Davison, Pennebaker, & Dickerson, 2000). All of the neurogenic communication disorders discussed in this text are associated with illnesses that are little known or understood by the public. This is particularly true with ALS. Public awareness of the disorder is very limited. Thus it is not surprising that support groups are considered to be a vital activity of local chapters of the ALSA. ALSA actually requires such a group to be instituted and maintained in order for local chapters to be recognized nationally.

For persons with ALS, support groups are essentially social communities that exist, in part, to allow individuals to tell their own stories and to hear the life stories of others coping with the impact of this disease. Most ALS support groups serve both persons diagnosed with ALS and their significant others. Remarkably, the experience of ALS is so life-altering that family members often continue to attend even after the loved one with ALS has died, and our particular local group was founded by the wife of Steve, who is quoted extensively in this chapter.

Support groups serve many functions (Shadden, 2006; Shadden & Agan, 2004; Shadden & Koski, 2007), as described in Chapter 4. For persons living with ALS, there is a need for information and resource sharing, as well as for empowerment in dealing with health care systems and in obtaining services. Given the potentially isolating nature of the disorder, there is also a need for embracement, for feeling part of a larger community and a larger narrative where one's struggles are understood. And of course, of paramount value is the fact that groups provide a vehicle for sharing the ongoing narrative of one's life before and with the disease. Because individuals are typically strangers when they join a group, they start with a clean slate in terms of the ways in which they present their narrative selves. Whatever self they present is completely supported and validated by other group members. There is no judgment, only acceptance. Often, the inquiries of other group members elicit more information about past roles and pre-ALS life story. And in a strange way, while the future is certainly not a cheery one, new group members see others dealing with ALS in varying stages in the disease's progression and still actively participating in their lives and engaged in interactions with others.

From the perspective of ongoing storying of self, it may be vital to see that the essential person continues even though the disease takes an increasing toll on the body. Attending group meetings month after month also allows members to see the narratives of others evolve, and this experience is true for caregivers, for loved ones whose lives are also changing with ALS. When a caregiver sees others coping with ALS in all its manifestations and stages, he is learning that there are many ways of living with ALS. That knowledge may be comforting, in the sense that there is no one way to be a good caregiver, nor is it possible to be the person you want to be all of the time.

It is common to find that ALS caregivers and family members feel they learn as much from persons with ALS as from other caregivers. The alternative is also true. "Learning" may be the critical term in the preceding statement. Because there are many similarities in the progression of the disease, those who have traveled further down the path can provide critical practical information about what to expect and where to get resources. Information may relate to anything associated with ALS—PEG tubes, ventilator issues, strategies for improving sleep. Sometimes, issues of empowerment are raised—for example, how do I get my local doctor to work more closely with the ALS clinic I attend in another state? This question does not require an informational answer so much as encouragement to persist in obtaining what is needed.

Group discussions are also important when members learn about new drugs or treatment trials. People tend to be more honest about the pros and cons, their hopes and fears, when they are with others who understand and have similar questions. In the northwest Arkansas ALSA chapter, group members are routinely supportive of others' beliefs, even when they are concerned about a person's treatment decisions. Support does not necessarily mean dishonesty. Participants offer concerns and raise questions, but they do so in a caring manner that allows the individual to remain open to their comments and that affirms the person.

According to Rappaport (1993), support groups can reduce professional centrism and link the lives of each individual to community-based processes. Thus, such a group may allow for both idiosyncratic personal identities and stories, as well as for a broader shared community narrative about ALS and people with ALS. Members may mobilize for political or fund-raising activities that enhance public awareness of the disease. Thus this group operates at all of the levels that Kovarsky, Duchan, Mastergeorge, and Nichols (2003) suggest are linked to identity: the individual, the interaction, the relationship, and the collective or cultural.

Rappaport (1993) also writes about the importance of being able to give back to others. One couple had been attending a support group because their son (who lives at some distance) had ALS. Initially, they felt a strong need to help others. At one point, when the situation with their son had been deteriorating, Judy wrote:

> . . . [we] are cutting down on our attendance at the support group meetings. We feel we are at a point that things are not really "ok" so we aren't really helpful to others . . . and we are like cousins, "once-removed" and we feel we are somewhat of a drag. We are a point that separating our being helpful in a sup-

port group is a negative for all. So, for now, we are keeping our energies at assessing where we can help others, but from the background.

The group facilitator was concerned, primarily because it seemed that group had not been able to reach out to this couple, to become enough of a community that they did not feel that they had to bring the "helpful" role to the meetings. Fortunately, Judy and Buzz did resume attendance. After several more sessions, Judy wrote:

> You can use us ANY WAY you want! We are already involved with how others should be treated—think that's why the Lord has allowed us this (and other) experiences. If we can't help others, it becomes worthless.

Hopefully the group is bringing them some sense of comfort and belonging. She goes on to say:

> We have been to the last two meetings —everyone seemed to want us there. They have been meaningful meetings— everyone is facing hard realities and we are like a clan. We've decided to always go when we can.

Communication Tools and Technology

As ALS progresses, PALS and their significant others become increasingly more dependent upon assistive technology to manage essential daily activities. Given the centrality of communication, one would expect a welcoming of AAC systems, often referred to as speech generating devices (SGDs) (Beukelman, Ball, & Pattee, 2004;

Hatakeyama, Okamoto, Kamata, & Kasuga, 2000; Murphy, 2004; Richter, Ball, Beukelman, Lasker, & Ullman, 2003). However, there is much we still need to know. Since there is a progressive decline in speech intelligibility with ALS, most individuals turn first to simple solutions such as a lightweight dry erase board to support communication interactions.

As communication becomes more difficult, there appear to be at least four broad types of response to AAC options. The first type of response is demonstrated by persons who appear content to allow loved ones to speak for them, relying on a lifetime of shared experiences and understandings to support this shared communicative process. Individuals within this group may also reject outright the concept of using anything to substitute for speech. It is difficult to determine whether this is a form of denial, or simply distaste for the idea that something computerized can replace the person's voice. As one support group member's mother was reported to say, "That's not me. I'm not ready to give up my voice. My voice is still fine." The daughter wrote that

> She is only able to be understood 10–15% of the time, speaking on a good day. She is adamant not only about no speaking device, but will not even write on paper, when we cannot understand her.

With such individuals, family members frequently exert increasing pressure to consider use of a device, but this pressure rarely does anything more than entrench the PALS' rejection of AAC. Over time, this rejection may change, but it will only do so if individuals are given the opportunity to reach decisions on their own, without outside pressure. As the daughter described above indicated,

I have the equipment, and I am working with it, so at least I know what to help Mom with, if she ever gets un hard headed . . . This strategy is the best that can be done—be ready with knowledge of the possibilities, for the hoped-for moment in time when the family member becomes willing to entertain the possibility of AAC and other technologies.

A second group of individuals with ALS are willing to explore various AAC approaches, but ultimately decide not to pursue these options. Jim's story illustrates this pattern. Within a few months of diagnosis, while his face-to-face speech remained mostly intelligible (supported by writing on a dry erase board), he was given the opportunity to explore a variety of AAC devices. Jim is highly educated and literate, and is known for his humorous e-mail communications with friends and colleagues. He agreed to experiment with communication devices, but it was clear that he was not particularly enthusiastic about the possibilities. In a follow-up visit designed to discuss AAC options, he shared the various ways in which he had "played with" one of the loaner devices. For example, he had spent considerable time reprogramming how the device said various messages (its pronunciation) to make it sound "Southern." However, he had no interest in pursuing an AAC system at that time.

Jim's wife's comments provide some insights related to Jim's disinterest in AAC. She notes that he was never someone who talked constantly, much as he enjoyed his e-mail communications with others. She also indicated that his successful use of the dry erase board might be an indication of his willingness to use AAC later in the disease progression, although this proved not to be the case. She states:

Jim was never a talker, he's not one of those people who needs to have his mouth open to prove he's alive . . . he's always been fairly quiet, speaking when there is something to say and I don't expect chatter and I don't expect a kind of narrative going-on about how the day has been, so it may have not be as major a transition for us because of that . . .

Jim also discusses his communication, both face-to-face and with e-mail, as in the following:

I can still type though slowly and with frequent mistakes as my fingers and hands grow more impaired. I am sending shorter messages, and not responding to some that I might have in the past because it takes so long and uses so much of my energy, which I'm short on these days. So if you don't get a message from me in the detail you would like, or don't get a response, don't take it personally . . . I'm really not conversing as much as I am partly writing and talking, depending on how well my listener can understand my speech. In any event . . . my communication now isn't as detailed as in the past.

These comments outline clearly Jim's perception of his communication impairment and explain to others how they should receive and understand his communications. There is no denial here, simply a choice to evolve with the changes in speech intelligibility. Even on one occasion in intensive care, while Jim was willing to use a communication letter board provided by nursing staff, he turned down the offer of a loaner AAC system for use in the hospital. However, as this chapter was being finalized, there have been changes in Jim's reaction to AAC options. It has become increasingly difficult for him to access the alphabet and word boards he had been using. Both Jim and Barbara now recognize how unsatisfactory these options are. Jim is no longer able to express easily any important thoughts and reflections, any topics beyond daily issues of pain, medications, and the like. Barbara describes this as a loss of nuanced communication, as well as a loss of personalized and unique communicative messages. Jim has recently expressed willingness to try using an AAC device with scanning at this time.

A third group of ALS patients are those who obtain an AAC device, at varying stages in the progression of the illness, and then rarely use it. Sarah is a particularly good example of this group. Before obtaining a device, Wade had a very clear sense of when he felt AAC would be useful to him and Sarah, pointing out situations like driving in the car, or to moments of communication breakdown when trying to understand her care preferences. His comments on this topic were quoted early in this chapter. He still attempted to encourage her use of AAC.

But when somebody comes to see her who hasn't been recently I get the Dyna-Write and put it all out and get her to write something—a greeting or something but she uses it really very little she uses those [points to erase board].

For Wade, it was important to have available a system that would allow Sarah to communicate more effectively as needed. However, the moments of communication breakdown that bothered him were very practical and concrete. When pushed to explain her seeming lack of interest in using her DynaWrite, Sarah persisted in saying that she was content to listen, and she maintained this perspective even when challenged by others who described this position as being a "copout." She also denied the possibility that she was simply being polite and gracious in a social context.

Sarah's behavior with the DynaWrite may shed light on why she was disinterested in using this system, particularly when contrasted with her handwritten communications on a dry erase board or pad. When communicating by handwriting, she was confident and relatively quick to respond. Throughout her life, she had been a person who valued the written word, and she was known for her beautifully expressed thoughts shared in notes to friends and family. In contrast, when using the Dyna-Write, Sarah appeared hesitant and cautious, extremely slow, and almost obsessively precise in typing her message. Others would begin to talk around her, often failing to note that she had completed her message and was ready to share it. When she did get her partners' attention, the conversation had moved on to other topics, and her comments seemed almost inappropriate, a fact that she appeared to recognize and dislike. Sarah was familiar with typing and with computers, so the fact that the device was computerized could not explain her caution. It is probable that the artificialness of the process left her feeling depersonalized and did not reflect her sense of self in any meaningful way. In contrast, writing was her "signature" form of expression in the past and one that continued into the present despite ALS.

While every situation is unique, Sarah's story illustrates the importance of attempting to understand the person's communication preferences and personal style. She participated actively in the initial process of selecting an AAC device, but was content to leave the device turned off in most social situations. The issue of artificial or unnatural communication processes using AAC is also highlighted by Chris in an e-mail after a support group meeting. He wrote:

> The one thing that stood out in my mind was on the heavy machine you said the person using it could bring up a general category hit the button and be ready to discuss the subject they had chosen. I have run across the fact that I or some in my condition using my machine do not get the opportunity to pick the subject. Usually we response to what the other people are talking about. I am sure there are times when we have to start the conversation but for the most part we type or hit a button in response to what others are saying or asking.

Chris himself used a dry erase board for several years, even after obtaining an AAC device (which did not work reliably). When his device was replaced with a more effective system, he began using it more often. After one support group meeting in which group members shared their AAC devices with those who had none, both Chris and others seemed more willing to participate in future sessions using their AAC systems.

Some persons with ALS initially welcome a device but find it does not provide the ease of communication they had expected. One woman was adamant about obtaining AAC as soon as she heard about the possibilities. However, the fact that the device required some programming to be useful and personalized led her to stop trying to use it, even though she received considerable support from SLPs and family.

Others become so frustrated with the complexity of the devices they receive or the mismatch between the device and their needs that they simply give up. The mother of one young man with ALS writes:

> The company will not have any success with selling this product if there isn't some sit down, hands on, technical support. It will ONLY work if the company's technical support meets the clientele at THEIR level—no matter WHERE that is. I mean physical level, too. [Our son] is looking forward to the device working. However, he says that right now, if asked by his support group, he would have to say that "customer service sucks!" She [wife] is getting tired and the kids have lots of last of school activities, so I think the device is on a shelf for the moment, while she goes to various functions and plays solitaire when she can . . .

The wife goes on to describe what needs to change:

1. If this is just a communication device, then it should be sold accordingly. No bells and whistle demonstrations.
2. If it is the bells and whistles they are selling, then it should come programmed or with detailed layman instructions. For all intents and purposes Larry cannot use the mouse and keyboard, plug in and out components . . . etc.
3. Customer support should provide live set-up and 1 or 2 training visits, phone or internet support is inadequate, frustrating, and extremely time consuming for all parties involved.

   Clearly this expense would pay for itself if the user felt good about the product and shared tha[*sic*]; conversely, an unhappy, unsatisfied, and frustrated client will share that too.

4. At this point we would not recommend [the device] based on their lack of patient education, setup . . . etc.

Several months after this first string of messages, the mother wrote:

The device is history. It sits in its box—unused and useless. The biggest disappointment is that it was such a dud—and so useless. Larry thought it would be a happy device—it wasn't!

In fairness to [the company]. the machine is not for an ALS patients in Larry's stages of the disease process. When the beginning is limb onset, and the end is bulbar, there is precious little to work with and the reality is that no one could use this device as it sits (or is advertised). It may be all right for an accident or stroke victim who is stable in their disability.

What is particularly disconcerting in this final message is the fact that it is clear that Larry will no longer be willing to try any other system. Technology that could have enriched his quality of life and sense of participation in his ongoing story has instead brought frustration and failure. No one living and dying with ALS should have to experience technology that increases their burden and sense of life disruption.

One final group of PALS seems to embrace AAC and related computer-based technology early on. For example, once diagnosed with bulbar ALS, Dave actively searched the Internet to learn more about his communication options, typically bringing questions about different devices to the ALS support group. He and his wife pursued an AAC evaluation while his speech was still intelligible, an important choice given the somewhat rapid decline in his communication skills after receiving the

device. In effect, Dave has been empowered by the device, and takes pride in his ability to understand its working and use its capabilities. He has programmed all kinds of long and short messages to share his thoughts, so the device is not a toy to him.

Before one support group meeting, Dave had programmed a series of messages that described in sequence the story of selling his tools at a yard sale. He told the story in stages, waiting for "audience" response before moving on to the next preprogrammed segment. He seemed to understand intuitively the rhythms and flows of conversation, creating his messages accordingly. What was particularly important was the fact that Dave made certain that he personalized his message to reflect his personality and style. For example, his version of the tool sale story emphasized his perspective as an accountant before retiring, including highly specific information about dollars earned. His wife then expressed her "warm fuzzy" version of the story, describing how deeply touched they both were by the church's help with this sale. At the end of this conversation, all group members felt as though they had been part of a truly spontaneous conversation in which both Dave and Jean were equally represented. The entire exchange worked because of Dave's determination to remain a viable communication partner.

Not surprisingly, Steve is another member of this fourth group of ALS patients who embrace communications technology and tools in general. One comment about finding the ClickIt software program was used at the beginning of this chapter. He wrote something similar in a different message, stating:

Oh joy!! Today I located a software package on the internet which will give me the capability to once again record my thoughts here with a modicum of effort. While the speed is pokey compared to what I once had, no longer will I waste prescious energy trying to use my two good fingers and one good arm to hit the right keys. I fell liberated, and thankful to once again use the right phrasing and word selection, not the most expeditious (or alternatively to use none at all).

For Steve, communication was vital, and he was willing and eager to use any and all tools that will allow him to continue communicating effectively. He thanked his employers for providing:

> . . . the specialized tools I need to remain productive. Because of them, I'm intellectually engaged and committed, and still able to add value.

In Closing

There is no right or wrong answer as to whether any person with ALS should use AAC, or indeed, as to what device is best. In the case of Steve, however, we can be grateful that he did use all possible technology to continue communicating. And we can be grateful to his wife Sylvia, who agreed to share his words in this text because, as she wrote, "I know he would have wanted it." While much of this text uses theory to interpret the actions and needs of people with neurogenic communication disorders, Steve shows us the power of language to preserve his narrative self and to affirm his life and life story, through past and present to its end.

At the time, he simply affirms the joy of the being alive in the moment.

This morning is the third in a row to tease me, whispering autumn. There is dew across the lawns and beds, themselves laden with late flowers and summer's last ripening vegetables. The high sky is of the variety designed to frame fly balls and kites, a hint of its depth given up only by the few strands of clouds scuttling along out of the east. I watched silently as Slvia arose during the night to close our bedroom windows against the cold.

Early in the year of his death, he is still exchanging messages with old friends, reflecting on time and on being at the beginning of forging one's narrative self and on how none of those experiences, those acts of communion, are ever lost.

> Of course you are well remembered, through the rose-colored lenses of a quarter century of time and space. [our times together] Long before the nicks, cuts and dings; before the triumphs and joys . . . before we had been fully shaped by the world and how we chose to walk through it . . . there are two young men working hard to succeed. Our adventures, foibles, laughter and tears—all are safely tucked away into eternity.
>
> All things considered, I've had a good, if abbreviated, run. How about you?

And 6 months before his death, shortly before he wrote that the endgame was in sight, Steve Kressen sent to many friends the following e-mail, born of a moment's emotion, and countless minutes of using what little of his body still moved to activate a switch to select letter by letter the words in the following message. In it, he captures the essence of his living with ALS, and the heart of his narrative self.

Those eyes of engaging, oversized,
    deep chocolate ammunition,
Already discovering their power to
    strike, surely to transfix as she
    grows
Are now flung open in maple sugar
    delight, flecked amber with
    expectation.

[My caregiver] has bathed me, dressed
    me, propped me at the desk.
He has poured today's ration of pow-
    ders and potions through my feed-
    ing tube.
More raptor than human, my fingers
    clutch at my synthetic link to the
    world.
My needs for the moment met, he
    bends down to lift [my daughter]
    skyward!

As she flies up and over his head,
    alighting in perfect piggyback
    position,
Her eyes meet mine and I am sparked
    apart from my melting, horrid frame,

At once the strong playful father and
    the giddy five year-old in a father's
    arms.

Those eyes, those eyes. I will not die
    today!

Postscript

During the writing of this chapter, Sarah lost her battle with ALS, but not before meeting her final life goal of seeing her autobiography of her early days published and shared with family and friends. After the manuscript was sent to the publisher, Jim also died, and while the copy edited pages were being reviewed, Chris and Larry died as well. It is possible that others who shared their world in this chapter will be gone by the time this book is in print. That is the reality of ALS, and the fact that death lurks around the corner simply makes the importance of supporting narrative self more poignant, more urgent, and painfully real.

CHAPTER 7

Life Stories in Parkinson's Disease

We have argued in this book that people use the tools of self construction to create life stories, and that these life stories (or narratives), in turn, create the self. In the previous chapter on ALS, it was noted that narrative self continues to be constructed, even when there is full recognition that the end of the life story will occur in a few years or less. Thus, for those living with ALS, the illness narrative is, in many ways, the final life story. That is not necessarily true for those who suffer from diseases that will not be fatal within such a narrow time frame. In this chapter, then, we are interested in how the construction of a good life story is affected by Parkinson's disease (PD). We look first at the impact of PD on communication skills and the life impact of the disease. We then examine the ways in which cultural, role, interactional, and biographical tools affect the construction of self for the person with PD and at how they affect the construction of a new life narrative that includes the fact of Parkinson's as an aspect of that story. We consider the effects of each of the levels of self construction on the new narrative, and also consider the question of how much of the new narrative must be an illness story. We examine the narrative itself from the perspective of

temporality, social others, and dignity and acceptance, and close with a consideration of communication tools that might help the PD sufferer write a new life story.

It is the basic argument of this book that people create their selves using the cultural, role, interpersonal, and biographical resources and tools available to them within a given context. These tools are carried in a metaphorical "tool box" (Swidler, 1986) and creating a coherent self narrative assumes both that we have available to us those tools that produce socially recognizable selves and that we have mastery over those tools. Because Parkinson's disease affects our ability to use the tools associated with both language and the body, in this chapter we pay particular attention to a person's *physical* ability to talk and to manipulate the body in an attempt to create and present a certain type of self narrative. As Frank (1995) points out: "Selves act in ways that choose their bodies, but bodies also create the selves who act" (p. 40).

Compared to ALS, the life narrative for one with Parkinson's disease (PD) is typically longer because the course of the illness is more variable and slower. Like ALS, the narrative *voice* is not jeopardized in the early stages of the disease, as the ability to communicate remains intact. However, the narrative *self* may be profoundly affected by changes in the motor domain, including dyskinesia, tremor, freezing gait (Abudi, Bar-Tal, Ziv, & Fish, 1997), and pain (Quittenbaum & Grahn, 2004), as well as an increased risk of falling. As the disease progresses, there will be an impact on spoken and non-verbal communication, including stuttering-like dysfluencies, static face (Pell & Leonard, 2005), dysarthria (including aspects of speech and voice) (Manor, Posen, Amir, Dori, & Giladi, 2005), and associated increasing difficulty in making oneself understood. Moreover, PD patients may feel that their ability to communicate deteriorates far in advance of actual physical impairment (Miller, Noble, Jones, & Burn, 2006), resulting in decreased self-confidence and agency. In part, this reflects a decreased ability to negotiate interpersonal interactions (McNamara & Durso, 2003). For those who have been diagnosed with Parkinson's disease, there is the understanding that at some point in the future, with no real predictability (Charlton & Barrow, 2002), there will be progressively greater loss of control over speech and bodily movements and the increasing prospect of the loss of independence (Bhatia & Gupta, 2003).

Thus, although the progression of the disease is slower than ALS or other types of neurogenic communication disorders, the impact of the disease on the individual's life is still profound. As Hodgson, Garcia, and Tyndall (2004) state: "Parkinson's disease leaves no system untouched." The consequences of PD are described in a variety of ways in the literature. For example, in addition to the physical and communicative challenges mentioned above, the PD patient will find it more difficult to negotiate the basic activities of daily living (e.g., rolling over in bed, writing a letter, catching a bus, brushing one's teeth) (Biemans, Dekker, & van der Woude, 2001) and will be likely to

suffer losses of jobs and professional standing (Caap-Ahlgren, Lannerheim, & Dehlin, 2002). Abudi, Bar-Tal, Ziv, and Fish (1997) identified four types of symptoms that are associated with Parkinson's disease in the literature: motor, mental, psychosocial, and nonspecific. Jenkinson, Peto, Fitzpatrick, Greenhall, and Hyman (1995) find "considerable impact of the disease on general levels of functioning and well-being" (p. 1) in their sample. In addition to the effects summarized above, Damiano, Snyder, Strausser, and Willian (1999) point out that there are also consequences for self-image, energy/fatigue, and sexuality.

Those with Parkinson's disease are aware that they suffer from an incurable disease that will progressively get worse, and they begin to lose a sense of who they have been and who they can be (Bramly & Eatough, 2005). Charlton and Barrow (2002) say:

> [PD sufferers] also perceived the effects of the illness as a threat to their identity, either by being labeled as a person with disabilities or a sufferer of a disease, or by acknowledging that they were no longer able to act in the ways which were characteristic of them. (p. 475)

In addition, changes in the person with Parkinson's disease have profound effects on their significant others, often leading to increased depression and decreased satisfaction with life (Aarsland, Larsen, Karlsen, Lim, & Tandberg, 1999; Calder, Ebmeier, Stewart, Crawford, & Besson, 1991). Depending on the symptoms of the PD sufferer, the significant other may also find it difficult to cope (Cifu et al., 2006). The PD sufferer may experience increased dependence on significant others because of physical changes associated with the disease, affecting previously established roles in the family (Bhatia & Gupta, 2003).

Thus, PD patients have lost some tools in their tool boxes that have previously been used to create their selves. At a time when they are facing frightening changes in their lives, they also face the loss of familiar ways of creating the self who copes with those changes.

In looking at the life story and construction of self of one with Parkinson's disease, we will focus on the case of Jerry Patnoe, a 66-year-old college professor of sociology and criminal justice who had been diagnosed with Parkinson's disease 2 years previously. Jerry is from Native American/ French heritage, originally from a working-class family, who attended a well-regarded university where he earned his Ph.D. He has been married three times—divorced once, widowed once, and currently living with his third wife. Jerry has eight adopted and biological children. He has always prided himself on his intellect, his education, and his virility. Now, while most of the symptoms of Parkinson's disease are being treated with drugs, Jerry still finds that there is considerable disruption of his ability to use speech and of his control over his body:

> I had been symptomatic for probably a couple of years and had paid no attention to it until my brother was diagnosed with Parkinson's—at that time, I then became aware of some of the problems I was having, which I had just written off as old age, prior to that. I had basically, tremors in the right hand, some muscle contractions in the right arm, balance problems, difficulty in walking. So from the first time I saw a medical doctor until I got the diagnosis was almost 11 months.

Upon receiving the diagnosis of Parkinson's disease, Jerry began to see himself as a different type of person, one who had gone from being "healthy" to one who had an incurable, progressive disease:

> So, on one hand, I . . . while I suspected I had Parkinson's, strongly, it was devastating, largely because I, um, I anticipated the worst. I mean while I thought I had a lot of knowledge, I went . . . on the . . . um, internet, it was fairly useless knowledge, it was much easier to awfullize, figure you'll be a vegetable in three years. . . .
>
> I, I guess I would like to say, particularly with most of the symptoms being under control, that it hasn't got a great deal of impact on my life, because I function quite well, but it it's constantly there. Just constantly. It's just [silence] no, I mean, it's very . . . constant is an exaggeration . . . only for brief periods of time, you know, can I remain totally unaware that I have Parkinson's, just routine moving about, I'll bump into a door jam or drop a paper, and that may just be basic clumsiness on my part, but it still translates as Parkinson's. . . . I used to have the comfort of thinking or believing that when I couldn't think of a word, it was sure signs that I was going into the early stages of Alzheimer's [laughter], but I don't have that anymore, so everything, whether it is a symptom of . . . whether it is caused by Parkinson's or not, that's what I have to attribute it to. And so, there's not a lot of escape . . .

Parkinson's Disease and the Self

Platt (2004) suggests that,

> If you live long enough, Parkinson's can decimate your sense of self. All the proprioceptive and social identifiers that,

without even thinking about it, add up to "You" suddenly no longer add up, leaving you wondering to whom this crazy body belongs. (p. 318)

Platt's comment sets the stage for the premise that people with PD must create a new self—one that takes the changes associated with the disease into account—and how these changes affect the cultural, role, interactional, and biographical tools used in creating a self. It can be argued that language and control of the body are two of the most important aspects of self creation, and because those are the two systems most affected by Parkinson's disease, we will consider their importance in the following.

Self and Culture

There are cultural norms about predictability and control of bodily movements and about speech. Because the person with PD may lose these very tools, he runs the risk of being seen and treated as a person with a lowered status. The older women with PD who were interviewed by Caap-Ahlgren, Lannerheim, and Dehlin (2002) yearned for their lost sense of self; worried about stigmatization; and particularly found the unpredictability of symptoms to be frustrating. They tended to restrict their social interactions in response to the lack of control over their bodies. They wished for a "stable body image."

In a different context, Garfinkel (1956, p. 421) talks about ceremonies in which a person's status is lowered through "public denunciation." In a modern society, we can think of the official diagnosis of a long-term illness as a similar status degradation ceremony. In fact, Jerry talks about his "damaged identity."

When the interviewer asked Jerry to describe himself before his diagnosis with Parkinson's, his response was about how he is vulnerable to being labeled as disabled and how he rejects that cultural label:

The biggest thing, if you had asked me before diagnosis, this is probably the biggest difference . . . if someone were to have asked me, describe the state of your health, I would have said good. I now have to say poor. I don't know if that's, it's . . . it certainly isn't good anymore and I find that very difficult, impossible to accept that you know I have this incurable disease, I just, I keep even today, if I have real good days, I'll still you know come up with, ok, maybe I've been misdiagnosed. You know I don't want to think of myself as being sick or with a disease. Or whatever you want to call it. I also have a great deal of, I don't accept it, it's like I have a disability. I just will not put that into my thinking, even when I have to use, because I'm having leg trouble or something, use my cane to get to my truck after work, I still won't use that word.

Clearly, having a disease that can be defined as a disability is very difficult to incorporate into his self concept. In fact, he has refused to incorporate that definition and so far, he is able to resist because he continues to have predictability of and control over his bodily movements. The interviewer asked Jerry to talk about his experience with Parkinson's in the 2 years since he was diagnosed. He said:

Well, living with it has been . . . I, I have very few obvious symptoms as long as I pay attention to dosage and all that type of thing, um, I time medication so that I know that while I'm, you know, at work there is a very small likelihood that I'll lose control. It has only happened once in a class that it got to the point where I had to literally stop, just stop, saying that we cannot go on, because I could not look that way in class. [The interviewer asked "What's 'that way'?"] I got the dyskinesia, jerking, and my head was snapping off to the side, and my hand was dancing up and my hand was clawing, I had a great deal of difficulty staying upright, so we ended the class quickly.

While Jerry can still typically present himself as a "normal" person, in cultural terms, if he times the medication accurately, he now must constantly take into account the possibility that he will not have predictability or control. If he attempts to present himself as normal, then he may fail in the attempt. And just as power and control are important in spoken language, they are critically important in the language of the body:

> People define themselves in terms of their body's varying capacity for control. So long as these capacities are predictable, control as an action problem does not require self-conscious monitoring. But disease itself is a loss of predictability, and it causes further losses . . . Illness is about learning to live with lost control. (Frank, 1995, p. 30)

The capacity for control is a cultural norm. Jerry acknowledges that if he cannot control his body, he will simply be incapable of creating the self "college professor" in a way that others will accept:

> . . . the physical, at least, what I typically experience, I, at least I have the ability to maintain some level of control over it

most of the time and I, if I didn't have that, I, I'd, God, I've had said adios a long time ago and I certainly wouldn't still be here on campus.

Self and Roles

Facility with language is central to the role of college professor and Jerry has been very proficient with this tool in the past. However, Parkinson's has now begun to interfere with his ability to speak. He describes this as "stuttering," since that is the most overt manifestation of his speech problems at present and is thus the most troublesome communication deficit. We will use his term throughout this chapter. Jerry finds that the increasing unreliability of language as a tool has dramatically changed his relationship to his role as a university professor:

> I make my living with my mouth . . . it's, rightly or wrongly, I've always felt that I could walk into a class . . . and I could do what I had to do in terms of lecture, exciting, entertaining, I could do that with my mouth. I can still do that to a great extent, but not as well, because I have to go through this thing of whether we ignore or whatever when I can't talk, so I know I'm not as, I know I'm not as good as I was. And it is so hard to go from knowing you are so damn good at what you do, wondering what the hell did I do? Did I pull it off, didn't I? Did it . . . that's just a a [stuttering] in a classroom, where I have power [laughter], power and authority, you know, social networks and power, uh, and that that that makes it the hardest . . . that's probably the hardest environment to deal with. Faculty meetings aren't real good either.

Arthur Frank (1995) says that "Serious illness is a loss of the 'destination and map' that had previously guided the ill person's life" (p. 1). The above quote from Jerry is a good example of Frank's point. In the past, Jerry believed himself to be very good at using the tool called "language" in his role as college professor—notice that he is emphasizing not the content of his words, but his ability to make sounds ("when I can't talk")—but that this tool is no longer reliable. Moreover, in the past, the situations in which Jerry found himself—the context called "college classroom"—were similar enough that he had no difficulty using this tool. Since college classroom is perhaps coterminous with the definition college professor, Jerry felt good about his self definition. In fact, these contexts were his "destination and map" and he felt at home. When asked, "Would it be fair, for you, to say that the difficulty with speech is more central to your self identity than the motor skills?" he responded: " . . . in my professional life, work, yes, it's central."

Self and Interactions

The ability to articulate clearly is an important tool in negotiating interpersonal interactions. In fact, we suggest that the act of talking is central to the creation of selves that are viewed by others as being powerful and efficacious in interpersonal interactions.

If self creation is, as we have argued, a negotiated project and if talk is essential to that negotiation, then the loss of the ability to talk will affect one's ability to use interactional tools in the creation of self. Jerry is painfully aware that if he presents himself to his students in ways that would previously have been unquestioned, now he may be unsuccessful in carrying that off. He continues to have the authority of the power relations in the classroom setting, but he fears that his control is slipping. He says: "I mean, I really think they are sitting there thinking, at some point thinking, why doesn't the old asshole just give it up instead of putting me through this?"

. . . I feel a lot more vulnerable . . . I don't have nearly . . . I . . . have lost sense that I'm in control. I'm also extremely bothered, particularly in classroom settings, which is basically, you know, a major portion of what I do to make a living, when I can't talk well. I have, I have to go to the . . . this . . . routine to offset what to me appears to be very discrediting. I, I have to adopt an attitude in the classroom that basically, like hey I don't know it or I have to make a lighthearted comment about it and a) I do notice it and b) it is not lighthearted and it, it hurts me because I know it's this fucking act I have to put on just to deal with . . . I don't know how else to deal with it.

They [the students] act like they don't see it or hear it. And I know, and that makes it, that does not make it easier because I know they see it, I know, I am not so foolish to believe that while I am doing this and doing the damndest, I can, I'm being evaluated, perhaps in ways I don't want to be evaluated with conclusions I certainly don't want.

Moreover, in the past, Jerry was able to take his facility with language beyond the college classroom and use it to his advantage in other settings. Platt (2004) discusses the fact that "a progressively ill person is often surrounded by health care professionals who have met the patient he has become but have only 'snapshots' of the person he was" (p. 315). So the interviewer asked Jerry if he felt that the medical establishment treated him as helpless or incompetent, and he responded: "Up to this point, I really don't have the sense of that happening to me. . . . They really haven't done that yet. But then, I'm the same person who told my cardiologist when I was in the hospital, to stop acting like an asshole." The interviewer asked: "And did he or she?" and Jerry responded, "He took great offense, and I said very pointedly that I said stop acting like one, not that he was one. I was describing behavior not person. Which only pushed the point of education further." The interviewer asked, "How did he react to that?" Jerry said, "He settled down real quick."

While content is important here, it is also clear that Jerry's ability to present himself as verbal and articulate is critical to the self he wanted to present in this interaction. Imagine this statement if he had been stuttering and therefore unable to articulate with authority. Because his role of college professor is a central part of his identity, as one who has considerable education and is particularly good with language, Jerry felt comfortable in interacting with high-status medical personnel on an equal basis.

So, in the past, Jerry has been able to negotiate the classroom and other interpersonal settings relatively easily. He has been able to present himself in a certain way—as being good with language, good at teaching. Now, because his speech is different, he fears that he is being evaluated in negative ways. That is, because he can no longer appropriately manipulate the tool called "speaking," he is not able to close the deal on the self he presents. This is painful not only because he loses control of the situation, but more broadly, he loses agency and his sense of self begins to get fuzzy.

In fact, Jerry has changed his interaction patterns, reducing them as much as possible to areas where he feels safe:

I think that's the biggest, the actual knowing, you know, that you've lost some of it . . . not, no, that it's been taken from you, some of that . . . In social circumstances, I have, unless it's you know personal friends, I do not go to social events. I do not go to the dean's receptions, or things simply because, no, I live in terror, I just acknowledge the fact that I will not be able to deal with it if I you know start slopping food, or dropping food, or stuttering, stammering. I can't, I don't, I won't be able to . . . I don't want to deal with it, so I just don't do it. My personal friends, yeah, that's ok, because they, they, I believe they can deal with it, take it for what it is.

This is to say that, with friends, Jerry can continue to use the tools that remain available to him, to present a self. However, it is not the same self as he was able to create in the past, even with friends. In fact, he sees himself as having lost agency—"it's been taken from you." The interviewer asked him, "If someone asked you to describe yourself now, since your Parkinson's diagnosis, how would you describe yourself?" He responded:

Oh God, when you ask that question, the first word that hit my head, which I resent being the first word in my head, uh, is diminished . . . I feel less than I was. And much of that has got, most of that, not much, most of that has not got anything to do with motor skills, . . . its because of the way I have to present myself, and I am constantly, . . . I have to present myself and work hard at presenting myself as if nothing's wrong with me. I have to pay attention, I have to practice my slow beginnings and soft starts and all that speech therapy stuff,

I have to pay attention, I have to pay attention to how loudly I'm speaking, because there's also some reduction in volume. . . . I've never in my life had to worry about whether are you talking too loud? You know, are you talking loud enough?

Jerry feels himself to be diminished because he has lost some tools for self-creation and he feels that he is in danger of losing some power in offering his self to others in social interactions. In his own eyes, he has lost agency.

Self and Biography

Earlier in this chapter we mentioned that, previous to the PD diagnosis, Jerry prided himself on his intellect, education, and virility. These characteristics are part of his biography—part of his physiology, history, and personal attributes. Moreover, because he had the appropriate cultural tools and knew how to use them, Jerry was successful in negotiating for the acceptance of these biographical characteristics in his interactions with others. For example, his Ph.D. from a well-regarded university gave him the tool to present himself as well-educated and smart. To demonstrate his essential maleness, Jerry stayed in good physical shape and walked with confidence. Now, while his intellect remains the same, his speech has been affected by PD and he can no longer either stay in prime physical condition or walk quickly and confidently. The loss of these tools has had profound effects on his sense of self.

One aspect that is very troublesome to me, in terms of how I think of myself, what I have to do now that I never had to do before. . . . I am attention seeking

attention loving, as long as it's attention, but all of a sudden, I don't want to draw attention to myself. That sucks. I view that very negatively.

Interestingly, Moore, Kreitler, Ehrenfeld, and Giladi (2005) found that those who had previously had an "androgynous" gender identity coped better with Parkinson's disease, presumably because the androgynous PD sufferer would actually lose fewer tools of self creation with the disease.

Parkinson's Disease and the New Life Narrative

In Chapter 4, we argued that narratives are life stories which allow people to describe and explain themselves. We have continued to emphasize the fact that narrative matters because storytelling is a uniquely human behavior. Our life stories allow us to create meaning in our lives, and these stories must evolve over time to accommodate life experiences and stages. Sharing of life stories means sharing what McAdams (1993) refers to as one's personal myth. The ongoing storying of life allows us to focus on self as storyteller ("I"), rather than self as a story dependent on others' telling ("me"). When neurogenic disorders destroy the ability to use communication effectively for narrative purposes, individuals lose the ability to express the active, self-creating I and become dependent on forces external to the person (other people and environments) for a definition of me.

A life story gives back to the person suffering from a neurogenic communication disorder the very thing that seems to have been taken away—agency—and allows the storyteller to continue to be the author of his own story. When asked to describe himself, Jerry reflects on several things that he used to have: he used to be healthy, he used to be able to walk into a classroom and dominate it, he used to be able to use language to acquire most of his goals. Jerry used to see himself as a person with considerable agency and power, and now he cannot ignore the need to create a new narrative:

> . . . the difficulty you know of maintaining the front, um, I think it's been one of the issues that were, uh, issues I've had to deal with . . . is recognizing the importance of that. It was always something that I could more or less ignore. Hell, I'm educated, I have a vocabulary, I know how to present myself. And all of a sudden, I'm having to deal with Goffman's notion of discredited identity— because I can't keep it hidden.

And yet, despite the fact that he cannot create the self he used to be, Jerry finds himself creating a new self with agency and dignity. While he recognizes that Parkinson's disease must now be part of any narrative he writes, he is also determined that he will be the author of such a narrative—it will not be written for him by others—and that his starring role will continue to be a person who creates his own sense of self, and who acts with agency.

In the following, we reproduce a lengthy quote that captures this sense of writing a new narrative, and then we talk about how the four aspects of the self are captured in this rewriting. We then address the issue of a new life story versus an illness narrative.

> The other day . . . ok, um, it was last Friday, I was outraged with the Rush Limbaugh comments about Michael J. Fox . . . oh Michael J. Fox had made a commercial about some individual running for office, in favor of stem cell research, and he was overreacting to the medication, and he went into dyskinesia. . . . Rush Limbaugh said he was acting or he deliberately didn't take his medicine, I was so angry about that, because frankly, did it make a difference if one is acting as if one has the symptoms of the disease one has, I find that fairly irrelevant, or if he had forgotten to take his medication, well who hasn't forgotten a pill. I did my class Monday morning without medication, I didn't take it the night before or that morning, just so they could see what it really looked like, and I wouldn't let them do anything, other than look. Of course, I had 110 quizzes to hand back and I dropped them, and several of the, you know, upfronters jumped up and I told them to sit back down, they couldn't do anything but watch.
>
> I got . . . no, I got my back up. In my own way, it was a statement for me. Um, it was a strong statement, it probably . . . I was so damn proud of myself. I mean, it was a very strong statement, I felt, in terms of [silence] . . . yes, I got this, this is what it looks like and now get off your stupid asses and start thinking. I don't care which way you go on anything, but know what the issue at hand is about, it has nothing to do with, the true issue as I see it, it's not got a god damn thing to do with a frozen embryo which is probably going to get tossed anyway, this is, this is how we look, there are all kinds of diseases like this, this is how we look, what it looks like. Students today, because students today do not see that and it's not that they they grow up in a . . . protected middle and upper middle class enclave, it's that we don't show our diseases anymore, we have medication that hides the diseases, we don't have the local restaurants where everybody

goes, society functions so differently, they just don't see it, they don't even know what the other side of the story looks like, all they know about is that Rush Limbaugh says that Michael J. Fox is acting so they can destroy embryos, well, there's more to the equation, more to the argument, and in spite of seeing pictures of little Timmy, you know, let's look at little Jerry, god dammit, I'm important too.

Interviewer: Isn't this just an extension of yourself . . . your self has always been involved in trying to teach students about reality and . . . media, I mean that is what criminal justice is all about . . . isn't this just an extension of that same self?

No. This is real personal. I'm going to let you see something only my wife has seen. [silence] It, it [silence] it's for me at that time, it was the strongest statement I could make that they simply . . . I'm here, deal with it. There are other people like me here, deal with it. I don't know . . . I was scared to death before I went into that because I had no idea how it would go. I just didn't know how badly, you know, I had no idea. I was damned proud of that one.

Interviewer: So how did it go?

I don't even know, they were probably more shocked by my refusal to let them do anything, um, because the other class that I had to cancel the other day because I just got started into the lecture, it was just a few minutes, medication, I mean I should have taken the medication earlier, I was getting a sense, just let it go too long, and so I went into dyskinesia, jerking and all that, which was fine, I . . . I could not at that point, because it was not scripted, I guess, deal with it, I just could not stand up there

and let them see the real thing. And Christ, they practically wanted to carry me back to the office. Well, it's a smaller class. I mean, honest to God, they were hovering about like they thought I was going to die or something. They were going to help me to the elevator. My room is directly across from the elevator. I said, no I can do this . . . I mean, I had taken the medication, I was just too late in . . . I didn't want to deal with it. I think, what I like most about all of this, this may be a topic, I mean given it all, the one thing I know yeah I still know, talking about a sense of self, I am still, a goddamn player, I will take it on. You know, I don't know, I was, I mean I adopted all those kids, I integrated housing areas, goddamn I am still doing it all my way, I will let my ass show, . . . I am not to the point where I surrender . . . I am not giving up. I have not got that in me. Um, I don't know how long I can keep it up, because at some point, you know, it's going to become very difficult or impossible to maintain any reasonable any sort of I'll call it required presence in the classroom, I mean at some point, I'm pushing the river . . . simply isn't going to cut it. At some point, possibly, I'm going to have to face reality. But it ain't here yet.

Jerry is writing a new narrative that includes agency and dignity and resolve. He is going to use the symptoms of his disease to make a point about people with neurogenic communication disorders, and he is going to take personal risk in doing so. He is demanding that his new, altered self be accorded dignity and acceptance. It is true that this is an illness narrative, but it is not a narrative of defeat.

In the writing of this new narrative, we see the beginnings of a new self for Jerry, one which incorporates both previously used and new cultural, role, interactional, and biographical tools. We see his effort to come to terms with who he is now, to compensate for the tools he has lost, and to create and negotiate for the acceptance of a new self, one with Parkinson's disease: " . . . I'm here, deal with it. There are other people like me here, deal with it." This is an illness narrative in the sense that it must incorporate within it a recognition of the fact that Parkinson's is now a part of the self— it will never be otherwise—but it is more than an illness narrative. It is a new life story. In the following, we touch briefly on the cultural, role, interactional, and biographical tools that are highlighted in this quote.

The New Narrative: Culture and the Self

Jerry recognizes that there are images in this culture about what it means to be old, to be sick, to be dying. He believes that the young in our society are not given cultural images that allow them to deal with these aspects of life:

> Students today, because students today do not see that and it's not that they they grow up in a . . . protected middle and upper middle class enclave, it's that we don't show our diseases anymore, we have medication that hides the diseases, we don't have the local restaurants where everybody goes, society functions so differently, they just don't see it, they don't even know what the other side of the story looks like, . . .

As a result, those who are ill and dying are set to one side and not allowed to have a self. In this one interaction that he has staged, he is forcing his students to come face to face with this cultural avoidance:

I think, what I like most about all of this, this may be a topic, I mean given it all, the one thing I know yeah I still know, talking about a sense of self, I am still, a goddamn player, I will take it on.

The New Narrative: Roles and the Self

The strength of this rewriting of the self comes from the fact that it took place within the context of Jerry's most cherished role, that of college professor. In fact, the risk he was taking terrified him, because his negotiation of self could have been refused and his new narrative therefore failed: " . . . I was scared to death before I went into that because I had no idea how it would go. I just didn't know how badly, you know, I had no idea." He called on all of the tools of his role, including power, to make a point to his students:

> I am not to the point where I surrender . . . I am not giving up. I have not got that in me. Um, I don't know how long I can keep it up, because at some point, you know, it's going to become very difficult or impossible to maintain any reasonable any sort of I'll call it required presence in the classroom, I mean at some point, I'm pushing the river . . . this simply isn't going to cut it. At some point, possibly, I'm going to have to face reality. But it ain't here yet.

The New Narrative: Social Interactions

Possibly our major point in this book is that the self is negotiated in interaction with others in social settings. Out of these negotiations, the person writes a self story or narrative, which must itself be negotiated, that is, presented to others for acceptance or rejection. If the story is rejected, the individual faces the loss of power and agency, and must rewrite the narrative or accept an imposed self. We have used the typical medical setting as an example of a situation in which a self is imposed on the person with neurogenic communication disorders by those with more power and status. We have here an opposite example. In this very specific interaction with his students, Jerry was able to make a statement about who he is and who he will continue to be. In the course of a few days, in preparing for this classroom interaction, Jerry decided on the self he would present, the negotiations he would make, the narrative he would write. He understood the risks, as we have mentioned above, because his negotiations may have failed. But the self story can be written in no other way. It is always in the single, specific interactional setting that one tries out a self and then keeps it or modifies it or changes it for the next interaction.

The New Narrative: Biography

Biography is biology, physiology, and the life story as written to date. Clearly, Jerry's biology—that fact that he is male, that he is 66—and his physiology—the fact that he has Parkinson's disease—are key elements of his rewritten narrative. Here, however, we would like to focus on the life story as written to date. In setting this stage of self presentation, Jerry references the aspects of his story that are critical to his sense of self: " . . . I mean I adopted all those kids, I integrated housing areas, goddamn I am still doing it all my way, I will let my ass show, . . . I am not to the point where I surrender . . . I am not giving up." What he is referring to is a lifetime of activism that he fully intends to include in his future narrative.

The narrative, then, is written as a story of the self, and the self is put together with cultural, role, interactional, and biographical tools. In the following, we talk about some specific aspects of the narrative itself, focusing on temporality, social situatedness and social others, and the need for dignity and acceptance. In this section, we also touch on the extent to which a life story is and is not an illness narrative.

Elements of the Narrative

Temporality

Life stories have a past, present, and future. When one has been diagnosed with a neurogenic communication disorder, the present and future stories are often (but not necessarily) illness narratives. The past was the healthy self, with an understanding of how to use cultural, role, interactional, and biographical tools to negotiate for acceptance of self in a given situation. The present is the self contending with changes and losses in those tools, and the resulting changes in negotiation and acceptance of the self. The future depends on the disability, but for people with Parkinson's disease, there is the understanding that the body will continue to decline. While time is important for all of us in writing our life story, time is a critical component of the life of a person who suffers from PD. As we have seen in previous quotes, Jerry used to define himself as "healthy," and that was an important component of his self. Being healthy gave him agency, gave him the ability to use and manipulate many tools, including independence. Now, he is losing that independence, and as he looks to the future, he continues to see additional losses in an area that is of critical importance to him, including his presentation of both physical and verbal selves.

Time is also important to his wife. When he was first diagnosed with PD, both Jerry and his wife turned to the Internet for information, but they quickly stopped. The Internet gave them the belief that the future was completely bleak—they would "awfullize" about how the life story would now progress. Because both Jerry and his wife had previously watched their spouses die from lingering diseases, this future was nearly impossible to contemplate. So, they have turned to more optimistic sources and are writing an illness narrative of hope. Nonetheless, any life story of one with PD will be tinged with the understanding that tomorrow may be worse than today.

So, to the extent that the new narrative must contend with Parkinson's disease as a fact of life, is it only an illness narrative? For Jerry, the answer to that question is clearly no. The temporal line of Jerry's life may have a sharp disjuncture at the point of the PD diagnosis, but it continues as the same line nonetheless. The diagnosis did not create an entirely new time line for him; he continues to use many of the tools he previously had in his tool kit for self creation and interestingly enough, he now uses the illness of PD as another tool.

For other people, the answer to the question might be yes. Sam J. has viewed his Parkinson's disease diagnosis as defining his life narrative, and this diagnostic label framed his storying of self for the remaining 23 years of his life. For him, the illness narrative was used to gain his wife's attention and focus, and he succeeded admirably. Needless to say, for his wife, her life also became an illness narrative, with most of her actions now related to Sam's PD.

In contrast, 46-year-old Rachel M. saw the PD diagnosis as an opportunity to create a new life story entirely. Having researched the disease, she realized that she had many more years, and she made active choices about new directions for herself during those years. At one point, she said to a speech-language pathologist,

> It's not that I'm fighting Parkinson's, it's just that I see it as an opportunity. I always wanted to go to med school, but I don't have enough years for that. However, I also wanted to write novels, but I never tried because I thought they would be lousy. Right now, it doesn't matter if they turn out lousy, it's just that I choose to spend my time writing while I can.

For Rachel, knowledge that PD constrains the time remaining to her became an opportunity for creating an entirely new narrative self, one that essentially ignored the disease while recognizing limits to the time available to her.

Social Situatedness and Social Others

As we have argued throughout this book, self creation is a social project. We have seen that Jerry has restricted his social interactions to those who will allow him to write his own illness narrative. He avoids those settings—receptions hosted by the dean, college faculty meanings, parties attended by strangers—where his agency and power will be diminished and his narrative will be written by others. While this demonstrates his—and anyone's—ability to create one's own story, it also shows how PD changes the life story. These types of interactions had never been particularly important to Jerry in the past, but if they had been, he would find it necessary to mourn their loss and incorporate into his life story a different view of himself, as one who is more of a "loner."

The impact of PD on Jerry's wife must also be considered. Her life narrative has now been profoundly altered as well and she is finding that some tools are no longer available to her. The roles that each has assumed in the family are changing and will continue to change. Jerry's loss of independence also reduces her independence. When I asked Jerry how his wife responded to his diagnosis, he said:

> It was very devastating to her, because well, we certainly hadn't had this in our retirement plans . . . and I think she too had at least this tendency to go to the worst the quickest, and saw life as we knew it ending in the next 16 minutes, and since then, . . . we both know that while I do have problems, I'm not progressing much at all, so if it stays as it is, it is certainly something we can live with for an extended period of time. We've made some living adjustments, particularly my reluctance to appear in public . . .

Moreover, Jerry's wife has always had independent sources of meaning in her life, and this will be an important factor in helping her to continue a life story that is not completely enmeshed in Parkinson's disease (Konstam et al., 2003). Nonetheless, for Jerry and his wife, their new life stories are fundamentally coauthored.

Birgersson and Edberg (2004) found, in their sample of six couples, that Parkinson's may result in the couple moving from "unity towards unity, from unity toward distance and from distance towards unity," and for Jerry and his wife, the move is from unity to unity. Again, then, we see that the new narrative need not be only about illness, and it need not be only about loss.

For some PD sufferers, there may be usefulness in joining a support group either in person or on-line (Lieberman et al., 2005). Groups are always important environments for negotiating self and may be important for people who need therapeutic intervention in mitigating the effects of the disease, such as speech and communication skills (Manor et al., 2005). Our focus here will be on support or self-help groups. Interestingly, Charlton and Barrow (2002) found that PD sufferers who do not join support groups may wish to avoid placing the disease at the center of their lives. In their sample, those who did participate in a support group incorporated the disease more fully into their life narrative. Charlton and Barrow (2002) say, "The discourse of non-members contained many references to a self-help group as a source of distress, while discourse of members identified it as a supportive resource." For some, the support group may provide additional tools of self creation; for others, the group takes the tools away. There is other research (Moreira & Palladino, 2005) that suggests that it may be more important to provide PD sufferers with hope than with facts. This ties into the issues of agency and control, to which we will turn next.

Agency and Control

Life stories must be written by the individual, even if they are coauthored with others. In Chapter 3, we suggested that agency is the ability to create a self and negotiate successfully for its acceptance. For someone with Parkinson's disease, this negotiation is all about control, primarily control of the body. To the extent that control is possible, Parkinson's disease need not be the major theme of the new narrative, and the illness narrative can be subsumed in what is simply a new life story. However, when control is no longer possible, agency begins to be problematic. One becomes vulnerable to the types of disability attributions that we have talked about previously and will discuss again in the next section. In many of Jerry's statements, we have seen the belief that when he can no longer control his body, he will walk away from his current roles. This will be a difficult moment for him, primarily because he will feel that he is losing agency. Remember that he said, " . . . the actual knowing that you've lost some of it . . . not, no, that it's *been taken* from you . . . " [emphasis added].

Jerry recognizes that he spends considerable time in presenting a self that either does not have the symptoms of Parkinson's or acts as if the symptoms are of no importance:

I'm also extremely bothered, particularly in classroom settings, which is basically you know a major portion of what I do to make a living, when I can't talk well. I have to go to the . . . routine to offset what to me appears to be very discrediting. I have to adopt an attitude in the classroom that basically, like hey, I don't know it or I have to make a lighthearted comment about it and a) I do notice it and b) it is not lighthearted, and it, it hurts me because I now it's this . . . act I have to put on just do deal with . . . I don't how else to deal with it.

The reason he "puts on this act" is so that he will continue to have agency in his creation of self, to prevent others from having the power to renegotiate his self, as someone who is disabled, who is not in control in the classroom, who is not the self he chooses to be and that is so important to him. He knows that if he cannot pull off this act, that he will lose the power to manage his relationships with his students:

And I know, and that makes it . . . that does not make it easier because I know they see it, I know, I am not so foolish to believe that while I am doing this and doing the damndest I can, I'm being evaluated, perhaps in ways I don't want to be evaluated with conclusions I certainly don't want.

When he can no longer manage these relationships, he will have lost the ability to negotiate his very definition of self in a role, in a situation, that has been the central theme of his life. As a result of this, he will have to begin a new life story. In the next section, we turn to that issue through a discussion of dignity, respect, acceptance, and understanding, which are all central to the ability to write one's own life story, that is, to have agency and control.

Dignity, Respect, Acceptance, and Understanding

A self narrative is always about dignity. However, we have seen how PD increases the probability that one will be viewed negatively, and we have seen how some PD sufferers reject the image of themselves as having a disability. When we are accorded dignity from others, we have agency. Lack of dignity takes away tools of self creation at all levels—cultural, role, interactional, and biographical. For example, if Jerry Patnoe's students no longer treat him with the respect typically accorded to a college professor, he can no longer be successful at using that role as a central aspect of his self. We have seen in previous quotes that it is at such a point that he will walk away from that role and that critically important aspect of himself altogether.

Interestingly, though, acceptance of the disease is not necessarily associated with the best illness narrative. As we discussed previously in this chapter, some PD sufferers do better if they write a new life story in which the symptoms of PD are not given the most importance in their lives (Charlton & Barrow, 2002). While this is still an illness narrative, the illness is not the major plot of the story. For others, making the illness the major plot of their new story allows them to access additional tools, such as those found in self-help groups. The important point here is that the person with the neurogenic communication disorder must be the one who decides what illness narrative will be written, and it is critically important that significant others, caregivers, and professionals recognize and facilitate that process.

Fundamentally, then, the person with Parkinson's disease or any neurogenic communication disorder would benefit from an understanding on the part of others about what the disease is, but more importantly, about the fact that disease does not take away our ability to create our narrative. Jerry talks about a future in which he could share his Parkinson's fully with his students, and they could interact as if it did exist rather than as if it did not. Currently:

> . . . I always, upfront, day one, I say ok this is what you may anticipate happening, so largely they will go through this very polite . . . they just simply ignore what is going on in front of them.

When asked what would be the appropriate way for the students to respond, he said:

> There is none—it's all in my head. No matter what they do, it won't be right. If they ignore it, I know they're . . . that's not true. If they laugh at it, I know they know it's not funny, and if they act as if oh well, shit there he goes again, that's

a negative, so there's no way, they can't win, I can't win. We certainly, ok, in my classes, we certainly haven't gotten to the point of where we can in all honesty not see the difference, or the problem . . .

When Jerry says that the problem is "all in my head," he knows that this is not true. What he means is that our society has not yet provided the average person with a tool that allows her to interact with people like Jerry in the same way she would if he had broken his leg—without the stigma of disability and the threat of lost agency. Such a cultural tool would be very valuable to those with neurogenic communication disorders, to their significant others and caregivers, and to our culture, as we will argue in our final chapters of this book.

In the next and last section, we turn to a discussion of those aids that might be provided by professionals such as speech-language professionals to help the person with Parkinson's disease continue to write his own life story.

Tools and Technology

Much of the treatment for Parkinson's disease involves medication and/or surgery. However, neither of these can remove all of the challenging deficits in communication and in other motor skills, nor can they resolve the cognitive challenges that some persons with AD experience in later stages of the disorder. As with ALS, tools of all kinds are available to those with PD. Tools such as canes and walkers may support independence in ambulation, but we have seen how people such as Jerry resist these aids because of the stigma of disability. Computers may provide access to a world of knowledge about PD and may also permit relatively normal communication through avenues such as e-mail. Personal speech amplifiers may be used to address problems of low volume in speech output.

Persons with PD are typically less likely to use AAC devices than those with ALS. While the reasons for this are not fully understood, one factor may be the relatively gradual decline in speech intelligibility, particularly when medications stave off the more severe symptoms. Another factor may be the fact that many with PD retain some intelligibility until the very latest stages of the disease progression. The onset of cognitive impairments may limit the ability of some individuals to use abstract AAC systems effectively. And finally, as with persons with ALS, individuals with PD and their loved ones place varying degrees of emphasis upon the importance of communication in their lives, just as all humans value communication to different degrees. In fact, it is possible that the choice to use AAC reflects choices, conscious or unconscious, to privilege the storying of self in moving forward with a new biography that includes PD.

We do not know whether Jerry will need and will use any form of AAC. That will be part of his evolving life story. Sam J., mentioned earlier, actively refused AAC even though his wife was unable to understand him because of deteriorating speech intelligibility and her own hearing loss. His refusal may be linked to his desire (probably unconscious) to exploit the illness narrative in securing his wife's attention. Jenny

R.'s concerns were only with AAC and assistive technology in general as they allowed her to pursue her new life goal of novel writing. Finally, Brenda S., a 72-year-old grandmother of four, sought assistance in obtaining and using AAC early on because, as she stated,

> What I want is to play with my grandkids. That's all. And I want to be able to do it for as long as possible. So if these speaking machines make that possible, I want one. And I don't care how funny it sounds, I'll just make the kids laugh and then I can hold my own with them.

Conclusion

As the story of Jerry Patnoe and examples from the lives of several others illustrate once again, the experience of a communication-impairing illness affects each individual and his loved ones differently. Although both ALS and PD are degenerative neuromotor diseases, they differ in terms of the nature, cause, severity of the communication breakdown, and time line of the disorder. These differences in turn influence the illness narrative and renegotiation of self. In the next chapter, we will explore the ways in which the challenges to the narrative self differ when communication is disrupted abruptly, typically due to a stroke, and when aphasia impairs the language system itself.

CHAPTER 8

Life Stories in Aphasia

MY APHASIA AND ME
by Massell I. Smith

Aphasia! A time of frightening darkness
Yet in this darkness, I have found myself,
Where an interesting new life has open to me
And inspiration has shown, honest friendship is real

Aphasia! You spark determination and humility
Awake my soul to the wonders of life
From the glory of the sunset, to the fresh morning dew
The unique experience of being alive

Aphasia! What crowded mind, unscrambled thoughts
The future looks grim, uncertainty sets in
But the intelligent mind refuses to cave in
So the struggles go on day after day
As courage endure and inner strength shines through

Aphasia! Never stop learning as babies do
Laughter's fill the room
As funny gestures and sounds act out words in my head
Elated I stand!
Joyful sounds and cheers can be heard all around
As successfully my challenges are met

Aphasia! One message is clear
Experiences in giving, is pure and a delightful joy
Receiving is equal and a blessing from above
So thanks,
Is forever spoken by these lips
It's the love and caring
Sent from the heart
And the smiles that shine through
The receiving heart

Aphasia! Humiliation you bring
My eyes are red, my cheeks are wet
Angry works burst forth as tears flow
Why should I be ashamed?
I never asked for your coming
Yet you are here to stay
But my stubborn will, restored self confidence
Invisible though you are
Our lives are intertwine as long has I live
Me and my Aphasia.

The narrative self faces unique challenges when confronted with aphasia. By definition, aphasia robs the person of facility in understanding and/or using those language symbols that are at the heart of the process we may call storying of self or self construction (Shadden, 2005). This loss of language stands in stark contrast to the type of speech impairment described in the previous chapters on ALS or Parkinson's. When speech alone is affected, and our muscles do not move in desired or predictable ways, we risk only loss of intelligibility. At times, such as in the early stages of neuromotor disorders, this loss of intelligibility is minor —an annoyance or nuisance more than a true barrier to the essential communicative exchange. While the natural presentation and negotiation of self in social exchanges may be affected by these challenges, the primary meaning-making tool—the language system—remains intact. With more profound impairments of speech intelligibility (as might be found in later stages of ALS or Parkinson's), it becomes more difficult to negotiate one's presentation of self, but as long as language skills are spared, there continue to be opportunities for self creation. Loved ones, even health care providers, often retain a belief in the underlying personhood of individuals with motor impairments.

However, with aphasia, the semiotic system of language is impaired; that is, the individual has lost the basic ability to use recognizable signs in interaction with others. The precipitating and frightening medical event is often stroke, and loss of language means loss of ability to share the experience and to affirm the ongoing self that exists beneath the outward impairments. Impaired language comprehension may also raise questions about competence. For the person in a wheelchair, with a cane, with a right facial droop or any one of countless markers of physical impairment, it is readily apparent that there is something wrong. One can see paralysis, one can hear slurred, distorted speech patterns. One's comfort with these differences varies, and different degrees of stigma attach to the apparent deviations from normal, but at least one part of the impairment is visible. In contrast, the language system is not as visible and the average person's understanding of aphasia is limited. Indeed, the idea of language itself is unfamiliar, except in terms of studying French in college or speaking with immigrants from other countries. If the basic concept of language is poorly understood, and communication is taken for granted, it is difficult for most people to come to terms with the impact of impaired language on social presentation and validation of self. Persons with aphasia but no physical impairment consistently describe their frustration with the well-meaning comments of acquaintances who say things like, "My Uncle Fred had a stroke and he couldn't get out and around like you. You are doing great, you're lucky."

Yet unlike the experience of persons with ALS, the life stories of persons with aphasia are those of recovery within the context of residual impairment. They are expected to move forward in life, but without the necessary tools for reframing the story and for renegotiating self. Loved ones are equally affected. They must provide care and support while sometimes lacking certainty about whether the person with aphasia remains unscathed beneath the surface of language and other deficits.

In this chapter, we will introduce a broad spectrum of individuals—male and female, married and divorced, retired and working at the time of the stroke—with a variety of occupations and interests. The biographical particulars of their lives, as well as their aphasia type and severity, make each person unique. The challenges to maintaining narrative self vary. Thus, these individuals cannot possibly represent the entire population of persons with aphasia, but instead serve as illustration of our focus on how people with communication disorders create narrative selves.

In Swidler's (1986) terms, the language system is part of one's cultural tool kit. Loss of this tool can be very isolating. In addition, loss of normal communication often leads to questions about an individual's competence, questions reinforced by early encounters in the medical community that underscore the patient's sense of powerlessness and incompetence (Mackay, 2003). With stroke, the initial effects of brain damage effectively challenge everything one has taken for granted in one's life, leaving

individuals to confront confusion that can only be expressed in chaos narratives (Frank, 2005). At a time when it is essential to be able to express this experience of biographical disruption and global impairment, those with aphasia have lost the communicative facility needed for this expression.

Current approaches to managing the life consequences of aphasia are strongly influenced by social models of disability and functioning and are often grounded in the *International Classification of Functioning, Disability and Health* (ICF) [World Health Organization (WHO), 2001]. This social foundation provides a powerful base for the themes explored in this chapter. Constructs of quality of life and life participation dominate current research and clinical practice, and caregivers and loved ones are receiving increased focus (Cruice, Worrall, & Hickson, 2006; Cruice, Worrall, Hickson, & Murison, 2003, 2005). The trend towards a social perspective on aphasia is moving us forward in looking at the narrative self in aphasia, but the inquiry has just begun. Sadly, we can only infer the challenges to narrative self experienced by those whose aphasia renders them virtually incapable of participation in typical communicative exchanges. Those whose words and stories have contributed directly to our understanding of the evolution of narrative self after onset of aphasia will be introduced as their contributions are shared. Thus, the rest of the chapter text will be informed by these and countless other individual clients who have graced these authors' lives, and by the spirited community of our support group that has endured for more than 24 years and has provided a true environment for narrative recovery.

As in earlier chapters, it is important to begin with the actual communication impairment and its impact on the lives of those living with aphasia, which we examine in the following section. After that, we will discuss how the four dimensions of self are challenged by aphasia, and how these in turn alter one's life story and influence the framing of one's illness narrative.

Aphasia and Life Impact

The first thing I remember was that it was the darkest black blindness very like a cave and then there was at some point a beam of light blue, yellow, and red I think, maybe green, like a shaft of light. And I think it's important for people to understand that there's no . . . it's simply a numb sense of observing without any feelings one way or another . . . it's like a camera . . . so for a long time, there's no sense of "oh my god I've had a stroke" or "I'm going to die." You don't think about those, and then I remember that in the darkness what looked like the top of telephone poles and I remember thinking that I could step a few feet from one of those to the other but again there was no sense of fear of falling, just observing. Then I began to realize that I was in a hospital but I really didn't know why I was there.

Welcome to Harry's world almost 11 years ago—October 12, 1997. As he begins his stroke narrative, it is clear this is a man of words, and images, and stories. He worked for many years as a case manager for the chronically mentally ill, serving as a passionate advocate, an instructor in dealing with life's daily challenges, and guide to taking control of one's life despite mental illness. We will rely heavily on the experiences of Harry and others as we explore the redefinition of narrative self post-apha-

sia. However, it is important first to establish some understanding of how the communication deficit in aphasia feels.

Language Loss

"I think it . . . but . . . but . . . where are . . . things . . . words . . . " (Ramon)

"Everyone needs to slow down . . . they hurt poor brain" (Jason)

"Reading was my . . . joy . . . now . . . work . . . too much work . . . " (Brenda)

These are familiar refrains from our clients with aphasia, capturing the essential nature of aphasic impairment. Understanding the language impairment and charting the recovery of language functions, however, reveals only the tip of the iceberg in terms of the monumental impact of stroke and communication loss on the lives of our clients and their families. As Wulf (1986, p. 14) states, " . . . such recovery is on the surface. Deep down is quite another story. True, it may be possible to write, to read, and to speak, though perhaps none of these abilities warrants close inspection. But internally?" Perhaps the iceberg is revealed better by the following quotes:

I don't . . . I not . . . I can't—all no, not—what is it I can? (Diane)

Everything has been taken away from me. (Dennis)

For some individuals, the aphasia is so profoundly impairing, the experience may be characterized as "living in a silent world" (Ritchie, n.d.). Ritchie has written at length on this experience for herself and her husband with aphasia, describing it as being "like a bomb falls on all your hopes and plans for the future and you are reduced by Aphasia from a person who could talk to a person who just 'talks in their minds' but nobody can hear them" (Ritchie, n.d.). She acknowledges the intense anger and frustration experienced by all who are living with aphasia, along with a perceived loss of competence.

Many persons with aphasia share this sense of frustration with the fundamental gaps between their thoughts and their words. Harry refers to this as "finding ways around the stumps with communication." Some individuals want to share the way the breakdown in communication makes them feel. Others simply disengage for a while. Harry says,

> Okay, I could hear when I spoke that I couldn't say the words the way I wanted to say them, and that was very confusing. I didn't know what aphasia was at that point. And in trying to speak it was very frustrating and confusing so I didn't feel the need of wanting to talk very much. I wasn't aware of that at the time. I just I didn't talk very much.

And Wayne notes, in the support group:

> I just go . . . smile . . . it's too much . . . I go away.

Another example of the impact of loss of communication is provided by Raskin's (1992) description of his reflections on the early days of dealing with aphasia:

> My most valuable tool, I thought, was making sense of the turmoil. I was wrong. My most valuable tool is words, the words I can now use only with difficulty. My voice is debilitated—mute.

He goes on to describe what his aphasia felt like initially:

> My understanding of simple conversation also seemed to be returning. I began to produce what I thought were words, but the puzzled look on the faces of my audience showed my that my long-awaited words were nothing more than gibberish. Then, little by little, people began reacting to my vocalizations. Imagine my relief at again being able to express my basic needs with a single word like "eat," "drink" or "toilet." Each utterance involved deep concentration and struggle to produce a somewhat intelligible word. Each "new" word was received with elation by my family and friends, motivating me to go on. A baby must be excited like that when he utters his first "mama" and "dada."

For persons with aphasia, communication can be challenging and exhausting. One risk in focusing interventions too closely on specific language deficits is the degree of effort that becomes associated with using language to communicate. If this effort cannot be sustained outside of the therapy room, communication may become associated with issues of personal success or failure, and these perceptions may actually begin to interfere with communicative success. Thus it is not surprising to find that the idea of comfort in communication appears in many contexts. For example, in describing his participation in an Aphasia-Talks project (Levin et al., 2007), Len states, "I was very comfortable—a safety zone. I knew that [other participants] couldn't find the words either. . . . They aren't going to judge me." And at the 2006 National Aphasia Association's Speaking Out! Conference, Tucker (2006) described the Adler

Aphasia Center as "a place where people can comfortably communicate. . . . And what we've found is when people are comfortable, they're willing to try to communicate. And the more that they try to communicate the better they feel. The better they feel, the more they try."

Communication also allows us to navigate the complex challenges of life's social actions and interactions, because it is fluid and capable of subtle nuances. Thus one major loss associated with aphasia, even in its mildest form, is a loss of resilience and flexibility, of resourcefulness and creativity, in using communication tools (Holland, 2007; Walsh, 2007). Pasupathi (2006) discusses the way in which communication affirms the texture of our lives in the small, daily exchanges, what he calls the *everyday self.* He highlights the fact that much of our communication occurs over breakfast, between loads of laundry, while reading the newspaper. These moments of small talk or chit-chat may not be major meaning-making exchanges, but they are the *communicative backdrop* for living out our lives, and thus our life stories. The simple act of sharing a conversational moment may be as important as a fully formed illness narrative in storying of the post-stroke self. Such moments are those in which people seek collaborative opportunities for recognition and validation. Certainly, they depend on the ability to effectively use one's cultural tool kit. At the level of chit-chat, changes in timing, in flexibility of message formulation, of responses to cues signal that something is "off" about the person's presentation of self. Even the best language therapies are challenged in addressing this loss of subtle facility in everyday conversation.

There is another communication level that is more difficult to describe. Liechty (2006) writes that, despite his recovery:

I yearn for the possibility of in-depth discussions with fellow professionals. . . . I would like to pursue a relationship with a woman, but it is hard to find things in common or build relationships when there are such great communication barriers. This applies to all of my relationships, not just with women. Although my family has been supportive, I find I need more than my brother, sister and mother can provide (p. 33).

What has been lost is the ability to function optimally in certain roles (whether professional or relational). It is certainly difficult to address this sense of void in the core of who we are and how we use language to frame those moments in which we share our multiple selves and receive validation. What is also challenging for persons with aphasia to communicate is a sense of what is important, what is valued, and why. Armstrong (2005) suggests that an inability to use language effectively for these functions may actually impair the ability or desire to engage in and contribute to previous social networks and current social activities (both personal and societal) and may also lead to the sense that the person with aphasia has little of value to contribute.

In recognition of perceived limitations, some persons with aphasia feel a sense of responsibility and failure when the language system breaks down, making communication with others difficult. Others attribute greater responsibility and burden to conversational partners and express frustration if the partner does not adjust communication appropriately. Harry speaks at length about the way others fail to accommodate his communication difficulties, attempting to provide guidance for those communicating with someone who has aphasia.

Simple things like talking too fast, not giving me time to process an idea and not making sure that their speed of speech is going faster. And that's a common problem with everybody, friends or therapists, of being unprofessional in not wait . . . pacing their speech to the speech that I need . . . it took me forever to find ways to tell people that I couldn't understand what they were saying and many times since my ability to speak and use affect of speech got in the way and people became angry or turned off by my interactions to them because I came across as angry and demanding. And I began to know that I was being demanding and inappropriate but I didn't know what to do about it. . . . I think I'm at the point now where I instead of saying "I had a stroke and you need to talk slower" to telling what I need in terms of volume. That's always a big issue. Even the doctors and therapists tend to get very loud when they're talking to me to the point that it's painful for my brain to have that much volume to . . . and it has to do directly with how many words a minute I can process. And the resistance that people have in meeting their needs as opposed to this person's stroke functioning. And I become very very aware of how selfish other people are in interrupting and disregarding the thought that I'm trying to make and their need to say what they want to say. [People] will assume that I'm trying to say a the rest of a sentence or a paragraph or a thought and the therapist interrupting to say they understand when they don't understand what I'm thinking . . . it throws my thoughts off like a railroad train switching tracks. So they don't seem to understand how hard it is for my attention to be distracted

with sounds any distraction. Someone else joining a conversation just throws me so far off track that I can't understand what the person just said because I can't process it because of the interruption and I can't understand the subject of that other person's thought.

For Harry, struggling with life with aphasia is in part the chronicle of the success or failure of his interactions with others. Early on, he was concerned about a perceived absence of friends and family, indicating: "I was confused as to why all of these many friends that I had were not calling or coming over." He immediately had prioritized the importance of relationships with others in the difficult task of reframing self interactionally.

Some stories of communicative "recovery" are tributes to the remarkable commitment of life partners, the determination to preserve and advance the viable self of the person with aphasia. In fact, some couples learn to share the communicative responsibility so seamlessly, others often forget the extent of the aphasic impairment. However, the negative impact of aphasia is also felt to a great extent in the interactional domain. As Harry indicates, "When I'm alone, I don't have aphasia." He goes on to say:

> But I spend more and more time alone because when I'm at home I don't feel like I've had a stroke. I think I can hear and function much better than I really can.

Just as some couples with aphasia are success stories, others seem to be unable to get past the aphasic deficit. Some become entrenched in the communication patterns established during the early weeks post-stroke, as will be illustrated by the story of Phil and Nancy later in this chapter.

In order to understand the impact of aphasia on the narrative self for those with aphasia, we must have an understanding of how this condition affects quality of life. Quality of life and related constructs are discussed briefly in the following section.

Quality of Life

Fundamentally, all strokes are life-changing, creating seen and unseen changes in many forms, including the emotional consequences of depression, frustration, and others. The life consequences of aphasia have been described in many texts and journal articles, as well as on the Internet (information and organizational Web sites, support groups, or patient forums). These studies will not be reviewed here. A greater understanding of the impact of illness in general has helped expand perspectives on the life consequences of stroke and aphasia specifically.

"Quality of life" is a highly individualized construct (LaPointe, 1999; Sarno, 1997), dependent upon cultural and social definitions and factors, as well as the person's mode of self-discovery and philosophy about life. Harry indicates:

> I spent a lot of time wanting to die, because the quality of life went from very very good to zip. And I even strategized in a rehab hospital how does one go about killing oneself. I think about life and what's important about that, and whether I would ever want to survive a stroke.

Quality of life and well-being are also linked to concepts such as a sense of self-worth or self-esteem. It is clear that interactional support for self-esteem is linked to feelings of agency, certainty, success, and a sense of belonging, all associated with

dimensions of self addressed in this text (Andersson & Fridlund, 2002). To understand a person's sense of self-worth, one must also understand the yardsticks against which he measures success and failure. For many, narrative self can only move forward after the individual begins to accept those experiences that had previously been defined as failures and to choose new arenas in which to succeed. Through these choices, new tools for self-negotiation can be created. Harry hints at this in the following:

> Sometimes I make failures with that, but I've also been able to give myself a lot of room to make mistakes and work on not feeling useless. And I do a lot of things around the house primarily to ease the burden for my wife but in the process it also allows me to feel that I'm contributing and being useful.

The concept of life impact of aphasia applies to all within the social world of the individual. The following poignant e-mail from a daughter living 200 miles away captures the essentially family nature of this problem:

> My father had a stroke about six months ago. His ability to speak is terribly affected, and he is so angry and depressed, we don't know what to do. Daddy has always been the heart of our family, and we aren't really sure how to help him. My mother is frightened and overwhelmed. I think Daddy gets angry with her and she sort of freezes up. My husband and I are trying to help, but we don't know how.

For this family, the only solution was to travel 400 miles round trip for 3 successive months to attend a stroke support group. From that group, and some family time with the speech-language pathologist, the father eventually reached a point of acceptance and actually moved forward with life.

We turn next to consideration of the impact of aphasia upon the self and life stories.

Self and Life Stories

The central premise of this section is that language is a core tool in maintaining a sense of narrative self, and that aphasia consequently creates a kind of identity theft (Shadden, 2005). The result is what Swidler (1986) terms "unsettled lives" and what MacKay (2003) describes in terms of a past self ("Tell Them Who I Was") that no longer bears resemblance to the post-stroke damaged person with aphasia. The experience can be described as a sense of disconnect between one's internal experience and knowledge of self (in part, biographical) and the culturally-defined, role-specific interactive selves that are presented to others post-stroke. This impact of aphasia on self is not restricted to the person with aphasia but encompasses all who interact with that person, as will be described in greater detail later in this chapter. When one person's language is impaired, this forces others to modify their language and interactive styles to accommodate the aphasia. The impact of aphasia occurs at the levels of everyday talk referred to previously as well as more overtly meaningful dialogues about needs, perceptions, and meanings.

Perceptions of self are hard to measure, so they are often probed indirectly through terms such as self-esteem, self-concept, and self-efficacy. We tend to make inferences about self through observed behaviors, interactions, and emotions. Another challenge in writing about the impact of aphasia on narrative self is the uniqueness of each individual's experiences of self, as illustrated in discussions with Harry. When he was first asked how his sense of self or identity had changed since his stroke, he appeared to struggle with this topic. In response to one probe, he described how his:

. . . feeling of being a child and an animal increased. One evening my psychiatrist was making his rounds and saw me in the cage, maybe crying with frustration that I couldn't use the bottle. And I was soaking wet and he saw this happen and at that point things changed. I didn't associate those changes at the time except that at one point I found a way to open the sides of the cage a little bit so I could sit up. And one of the nurses came in there and reprimanded me for doing that and I just felt hopeless at that point. I was being controlled without knowing why or what I'd done wrong.

At this stage, Harry remembers treatment as demeaning and infantilizing; it is clear that others are responsible. Later in the same interview, he indirectly addresses changes in self when he describes himself before the stroke, then focuses on how others treat him now. In all instances, his need to validate himself is clear.

On a separate occasion, over lunch in a restaurant, he began to discuss his constant battle for recognition from others, whether friends or strangers. For the first time, he explored the fact that he was still fighting against the aphasia, still demanding attention that validated the pre-stroke Harry, the biographic particulars that had made him "who I was." He went on to say he was trying to reconcile two "histories—who I was and starting over with who I am." Harry described the challenge of having to switch gears, as though there would always be a disconnect between his past and present self. Yet narrative self is dependent upon linkages from past through present to future. His struggle in reconciling past and present self has consequences for his wife. Until he finds some continuity in his projection of self, it is difficult for her to provide those interactive responses needed to recognize and affirm that self.

Another example of the difficulties of discussing self can be found in the following e-mail from the wife of a stroke survivor, after the topic of self-esteem had been raised. She wrote:

> And you are right about self esteem being a huge issue. One of the biggest things that I noticed with Jeff is having all the filters that he developed over the years to protect him and his identity stripped away leaving him vulnerable. I think he has done quite well under the circumstances, but some of his fears are too strong to get past sometimes. I have to give him credit for being willing to put up with me and at least trying different things. . . . He is not the most aware individual of his physical and mental cues. He tends to describe things in the most general of terms. As you can imagine, trying to get to the root of something can be difficult.

These comments are intriguing because the wife actually brought up identity issues when asked to reflect on self-esteem. It is also interesting to note that she refers to Jeff's premorbid style of self-reflection and communicating, highlighting the importance of understanding the person before the onset of aphasia if we are to understand her after.

Sometimes brief observations (in this case, offered spontaneously by a person with fluent aphasia) capture the global impact of aphasia. Dennis was introduced earlier in Chapter 4 of this text. Over the course of several stroke support group meetings, he talked about his struggles with the total destruction of his life story as the result of a brain hemorrhage 3 years previously (when he was 39). He articulates his sense of loss of core self with remarkable and poignant clarity.

> They keep telling me to let go of Bob—he's dead and gone—but I miss Bob.
>
> I died 3 years ago—that's what the doctors said should have happened, and I do believe I should have died. Well, I did die . . . I went away.
>
> I don't look at myself as a man anymore. I'm erased.

Although these quotes suggest that Dennis's primary "battle" is with a perceived loss of some core or essential self, his story contains elements of all four dimensions of self described in Chapter 3. The connectedness of aphasia with multiple dimensions of self is also seen in the following statement from Raskin (1992):

> I now realize that my vocation in life has changed. Now I represent the one million Americans who cannot speak for themselves. My plight and theirs are one: to inform the public that those of us who have lost the ability to invent fluent phrases or sentences have not lost the ability to think. We retain the skill to communicate our thoughts and feelings, whether through writing, picture boards, pantomime or facial expression. We can still speak! We hope that you will listen with your ears, with your eyes and always with your heart.

In this quote, Raskin highlights his new sense of responsibility that goes beyond the work of reframing self *interactionally* to consideration of self structurally (in new roles) and culturally (at the level of public awareness and policies). He pleads for awareness and understanding, reaffirming the fact that aphasia does not destroy the person or diminish the person's need for communication with others. Elsewhere in the same document, he provides his biographic particulars, including the fact that he is a person with aphasia.

In the following sections, aspects of self related to culture, role, interaction, and biography will be considered through the lives of persons living with aphasia. Often, these four dimensions are difficult to separate, and they are always interwoven with the life stories and illness narratives that people share.

Self and Culture

Persons with aphasia are often confronted with issues of self and identity at the cultural level. Successful presentation of self requires society's implicit or explicit assumptions of what characterizes successful individuals in any culture. In the American culture, for example, those attributes most valued are independence, power/strength, material affluence, and competence, among others. Thus at the level of cultural values, the person with aphasia has an uphill struggle for acceptance and validation, because she has few of these attributes (except possibly material affluence). Almost immediately, stroke survivors are also confronted with the loss of status associated with being a patient in a medical environment that defines ill persons as those who are dependent, incompetent, and without control. In understanding self construction at the cultural level, therefore, it is probably most important to recognize these cultural values related to illness and disability, as well as the associated stigma.

Issues of disability and identity or self were alluded to in Chapter 3 of this text. In recent years, there have been several studies exploring social/cultural values related to stroke, aphasia, and disability (cf. Clarke, 2003; Mold, McKevitt, & Wolfe, 2003; Moss, Parr, Byng, & Petheram, 2004). In all studies, there is consistent evidence that public images of disability related to aphasia (and stroke) may interfere with access to services, sense of well-being, and negatively-framed identities carried forward in illness narratives.

One issue in reestablishing one's sense of personal agency relates to the stigma sometimes associated specifically with brain damage, particularly impairments of the less visible cognitive or linguistic skills that define us as persons. Kate Adamson is quoted by Moran (2006, p. 37) points out, "Everyone has a disability. Some of them are visible, some of them aren't. It's all about what we can do, not about what we can't." On-line posts often tackle this difficult issue of disability and stigma. As one person wrote, "Too often people are not given a chance—we just assume that this particular disability means that 'you can't' rather than looking at what YOU CAN do."

The idea of social/cultural stigma associated with stroke and aphasia also leads some to try to validate the disorder. In a presentation at the Speaking Out Conference, Harry Alter (2006) talks about the "country of aphasia," "aphasia people." Others try to develop images that capture their challenges in more familiar terms. For instance, Harry refers to "getting around the stumps ways of functioning in daily life at home or outside." But at the most basic level, Wulf, 1986, p. 13) asserts, "Every aphasic needs to know there is something he can do, even if it's watching birds."

Time and again, people living with aphasia and advocacy groups highlight the fact that most people know little or nothing about aphasia (National Aphasia Association, n.d.). One on-line discussion group participant wrote: "No job after aphasia is common—because people don't know about it." Another pointed out, "There are more people with aphasia than Parkinson's, but we don't have a Michael J. Fox that stands up and talks about it." Lack of awareness about aphasia is one small component in the more overarching cultural challenges created by negative perceptions of illness and disability.

Another consequence of lack of public awareness of aphasia is the tendency for friends, family, and strangers to make inappropriate judgments about what the person with aphasia can do. A new member to a stroke support group expressed her fear of telling people she had had a stroke, because she would be seen as incompetent. This was a particular concern with respect to driving. Although she knew she was competent in her driving, she was afraid she would be blamed in an accident because of her stroke. Others apologize frequently for their difficulties. It is common to hear persons with aphasia say, with some embarrassment, "I used to be able to spell," or "I used to read all the time."

Some try to develop images that capture their challenges in more familiar terms. For example, for 10 years, Harry has been angered by the cultural misperceptions of his aphasia and by extension his competence. At one point he suggested, "They build ramps to buildings. Why can't they make the waiters study aphasia and change the way they are with people like me." Harry's pre-stroke perceptions of self were very strongly anchored in culturally validated domains. It was important to him to be important in the community, and he expected cultural validation. Thus it is not surprising that he struggles with self validation within the broader

community. Others also resist the cultural norms that suggest they should accept their dependence and role as incompetent.

For example, Doreen is a 75-year-old woman who experienced an extensive left hemisphere aneurysm rupture and who was profoundly impaired during the first months after the stroke. Her language recovery was relatively rapid, and she appeared to have little trouble dealing with the fact of her new life that included some degree of aphasia. In fact, her approach to treatment was systematic, thorough, and rigorous. She welcomed homework and independently began writing and reading on her own. During a therapy session about 5 months post-CVA, Doreen began to describe having a "sad day" accompanied by what she referred to as flashbacks to her time in a geriatric psychiatric unit. All of this monologue is transcribed below. Portions will be referred to throughout this chapter section.

. . . because I was saying I don't think it's because this happened because of you. I don't think it's because that you knew how I was feeling, what was going on with me. You didn't know about it. And that made him feel better. Except that I said, I just want you to make a promise that I will never have to stay in a place like that again ever. You get somebody to come to the house to take care of me whatever it is. because I don't need to be in a place like that to. I mean it doesn't makes me feel bad, it makes me feel terrible. Because xxx he would come in and maybe 20 minutes in the evening. and that was it. He never brought a dinner over so we could read together. and I'd say maybe they'd let me walk, you could . . . take me for a walk around . . . nearby or something like to let me know I'm a real . . . really alive person. I just felt and you felt like you first everything's locked up. and and all this like I'm in prison a real prison, you know, this is a real prison. and that's it. really made you feel bad. I wasn't the only one. this this this wasn't a happy time in any respect. Well it isn't like feeling in control. it's just that this is me my person. This is what I'm doing . . . and then eating real food and uh all this sort of things would just save your life. you have a life. you you just feel like you don't have a life. I felt like I was in prison. and when I get out of here I'm going to save things and run away someplace. So I because I knew Dave was not thinking I was real. but he still feels I was this person that would Pffff any place any time. And um that he had to watch, be careful, watch watch. If he just had come, brought a paper, read the paper to me rode. Well you're not supposed to be able to do anything. You're supposed to be just sitting there.

In the context of cultural self, Doreen's comments about her environment and her treatment in that environment are particularly relevant here. She felt she was in prison, treated as a nonperson, assumed to be incompetent and docile. Her comments also relate indirectly to self as structurally defined through roles, to which we turn next.

Self and Roles

For Doreen, the roles implied in the above transcript relate to being a wife, being a homemaker. In these roles, she would be accorded recognition for the person, the self that she is. Instead, she felt that her husband could no longer perceive her from these perspectives, and that absence is profoundly disturbing. Dennis also struggles with roles and self in his attempts to move

past his stroke and aphasia. Part of his projection of self pre-stroke was the role of competent, responsible, powerful professional in his job. In a support group, he referred repeatedly to all he had lost in the public persona he projected in his job. For him, the loss of these structural/role governed aspects of self leave a tremendous void in his narrative self, and he has not yet been able to determine how to fill that void. He has not yet been able to give up his pre-stroke structural self.

Harry has struggled constantly with alterations in life roles and their implications for his sense of self. Of particular interest has been the difficulty he has experienced with knowing how much or how little to talk in the stroke support group that he originally cofounded years before his own stroke.

. . . but there's been a long transition where the group needed for me to kind of back off and I was still trying to be a co-leader. That's created some communication problems within itself because the other members wanting to take more power or authority in running a conversation and me still trying to lecture or teach. And that's still a problem. I'm trying to back off with talking so much but I have a real problem in finding a way or seeing the signs that say I'm talking too much. And that's hard— I need to be able to talk . . . to help the group through my talking.

For many, work and family roles are those most altered by aphasia and thus those with greatest potential impact on self. For one couple, the husband's stroke occurred shortly after they moved to a new state and a new job as pastor of an area church. Roger found it difficult to acknowledge that his aphasia and other cognitive deficits might leave him unable to "do the job" of serving as spiritual leader. He and his wife were only able to move on with their life story when Roger was asked to share his illness experiences with other pastors, or in their terms, "to tell our story." Only then could he make a decision to retire officially from his home church.

In the life stories described in this chapter, there are numerous examples of how roles are powerfully linked to sense of self. For example, when creating a personal Web sites to tell the story of life with aphasia, most persons include clear statements of previous roles—occupational, familial, recreational, and others. There is no question that we define ourselves in part through these roles.

Self and Interactions

The interactional component of self reconstruction is described in many articles (cf. Ross, Winslow, Marchant, & Brumfitt, 2006; Simmons-Mackie & Damico, 1999, 2007; Sorin-Peters, 2003) and receives prominence earlier in this chapter, particularly in discussions of psychosocial consequences and quality of life. It is the interactional domain that is clearly affected as people begin to reconstruct their life story post-stroke, because the role of language in the cultural tool kit is most evident when we relate to others. Family and friends are most likely to express concern about the impact of aphasia on relationships. In one e-mail a friend wrote about her mother's stroke: " . . . she is left with sufficient communication problems to affect her daily life (particularly in her sense of identity with her husband)." After a life of being the consummate communicator, Harry struggles to find successful interactions.

Most of the quotes in this chapter relate in some fashion to self and interaction, but only the example of Phil and Nancy will be used here. Phil's recovery of speech-language functions began many months after the initial stroke, because of a series of life-threatening medical events that intervened. More than a year post-onset of aphasia, he began to achieve increasing success in communicating his messages and responses in therapy, using multiple modalities and considerable clinician support. The give-and-take of the conversation began to appear relatively natural; only written transcripts revealed the considerable verbal impairments that still remained. Yet Phil's wife Nancy continued to see him as incapable of any meaningful communicative interaction and became angered with the clinician's reports of relative success in treatment. She was asked to observe one session; during that observation, she focused exclusively on all the things Phil was not doing, commenting that the clinician was sweet to help him the way she did.

The observation session was discussed with both Phil and Nancy. It was clear that Nancy still saw him as dependent and impaired, as he probably was immediately post-stroke. When encouraged, Nancy would try to prompt or support Phil's responses to questions, but she did so with an apparent sense of disengagement and no confidence in the process (e.g., "They tell me I should ask you to try to find another way of saying it. So . . . I don't know, what do you want to do?") What was more revealing was Phil's refusal to participate in this discussion. He made no eye contact with Nancy, looked frequently at the clinicians with an expression of irritation, often rolling his eyes at his wife's comments. He made no effort to respond to her awkward attempts to help but would use multiple modalities to communicate with the clinicians. Clearly this couple had lost a sense of interactional self, and both had disengaged from any attempt to share who they were and what they were feeling or thinking. "Fixing" Phil's language deficits will not resolve the much greater underlying issues of self with aphasia.

Self and Biography

One of Dennis's stronger comments in his first support group meeting was,

I look in the mirror . . . well, I can't . . . I just started to be able to . . . I don't know who that person is.

While this comment can be interpreted on many levels, it is certainly a statement about biographic self. Further, when he states that "I don't look at myself as a man anymore," he is also making some reference to biographic self. In an article in the *New Yorker* magazine, famed neurologist Oliver Sacks (2005) quoted Scott Moss, a psychologist who became aphasic at age 43. Scott describes the experience of global aphasia: "The part of myself that was missing was [the] intellectual aspect—the sine qua non of my personality—those essential elements most important to being a unique individual. . . . For a long period of time I looked on myself as only half a man" (p. 1).

The experiences of having a stroke and developing aphasia do not necessarily change one's biography completely, as one's age, gender, family facts, and childhood history remain the same. However, aphasia does alter one's relationship to one's biographic particulars in the present and in the future. For example, for the individual who acted in theater as a hobby before the stroke, the biography will need to be rewritten, if only to state that part of the biography is now, "used to act in plays" as opposed to "loves to act in plays." One's new biographical self is also one defined as "a person with aphasia" or "living with aphasia." Some of these changes have relatively little impact on the individual's narrative self, but others have profound implications for the life story of the future.

Having acquired aphasia does not alter the ability to acquire new biographic particulars. For the family that traveled hundreds of miles to attend a support group, the most celebratory e-mail from the daughter was one in which she gleefully described her father's new hobby of playing the piano. In addition, there is an intense human drive to share one's story, one's biographical self. Numerous stroke survivors have written full-length books about their recovery process, and these efforts appear designed both to help others and to validate the competence and ongoing narrative self of the author (cf. Berger & Mensh, 1999; Buck, 1963; Douglas, 2003; Hofvander, n.d, Liechty, 2006; Mills, 2004; Newborn, 1997; Wulf, 1986). The popularity of such autobiographies can be attributed directly to the fact that they affirm the fact that the life story continues. The sharing of written words also provides an opportunity for interactive self construction. Increasing participation on Web sites and in on-line discussion groups underscores the need to tell one's story, to share one's biographical self.

Having considered the ways in which aphasia affects the tools of self construction for storying the self, we turn next to the example of Mike, and how he put these tools together in a narrative with a past, present, and future.

Constructing a New Narrative Self: The Story of Mike

Mike was a successful married physician. Approximately 4 years ago, he experienced a mild stroke, followed 1 week later by a massive stroke that damaged significant portions of his left hemisphere. The impairments resulting from the second stroke were extensive—virtual paralysis of the right side of his body, moderate receptive aphasia, and a severe nonfluent expressive aphasia. Based only on reports from Mike and his family, it appears that his language deficits could be characterized as a mixed nonfluent aphasia.

From the beginning of our involvement with Mike, it became apparent that sharing his life story was extremely important to him. During the years of recovery, Mike was able to rework his life story from one of chaos, trouble, and disruption to a very different narrative self in the present. Initially, the stroke was the endpoint of his narrative. Thus, his communication about self was oriented exclusively to the past, either pre-stroke in his role as respected physician, or centered on the narrative of his stroke and its consequences. He wanted people to know him as competent, but he also focused on his loss of competence and agency as a result of the stroke. Over time, Mike reoriented his life story to incorporate a healthy focus on the present—his children, his home—and the future, making plans to attend the Michigan intensive treatment program again, planning trips, and so on.

What is most remarkable in this evolution (more than 3 years post-stroke) is Mike's renegotiation of his sense of narrative self and his reconstruction of his life story through the past through the stroke into the present. He has managed to reweave the threads of this story so there is no biographic disruption, and he is consequently more comfortable with himself in his present life. While all who successfully continue their life story after stroke accomplish these same things, Mike has done so in a very explicit fashion, and part of his ability to continue his life story has involved finding ways to overcome the communication impairment that removed the tool most commonly used in the story of self.

Mike's story is one of reconstructing the self in all dimensions described in Chapter 3. We give some brief examples in the following.

Cultural Tools and Resources

As told by a family member, one reason Mike suffered the second stroke was his wife's refusal to authorize a medical intervention because it was costly and, after the strokes, she reportedly began plans to divorce him and obtain many of his financial assets. Eventually, she sought to have Mike declared legally incompetent. She was initially successful in these efforts, since Mike was unable at first to obtain records of his own medical treatment because he was not judged competent to frame this request. While it is true that Mike had severe physiological impairments in his ability to speak, his competence remained unaltered. At the cultural level, though, the stigma associated with the inability to form words was enough to convince the court that Mike was not able to manage his own resources.

Roles

During his recovery, it became apparent to Mike that his former profession as anesthesiologist could no longer be part of his narrative self. When his life as a physician was discussed, he would typically shake his head or say things like "no more" to indicate this was no longer part of his life story. However, he continued to have a strong need to take control of his life and to be productive. He began volunteering at the local library, eventually creating a computer inventory of all their books. He also began a process of organizing his personal possessions and planning the construction of his own home on the land owned by his brother and sister-in-law. Thus, he created for himself a set of new roles to replace the one he could no longer assume.

Interactions

Eventually, during his recovery, Mike moved to the home of a brother and sister-in-law who began to explore additional resources for helping him deal with the consequences of his stroke. That led them to a local stroke support group, and ultimately to additional speech-language therapy. When Mike first joined the support group, he communicated almost exclusively with single content words and short phrases (including heavy reliance on the phrases *oh gosh, stroke, I'm sorry*), as well as use of his notebook to answer frequent questions. He said "stroke" with extreme frustration and disgust when he was unable to find the word he wanted. He also used "I'm sorry" with frustration and embarrassment. Mike truly appeared to be apologizing for his damaged self. He also relied heavily on his family, particularly his sister-in-law, to coconstruct his story and his personal portrayal to others. Now, he rarely says "I'm sorry," except with strangers. He still says "stroke" when he experiences aphasic breakdown, but the word is said in a casual, matter-of-fact fashion and he immediately continues his communication. In early therapy semesters, treatment goals had included increased initiation of communication and improved focus on others. In a recent communication group, Mike often began or changed topics, taking on a quasileadership role. He also listened more closely to others' communications and asked questions or shared comments. He even shared his own communication support materials in order to help others participate more effectively.

Mike's reconstruction of life story became most apparent in his most recent involvement in a communication group that focused on sharing personal likes, preferences, and interests along with stories of the past. In the group, participants agreed on a topic for the next session—favorite foods, hobbies, best vacations, and so on. In the time between sessions, they were asked to reflect on the topic and be prepared to share with others during the treatment session, using any and all tools that will facilitate this sharing. Mike began bringing complex scrapbooks in which he had documented—in writing and with pictures and other artifacts—different events in his life. In sharing these scrapbooks, he was able to link his past and present seamlessly and highlight future events and activities. In a very symbolic way, he demonstrated to others the importance of moving past the biographic disruption created by his stroke and aphasia by building these events into his extended life story; in other words, he demonstrated agency. Mike also received social validation for his sharing. Both graduate student clinicians and other persons with aphasia in the group were fully engaged with his stories, and other stroke survivors were able to build on his scrapbooks to initiate information about their own lives.

Biographical Tools

As we mentioned previously, after the second stroke, Mike's wife started proceedings to divorce him and have him declared legally incompetent, and she was successful in doing both. So, in the beginning, Mike's illness narrative focused principally on trouble, disaster, and chaos, with two major themes: his wife's abandonment and the severity of his impairments. After about a year, however, Mike began to focus on recovery of his functions and he became determined to overcome the stroke. Thus, his initial concern was with his biography, both in the sense of his biology and his previous life story. As he moved on, these aspects of his self, while still important, became less central. Emphasis upon elements of the biographical self also appeared to shift, most immediately apparent in the increased frequency of his discussions about and contacts with his children. At present, when asked about his previous profession as a physician, he expresses some regrets but he has clearly moved past grieving for that particular piece of his biographical self.

In recreating the post-stroke self, the resources at the cultural, role, interactional, and biographical levels are used to construct a new life story. This life story will initially be an illness narrative. We turn next to how these narratives may be constructed and what importance they may have for the person with aphasia.

Life Story and the Illness Narrative

"Life participation means getting on with the life story" (National Aphasia Association, n.d.). This simple statement captures the essence of this text and of the dilemmas that confront many. Under normal circumstances, our life stories unfold naturally, through shared communications and activities. Each life has biographical particulars and autobiographical memories that are being constantly refined to be consistent with the narrative self we present to others. We filter life experiences through this narrative lens, and when we confront "trouble" (anything that places us into crisis or deregulates our carefully won equilibrium), we rework our life stories to embrace and explain these events.

In this sense, Eriksen (1963) attributes to humans the status of creator. We use communication to craft a self that is complete and purposeful primarily because it is embedded in a coherent and meaningful story. Thus, the direct, immediate, and devastating effect of abrupt loss of language skills takes away the very tool we need to move forward with our lives. Oliver Sachs (2005) once wrote in the *New Yorker*, "Nevertheless, a feeling remains in the popular mind, and all too often in the medical mind, too, that aphasia is a sort of ultimate disaster, which, in effect, ends a person's inner life as well as her outer life" (p. 2). The challenge is to allow persons touched with aphasia to find new ways to story their past so others can understand it, to share the present with particular attention to the telling of the experience of stroke and aphasia, and to begin to communicate about a future.

For some period of time, post-aphasia, the new life story will be an illness narrative. As noted earlier in this text, "illness is a call for stories" (Frank, 1995, p. 55), a wake-up call to those who assume independence and agency are markers of success. At the relatively rapid pace of many persons' lives, an illness that occurs abruptly, without warning, can be overwhelming. For stroke survivors, a stroke and its immediate consequences create an immediate and dramatic narrative disruption in their lives, a kind of "narrative wreck" (Frank, 1995, p. 55), particularly threatening to one's identity, self-respect, and life plan (Brody, 2003). Shadden and Hagstrom (2007) underscore the centrality of meaning-making in the ensuing recovery process, as reflected in renegotiation of narrative self. Part of this process is the sharing of the illness story that allows others to understand and acknowledge the events that have transpired. This sharing is critical in helping the individual make sense of events, as well as recognizing and assigning meanings to the perceived challenges to sense of self and disrupted life story. Sharing can also counteract the experience of being an impersonalized statistic or diagnosis. Finally, the reframing of the story of one's illness provides a critical bridge from past through present to the future (Shadden & Hagstrom, 2007). Conversely, the loss of ability to share our past can have a profound impact, whether that past is conveyed as a significant life-changing event or a simple retelling of anecdotal episodes.

Illness narratives as stories are shared in many contexts, including on-line forums and published stories (e.g., Patients Like Me, Dementia Rescue, Aphasia Group on Yahoo). Members of on-line discussion and support groups often seem to recognize intuitively the importance of the sharing of stories in the context of the ongoing and changing storying of self. Illness narratives also incorporate life elements beyond the aphasia story, as seen in Harry's elaboration about his failing heart.

> I began to realize while I was in the hospital that I was dying. I was becoming more and more weak and a awareness . . . that I was aware that I was dying. And I talked with my wife about that and she had observed that also and so there at that point they felt that we had to take the open heart surgery at that point.

In stroke recovery narratives, there are some common themes. Rittman, Faircloth, Boylstein, and Gubrium (2004) highlight two salient features of post-stroke transition and self construction, the fact that " . . . the process (1) occurs over time and (2) involves changes in identities, roles, and behaviors" (p. 260). Almost always, there is story of biographical disruption—by illness, and more specifically, stroke. There is often a parallel theme of biographical accommodation—stroke survivors describe the work

needed to construct a meaningful lifeline in the face of this catastrophic illness. Narrative mechanisms used in constructing the stroke event include (a) use of typification to construct the body during stroke, (b) portraying stroke as an internal communicative act, and (c) explaining stroke as a physical sensation with mechanism used to minimize body concerns.

Illness narratives also change as individuals attempt to give them meaning within the context of the broader life story. If there is a basic human drive to be able to tell one's story, there is probably also a need to fill in any gaps in one's life story, although we all differ dramatically with respect to our memory of events. Harry's experiences illustrate this well. He has consistently described his earliest memories in a rehabilitation facility, saying:

> Several times some of the nurses or a doctor saying "Harry you really have to start your rehab" and I had no idea what they were talking about but I began to wait for something to happen and they didn't understand that I didn't know what they wanted me to do. And I couldn't speak so I began to just feel confused but again not with much feeling one way or another.

However, about 3 years after his stroke he began telling a new illness narrative about his earliest perceptions, as quoted earlier. This evolving illness narrative was strikingly similar to the tape-recorded comments of Larry, a young man with a traumatic brain injury who described how it felt when he initially came out of his coma (Shadden, Raiford, & Shadden, 1983). Harry had heard this tape many times prior to his stroke. While it is possible that their experiences were indeed that similar, it is also possible that Harry's brain unconsciously sought a way to fill the memory void and used this information accordingly.

In addition, he began to weave into his illness narrative images of his pre-stroke self as a competent professional. His stroke occurred while he was asleep on a Sunday; his wife came home to find him trying to make a cup of coffee, very confused, talking in jargon. Yet about 8 years post-stroke, Harry began to share the following story:

> I had been told several months after the stroke that . . . and by the way I had that stroke while I was doing that training for the police that day. One of the chief of police who was the training officer at the time said "All of us, Harry, realized that you had a stroke while you were there." Apparently I drove back home I don't remember driving back home but that's how you found me when you came home and realized that I had had a stroke at that point . . . it was several years after that training day when the police officer I I think I asked him had I had a stroke at that point and he said "Yes we realized that you had had a stroke" so maybe that happened on a Friday or something and and I was impaired during that period. I don't know but anyway . . .

While it is true that he had provided such training several weeks before the stroke, and equally true that he was probably already experiencing some neurological problems, there was no connection between these events. Harry seems to have bolstered his sense of self as competent, respected, and important by linking the stroke with an activity of professional achievement. An important question that remains unanswered is—from the perspective of moving forward with his life story, should Harry's version of the story be corrected? Should Harry be corrected? Should others volunteer the correct version of his stroke narrative? Or is it more important to let him manage his story in ways that will let him move on, regardless of his accuracy?

Moss, Parr, Byng, and Petheram (2004) underscore the importance of being able to share one's illness narrative, asserting that part of this process is learning to think differently. Indeed, they state that "striving to be one's old self is a futile undertaking" (p. 754). In Dennis's situation, he reported that others had told him to let go of his fixation on his life before the stroke, but he has been unable to do so. His instinctive clinging to the person he once was is not totally inappropriate, since that person is the starting point of the illness narrative. However, the challenge is not to eliminate the past but to weave past with present narrative so that a future can be imagined and pursued.

In order to develop a better understanding of aphasia narratives, Moss et al. (2004) asked people with aphasia to explore a variety of Web sites, including those associated with aphasia, stroke, and disability, and then create their own narratives. Many of the Web sites conveyed an institutional or organizational perspective that potentially excluded those with aphasia. The importance of helping persons with aphasia to create and share their unique illness narratives was highlighted, particularly since identities in the context of aphasia are "mercurial and difficult to pinpoint" (p. 753).

Stroke and aphasia may change the way persons view themselves and their sense of agency and power, and must be understood against the backdrop of other individual circumstances (Mold et al., 2003). One cannot consider the future if one is unable to understand the impact of an illness on one's previously defined life course and on the current context for self construction.

There exists a literature of formally elicited stroke narratives that provides some insights into the illness experiences of stroke survivors. McKevitt (2000) has suggested that formally eliciting stories about having a stroke may create positive outcomes by emphasizing "the creativity of the human capacity to communicate, engage and order" (p. 80). He also suggests that elicited illness narratives may allow individuals "to make sense of suffering, setting a physical experience in a social and moral context." In four interviews conducted in London and in Riga, Latvia, with persons 1 year post-stroke, clear narratives were only elicited in two instances. In a third interview, the primary barrier was the presence of communication problems. As McKevitt (2000, p. 94) states, "Highlighting the accounts of the articulate obscures the difficulties faced by the less articulate, urged by an unknown professional to give expression to their experiences." In the final interview, the strong resistance to telling the stroke story was construed as a possible indication of the person's expression of individual agency in the choice not to share the narrative. McKevitt also notes, "If narrative is about reconstructing a whole with an attempt to reach an understanding of the story, discerning, creating, and representing some meaning in that story, then perhaps some individuals feel that there is no meaning to be discerned or invented" (p. 92).

In other stroke narratives, the storying of the experience appears to be important to one's concept of self evolving through time (Sacks, 2005). Periods of illness may actually become markers of the chronology of a person's life (Charmaz, 1983, 1993). So the narrative frames change, and the storying of self must be linked strongly enough to reality to make life participation possible once again. Most humans tend to see their life course as organized and temporally linear (Faircloth, Boylstein, Rittman, & Gubrium, 2005; Faircloth, Rittman, Boylstein, Young, & Van Puymbroeck, 2004). With this linearity come expectations of life stages, chang-

ing abilities and even disabilities, and the end-stage landscape of aging.

This association of stroke with end of life is an unfortunate reality in the health care world. Faircloth et al. (2004) suggest that the medical community in particular sees older stroke patients in terms of an old age trajectory, one associated with decline and even the assumption of illness and disability. However, older stroke survivors perceived their illness trajectory as one linked to a hopeful future, one in which there is a future self (even if different) and one in which hope plays a role. There is an expectation of regaining control or power in life, the idea of a recovery trajectory (Faircloth et al., 2004).

By definition, the sharing of a stroke narrative relies in part on written or verbal language. Thus research on stroke narratives often excludes the perspectives of persons with aphasia who cannot participate in the narrative process without additional supports (McKevitt, 2000). Armstrong and Ulatowska (2007a, b) are among the few who have actively elicited illness narratives from persons with aphasia. While their interest lies primarily with the evaluative language used to express feelings and opinions in such narratives, they also note that illness narratives can function as a coping mechanism. In effect, when we verbalize experiences from our own perspective, the process of verbalizing shapes these experiences, our reflections, and our perception of their significance in our life. They suggest that, in sharing these stories, we engage others in the interaction, shaping the experience to communicate more than the events, perhaps to encourage or evoke a particular listener response. Evaluative language, particularly in illness or self narratives, is important in presenting ourselves *in relationship* to our communication partner.

In the following section, we talk about some important components of a successful illness narrative: temporality, life span, control and agency, recognition and respect, acceptance and understanding. Following that, we will consider the importance of social others in the writing of the illness narrative.

Temporality: Past, Present, and Future

It was noted earlier that Rittman et al. (2004) identified the element of time as one of the two salient features of self-construction post-stroke. Almost always, there is a story of biographical disruption—by illness, and more specifically, stroke. There is often a parallel theme of biographical accommodation—stroke survivors describe the work needed to construct a meaningful lifeline in the face of this catastrophic illness.

Clearly, narrative processes cannot be understood without consideration of the temporal dimension. Unlike any of the other neurogenic disorders discussed in this text, for persons with aphasia, time represents the possibility of recovery, a recovery trajectory, as well as a long-term sentence to living with this condition. Time may mean more opportunities for therapies, or may reflect the very real limitations on services imposed by the health care system. Time may represent days, weeks, and months seeking a way to fill the hours with meaningful activities. If the person with aphasia was employed prior to the stroke, time may also raise challenges about returning to employment or retraining for an alternate job within the competence of the individual. Time determines whether a person continues to write an illness narrative or moves on to another life story.

With stroke and aphasia, time is an unknown quantity. There is always concern about the possible recurrence of a stroke,

although this fear tends to lessen over time. When health professionals are asked questions about recovery, both extent and time frame, they often find it difficult to answer definitively, because each person's experience with stroke is unique. While no one wishes to hold out false hope for recovery, it is equally damaging to paint a dismal picture of limited options for the future. Either way, it is difficult to move forward with one's life story when it has been so abruptly disrupted. Those who succeed in moving forward with a life narrative are those who have learned to accept some of the unknown.

Temporality is associated with the concept of coping with an illness or disorder such as aphasia. There exists an extensive body of literature (not reviewed here) addressing the topic of coping with aphasia —for individuals with aphasia and for their significant others—and possible changes in adapting to such major life changes (Livneh & Antonek, 1997; Lubinski, 2001; Luterman & Luterman, 2001; Lyon, 1998; NAA, n.d.; Norlin, 1986; Sarno & Peters, 2004; Tanner, 1999; Tanner & Gerstenberger, 1988). Coping is usually described as a process of accommodation to and acceptance of change (Lazarus & Folkman, 1984; Parr, Byng, Gilpin, & Ireland, 1997). Parr et al.'s (1997) aphasic respondents particularly emphasize the need for active reframing of reality in the light of aphasia. The process of coping with aphasia is characterized in terms of taking on various rules that define self in the recovery process. Again, the emphasis is on reconstruction of a sense of self and an account of the new world, the aphasia. Without such an account, our aphasic clients may justly exclaim: "My aphasia is forever. What does that mean?" (Wulf, 1986, p. 172).

Most persons living with aphasia would agree that a stroke and aphasia must eventually be incorporated into a sense of self in the present and future (Tucker, 2006). As Adamson (quoted in Moran, 2006, p. 37) states, "There is a secret to recovery from stroke or any other major life problem: Willingness. Willingness to face the facts of what is happening today, and in spite of that, to have the stubborn willingness to continue to fight." Ten years after her stroke, Kate Adamson is still fighting. What is important is the idea of life moving on, not getting stuck in the illness component.

One important component of the illness narrative will be a reference to a past, as a trajectory for the present and future. For example, on an aphasia group on Yahoo, Andrew shares a story of his past or pre-stroke professional identity as a competent and successful optometrist, along with a clear statement of the impact of lost reading and writing language tools that were associated with this identity and his sense of needing help finding a path to the future. And on a Queensland Aphasia Group Web site (n.d.), Arthur's story captures the way in which a life story can be reconstructed to keep past, present, and future consistent with one narrative. His posting also encompasses the four dimensions of self discussed throughout this text.

My name is Arthur Thompson.

I was born on the Isle of Man.

It is situated in the middle of the Irish Sea.

Before my stroke, I was an international project officer.

I was involved in the construction industry and I worked all over the world.

My most interesting time was working in Africa.

I had a stroke in 1996 which left me totally speech paralysed.

For the first time in my life, I now have the freedom to spend time on myself . . . and on the things I really want to do . . . instead of working.

My wife Nina and I established the "World Reforestation Project" in 1991.

My interest and Aim is to promote the WRP.

As I do not speak, I use a voice simulator. This is controlled through my computer. This allows me to communicate.

Thank GOD for this wonderful technology.

I make speeches to Service clubs and sailing clubs etc.

My hobbies are: sailing, photography, creating drift wood designs and things environmentally friendly.

Some persons with aphasia remain locked into their past, unwilling or unable to move their life stories into a present that includes the aphasia. In Dennis's story, told earlier, his past represented the height of professional success and responsibility. At age 40, he was approaching the peak of his career, and this fact was a critical part of his image of self. Thus it is not surprising that he remained almost obsessed with the loss of who he was 3 years ago and with his relative youth. At one point in a support group meeting, he indicated that he was embarrassed to go out because others who knew him before would see him and pity him or humiliate him. For him, participation in the support group has begun to provide him with important validation in the present, although the future continues to seem filled with hopelessness. In part, his transition into some present tense storying of self can be attributed to the response of support group members. When Dennis has discussed his past, members have acknowledged the importance of his professional success and recognized him for that. However, they are much more interested in his present, the self who he projects in the meetings, and he is constantly validated for that self. Often, group members have told Dennis what they see and hear when he is sharing. It is clear that he is surprised by the positive feedback based on his present self.

Like Dennis in some ways, Harry is struggling to move beyond the narrative self of his past. He describes that past in terms that capture his sense of power, of agency, of competence in his professional successes as a case manager for the chronically mentally ill.

> Well I was working very active in my job and friendships and theatre and very active in the community. I was working with groups of people on issues like assertiveness skills in the community, stress, groups about people divorcing and how to get through that. . . . And I felt very successful in doing that and lots of feedback of success and being successful at my jobs. In working with mentally ill people at that time, I retained my ability fully intact in how to interact with mentally ill people and help them. There was a feeling of success in several areas.

Keep in mind the fact that Harry continues to have auditory comprehension challenges that limit his ability to engage in sustained communicative interactions. In interviews for this text, Harry was unable to talk directly about the self of the past versus the self of the present. However, in a separate informal conversation, he began to share his feelings about his present self, describing the challenge of "reorientation of self" as a "huge and varied process." He went on to say that "I remember who I am and I'm having to almost start over with who I am." In fact, the impact on life story is most evident in Harry's statement that "It is hard to deal with two different histories—one of remembrance and the other is starting over—there is disorientation."

In this conversation, Harry also began to talk about some of his present perceptions of self, including his sense of "frailness" that is manifest in small everyday challenges like dropping things. It is interesting that he focuses on a physical challenge, given the fact that the majority of his challenges are cognitive and linguistic. He also said, "I see myself now as an 'old handicapped personality.'" Although age has never been an issue in the past, it is one now in the context of his stroke-related disabilities. Finally, he acknowledges that he has trouble focusing on what he is, on his strengths, while at the same time having a "standard reaction to people who treat me as less than I was or they are." Clearly, Harry's life story is somewhat stuck in the past, and he uses stories to focus the attention of others on that pre-stroke past self.

Life Span

Harry's altered perception of self to include a critical component as old and frail reminds us once again of life span issues in coping with aphasia. Acquisition of aphasia at 33 years of age is vastly different from the experience at 83 years of age. One is not in any manner "worse" than the other, but the expectations associated with different life stages affect one's response to the disorder. For example, younger persons with aphasia may be those with active careers and work lives, and with children still in the home. Older persons with aphasia may be retired but active in different types of family interactions, as well as community roles and groups. If one could hypothetically envision a 33-year-old and an 83-year-old as experiencing the same aphasic symptoms, society would typically view the impact of the aphasia on the 33-year-old as much more devastating. Further, in virtually all contexts, the younger person would be seen as more competent and capable of achieving greater independence than the older person. In the health care environment, age may influence access to health care and the quality of daily communicative interactions. The latter is particularly alarming considering how important social interactions are in the process of self definition.

When confronted with the fact that aphasia will be present for the rest of their lives, some younger persons view this as even more reason to improve. Others, such as Dennis, view this as a life sentence. At his first support group meeting, he indicated: "I became unconscious feeling like a 22-year-old and woke up feeling like an 82-year-old and I still feel that way." As he looked around the room and recognized that most of those present were considerably older than he, it was clear that he was struggling with how to belong (and perhaps whether he even wanted to belong). He was comforted to learn that there were many who had survived 10 to 14 years post-stroke, but that reality also filled him with a kind of terror, faced with many more years of "nonexistence." Acknowledging this fear, he noted: "If I were older, it might be okay. I just can't face a long future with all of this" (pointing to body and head).

Younger persons with aphasia (or their significant others) often emphasize their age when first sharing elements of their life story, often with a sense of outrage at the unfairness of the illness. Such life span issues must not be ignored in managing aphasia and its life consequences. It is also important to explore the individual's perspective on her life story. We must remember that, with advanced age, people sometimes refashion their personal myths to ensure that there is something of significance and importance that has occurred with the living of their lives. This brings us to the topic of control and agency.

Themes in Illness Narratives

Control, Agency, and Related Constructs

When they first came in, they were defining themselves by their disabilities. After a few months they're excited about their capabilities. These are things that they were doing—they weren't even doing this before the stroke. Their whole self esteem has improved (Tucker, 2006).

While on the surface, this quote appears to be about self-esteem, it is also tapping into a more fundamental issue of the importance of a sense of competence and agency in the process of writing a new life story. Some of the contrasting terms used to describe this domain include disability versus ability, incompetence versus competence or mastery, stigma and exclusion versus acceptance and inclusion, weakness versus strength, and dependence or powerlessness versus independence, agency, control, and autonomy. While there are probably theoretical distinctions between these paired terms, they can be viewed as reflections of an underlying construct related to agency. Certainly, agency is threatened when aphasia impairs an individual's ability to communicate. In fact, issues of competence or incompetence are always close to the surface for individuals living with aphasia.

Aphasia's abrupt onset and associated problems allow no time for adjustment to gradually dwindling skills. Instead, the person with aphasia is confronted with the challenge of "getting better" in the limited time frame dictated by the medical community (which often offers the hope of recovery only for 6 months or a year). They are also exposed to a medical environment that tends to depersonalize people and that emphasizes weakness, disability, and dependence, the "sick" role rather than the "healthy" one (Kovarsky, Duchan, Mastergeorge, & Nichols, 2003). Not surprisingly, most persons living with aphasia continue to struggle with their sense of competence in the months and years post-stroke. Challenges to one's sense of control and autonomy range from the frustrations of being told that driving is no longer an option to the very real inability to express one's needs and feelings in important situations. Attempts to rebuild narrative self based upon perceptions of disability and incompetence are doomed to failure.

Most of the people living with aphasia who informed this chapter have commented on their sense of incompetence and powerlessness. It is in many ways a universal refrain. Doreen stated,

Well it isn't like feeling in control. It's just that this is me my person. This is what I'm doing.

Both Dennis and Harry refer to the perception that they are being treated like children. Harry's elaboration on these experiences is a direct reflection of his premorbid strong personality and his need for a sense of agency and success.

And one of the nurses came in there and reprimanded me for doing that and I just felt hopeless at that point I was being controlled without knowing why or what I'd done wrong . . .

I . . . as the therapy went on I remember at times becoming angry and frustrated—frustrated for some of the complaints of beginning to feel like I was treated like a child. There was one instance when I was being taken down a hall or a runway or . . . at the end one of the nurses dragged me by the shirt and started pulling me faster than I could go. That made me angry and that was combined with that childish "now Harry you have to do this . . . " and suddenly this strong, or relatively strong feeling of anger or indignation. And I pulled back and said or thought this at least, "I'm not a child." At the time I didn't understand what happened next. I was put into a room with a cage on top and I didn't know why they had put me in there because it was really uncomfortable and felt not just like a child but like a caged animal without knowing why. Much later I associated that with the nurse pulling on me and me pulling back, it was like shrugging away. And maybe I was told as being resistive or something like that.

Spirituality and Religion

Themes of control and agency are probably also linked to other common topics in the illness narrative. For example, in some cultures, it is common to find stroke survivors and their families discussing the comfort of their faith and the way in which the spiritual parts of their lives allow them to move forward. For these persons, spirituality is one part of the cultural tool kit that remains unscathed and can be brought to bear on one's new life circumstances. A belief in a divine spirit can be important in coming to terms with life changes that appear to rob us of agency. However, there are also some who struggle to reconcile the way in which their world has been turned upside down with respect to a belief in a caring, involved God. Harry reflects on his beliefs and his mortality, saying:

> Having grown up with a belief system of a God and a caring God, I, while I was in the hospital, was not aware of my concerns about that . . . I began to . . . I had a thought of one of the psalms of the valley of death and feeling that there was so much sense of being loved and taken care of for most of our life and then begin to realize what my theology was doing. And I began to get angry and frustrated at the idea of a god that had lied to me about god being there to take care of me . . . and I think some of that had to do with a long-term feeling of being abandoned as a child and that . . . god had abandoned me.

Liechty (2006, p. 33) also notes: "I had difficulty identifying and interacting with the sacred, and again I felt isolated." And in a support group meeting, Dennis raises questions about whether or not God intended what happened to him, whether or not he was supposed to learn something from this experience. The group discussion was tentative, given the fact that no one wanted to dismiss faith or faith-based belief systems. At the end of the discussion, Dennis indicated that he and God had made peace. Later, in talking alone with the group facilitator, he acknowledged that he had not been totally honest, and that he had indeed been very angry with God.

Recognition and Respect

Agency and control may be internally perceived but they are also essentially socially validated phenomena. Not surprisingly, in all of the narratives that provided the data for this chapter, a common refrain was the need for the recognition and respect of others in coping with aphasia. While all humans need the respect of others, it becomes even more important when an individual suffers loss of one or more skills that she considers to be part of who she is. Clearly, communication is one of those skills. Persons living with aphasia often share stories of not being respected in various circumstances, including interactions with health care providers, friends and family members, and strangers. Dennis talks about "giving a hard time" to a speech-language pathologist, explaining "I'm still a grown man. I don't deserve to be treated like a child." Others note that disrespect or outright dismissal isolated them when they most needed the support of others. Harry speaks of respect frequently:

> There was an awareness fairly early on that I began to realize that I wanted to be respected and treated as an adult because there was the awareness that I was a mature man and of an expectation of being treated as an adult . . . At first I couldn't get to the bathroom and when I found a way to slip through the cage a nurse came there and scolded me as I said and I said to her, "I am a grown man, not a child," and I felt humiliated and scolded at that point. And . . . it was interesting because the nurse stopped and thought for a moment and said, "I understand that now, Mr. Shadden."

His sense of the loss of respect during the months post-stroke leads him, in virtually every social encounter (even with virtual strangers), to challenge others to acknowledge him as his pre-stroke self—funny, smart, competent, life experienced. He demands respect for the pre-stroke past, even though the present Harry is different in many ways.

Recognition and respect can become issues within families, since doubts about the competence of the individual with aphasia may permeate all interactions and life plans. Doreen talks about how others, including her husband, did not seem to realize she was aware of what was going on, " . . . don't think they thought I had any [awareness]. This this this wasn't a happy time in any respect. Well it isn't like feeling in control. It's just that this is me my person. This is what I'm doing." Clearly, the perceived lack of respect angered her.

Acceptance and Understanding

Recognition and respect are associated with, but not equivalent to, acceptance and understanding by others. Regardless of the source of acceptance, it is extremely powerful when people are struggling with the isolating consequences of aphasia. Marie Putman writes a column in a local newspaper. Her husband's stroke was, on the surface, relatively mild, and they had been living with its consequences without any real support. About their first support group meeting she writes:

> But it was our first visit to a stroke support group that gave the hope and help we needed. Here were people who understood, not only his physical limitations, but his emotional needs. They allowed him to talk, to tell his story. They listened and verified everything he was feeling (M. Putman, personal communication, March 11, 2007).

She goes on to say:

> The moment we walked into that room, we found hope. A group of people who

had been there let us talk. They smiled and nodded their heads. Yes, they would say again and again to our confused questions. You've found the answer, they confirmed. Stroke does cause depression. As we saw men who bore the evidence of a crippling stroke, some as many as ten years ago, we began to believe, you can continue to improve. And you don't have to live in terror about statistics which give percentages of having another stroke . . . The group gave us literature and information. But most of all they gave us understanding. When we would go into our separate groups my small group of women encouraged me to talk. How do you feel? What are you going through? I remember how much I felt like crying that first meeting. I was no longer alone or had to feel isolated and keep my thoughts and feelings to myself. Talk. Talk. Get it out. Those sweet caregivers didn't make me feel guilty. They understood because they'd gone through it before me. Month after month, we received the same loving consideration. Our needs were important (M. Putman, personal communication, March 11, 2007).

While Marie's words related specifically to the power of support groups, they also identified the importance of being understood and accepted in living with aphasia. On the Aphasia Hope Web site, David Douglas Allard also writes about the power of friendship.

> When my friends came over to see me and they saw me with tubes attached to my body they smiled. I smiled back. They reminded me that they still held a place for me in their heart and souls. They started to talk. I listened but I could not follow them. I had to say

something but no matter how I tried the words just would not come, so I curled back and listened quietly.

That is how I came to understand my own life better

And Barbara Newborn (1997) writes: "On the whole I've learnt to come to terms with myself. Everyone deserves the chance to be accepted for themselves."

Dennis also has issues of acceptance. He is afraid of everything and everyone, and his fear is associated with experiences of being rejected by former peers. Ironically, Dennis believes that older people might understand his experience better, but they probably will not want to be friends with a younger person like himself. So he feels totally alone, isolated from those he would consider peers and from those who might grasp what he is feeling.

Finally, the previously described family who traveled 400 miles to attend a support group illustrate themes of understanding and acceptance. Prior to attending their first support group meeting, the family met with the group facilitator. Throughout that meeting, each family member gave full attention to the father's efforts to communicate, because they knew his communication was at the heart of who he was. They knew that they needed to find ways to help the father/husband, because his aphasia had disrupted the life stories of the entire family.

These stories illustrate that selves are fundamentally social, as we have argued throughout this book. One can have a sense of persistent self, but without a "looking-glass self" (Cooley, 1902), we may feel that we have no self at all. Certainly, to have a self with agency who is able to rewrite a post-stroke life story and eventually to get beyond an illness narrative, one needs the validation of others. We will see the importance of these themes in the following.

The Importance of Others in the Illness Narrative

Ideally, if there were a simple way of predicting which people matter in the lives of persons with aphasia, and what social situations are important, treatment could be much more focused. Cruice, Worall, and Hickson (2006) explored the regular social contacts and activities of older persons with chronic aphasia, contrasting these with healthy older adults. For adults with aphasia, there was a considerable range of social contacts and activities, but the actual number of contacts was fewer and less satisfying. Thus each person living with aphasia has priorities about which people are most important and what activities are most valued.

Most families living with aphasia describe some degree of abandonment by friends and even family members post-stroke. Some social others feel uncomfortable with the communication barriers created by aphasia. An even more common experience is the negative response of strangers—restaurant servers, sales clerks, and so on. Often, the person with aphasia is simply ignored, and the loss of communicative connection and even basic eye contact and recognition conveys a powerful message of stigma and incompetence. On other occasions, the conversational partner may begin using a kind of "elderspeak" (Melton & Shadden, 2006), increasing loudness, exaggerating intonation, simplifying statements, and repeating, without giving the person time to process. Again, the person with aphasia feels diminished by these interactions.

What may be most important is understanding the lived social experiences of each individual. Wayne, a long-term stroke survivor, enjoys social experiences, valuing the bonds with others and deriving satisfactions from the interactions. He appears to feel accepted by others and at peace with his aphasia, at least most of the time. In contrast, for Harry, every moment around people is a challenge and there is little discrimination between people and situations. The stranger passing on the street or the hotel clerk appears at least as significant as family and friends. This indiscriminant need for recognition sets him up for failure, and he is often disappointed in his social contacts, and people's responses are frequently nonvalidating. It is a tribute to his powerful personality that he continues to experience some successes in this rather random process of seeking social validation.

Those social contexts, situations, and people that matter often change in the months and years post-stroke and -aphasia. An individual who is frustrated by being ignored in public settings at one time may accept and ignore such encounters 6 months later. Certainly, Harry has gone through a number of stages characterized by which social others matter at different points in time. About one early time in the hospital, he says,

> I was not unhappy about the care of the nurses. It seemed like they were doing their routines and doing their jobs but nobody coming around to be friendly. And it didn't seem to bother me at the time, I was so out of it.

Several years later, when hospitalized for an unrelated problem, he became infuriated with the nurses' failure to make the time to communicate with him.

Clearly, family interactions are priorities for most persons with aphasia. The failure of a family member to recognize and accept the new reality of a person with aphasia may be hurtful in the early months post-stroke. Over time, as life stories evolve and one's sense of identity is renegotiated to encompass living with aphasia, the behaviors of the same family member can be put into perspective and are consequently less painful. Those who work and live with persons with aphasia must constantly take stock of these changing perceptions and realities.

Loneliness, or at least a sense of being alone, is common. As Harry suggests,

> There may be a theme of aloneness—not sure I became aware that I was spending time alone and I did care about that.

Doreen also speaks about feeling alone. While she sees herself as independent, a loner who does not need many people in her life, she is also frustrated and perhaps hurt by what she perceives as her husband's failure to be there for her, particularly while she was hospitalized.

> He never brought a dinner over so we could be together and I'd say maybe they'd let me walk, you could take me for a walk around . . . nearby or something like to let me know I'm a real . . . really alive person.

When we talk about others in the construction of a post-stroke narrative, however, we must pay attention to the fact that the narrative is typically cowritten with a significant other and often with other caregivers. It is important to understand how aphasia affects these people as well.

Perspectives from Caregivers and Significant Others

Aphasia is indeed a family illness (Buck, 1963, 1964). When the life story of a loved one is disrupted, along with the communication tool needed to make sense of that disruption, a similar disruption in life story and narrative self occurs in the lives of caregivers, often spouses or adult children. As Marie Putman (personal communication, March 11, 2006) writes:

> You can be a joyful caregiver if you know it will only be a few weeks. But most illnesses go on for years, and the time is unknown. That's the hard part. An ill person increasingly becomes dependent on the one taking care of them; they find it harder and harder to make decisions or go places alone . . .
>
> Jerry is reading everything he can find on the subject. But Jerry is so alone. And so am I. It's scary. We want answers. I complain and withdraw some more. My Christian sisters pray for me. My family and friends care. [In the stroke support group . . .] Month after month, we received the same loving considerations. Our needs were important.

Communication deficits can have a major impact on the care providers' "lived experience" of the relationship with the stroke survivor (Sundin, Norberg, & Jansson, 2001). Marie calls attention to the erroneous assumption that quality of life impact is related directly to severity of aphasia, writing:

> People often say, 'Oh, that person only had a mild stroke.' Don't believe them. Even if it's a doctor saying that. A stroke is a stroke. It not only affects the patient but the family as well.

In one case study, Shadden (1999) reported that daily caregiver fatigue and stress influenced the post-work communicative exchanges between spouse and person with aphasia. Specifically, high daily stress was associated with more spousal initiation of conversational turns and comparable levels of transactional and interactional behaviors. In contrast, high levels of fatigue were associated with higher levels of responding (vs. initiating) behavior and more transactional than interactional communications. These results underscore the complex interaction of factors that influence spousal communication with a person with aphasia.

Some (perhaps many) caregivers live with the fear of being judged for their behaviors and decisions in caregiving, and many recognize that their daily lives are poorly understood by others, even family members. For example, one new support group member shared the story of her husband's five strokes. With great anger, she described how none of the therapists helped him at all. Her husband was in a nursing home, and she proceeded to explain that "he doesn't mind. He understands" with respect to this placement. Further, she elaborated on the fact that her husband appeared unmotivated to improve, and indicated that the stroke must have affected his "don't' care" brain. It is apparent that she continues to struggle with the decision to use long-term care, blaming others and the stroke for putting her in this position.

While Doreen focused repeatedly on her husband's perceived failure to treat her as a person, her husband literally felt hopeless in the early weeks post-stroke. A relatively private person, he began sharing some of his concerns and feelings about his wife's behavior with colleagues, friends, and professionals, seeking help in understanding what was happening. Just as she blamed him for refusing to recognize her and validate her as the person she was and still is, he had no tools for relating to the person she had become, however briefly.

While it is easy to take sides in such situations, there is never a clear right or wrong, good or bad, culpability or blamelessness. The only way professionals can help people living with aphasia, including significant others, is by focusing on their life stories and on the manner in which the aphasia has disrupted the self and its narrative expression at all levels. Professionals must probe what caregivers have been told and what hope has been offered (or withdrawn). While stories of caregivers are those of both true emotional heroism and despair, the vast majority reflect good people doing the best that they can with a difficult situation. Further, there are many more stories about significant others helping the person with aphasia coconstruct their life stories and repair the narrative self damaged by loss of communication. These stories are told less frequently, but we have much to learn from them (Sundin et al., 2001).

Bill suffered a massive left hemisphere middle cerebral artery stroke that left him without speech and with extremely limited mobility. Despite these facts, Bill and his wife Rachel consistently displayed their love and support for each other over many years post-stroke. At a support group meeting, Rachel was asked how she managed the difficult changes in their lives. She appeared genuinely surprised by the question. After some reflection she said, "I don't really feel that anything important has changed. We've been together for 52 years, and he's still the same man I married. And he doesn't need to talk for me to understand what he is thinking." Bill was then asked how he coped with not being able to communicate through words. He pointed to his wife and began to cry. When the facilitator asked if he was upset because of communication difficulties with his wife, he shook his head no, and pointed to his head, then hers. Rachel immediately said, "It's what I told you. We don't need words." Bill smiled and patted her hand. This is a wonderful love story. It also underscores the primary theme of this text—the need for validation of narrative self. Rachel and Bill continued to maintain their shared life stories because they continued to see the essential self that had continued despite the stroke.

Clearly, others matter in the framing of the illness narrative and the ongoing storying of self. In some instances, support may be derived from engagement in larger groups and communities that provide a mechanism for social reframing of self.

Groups and Communities

A sense of community is important in the social grounding of the experience of aphasia. The power of community is evidenced in the success of facilities such as Connect (London, UK), the Pat Arato Aphasia Center (Toronto, Canada), and the Aphasia Center of California. Each of these facilities and agencies provide, in addition to special services and programs, an environment for belonging. Thus, a community can be as small and casual as the Friday morning coffee hour of four retired men in a retirement community or as large and extensive as the National Aphasia Association's membership and outreach. Membership in groups and communities can also be formal or informal. Groups and communities allow us to share who we are in the context of a common agreed-upon reality (Shotter, 2003, 2005). Within groups, countless "minute social systems" (Goffman, 1959, p. 67) exist, and these systems are organized to support the self-expression that is critical to storying of self. Thus, groups provide environments in which we can become interactively responsible to and for others (Shotter, 2003. It is not surprising that Alter (2006) has referred to the magic of groups and others have described these in therapeutic terms (Shadden & Agan, 2004; Shadden & Koski, 2007).

Stroke and aphasia support groups have proliferated in recent years. There are also growing numbers of on-line stroke and/or aphasia discussion groups and forums (e.g., the Stroke Network, http://www.strokenet work.org). One value of on-line support communities is that they provide social connectedness at almost any time, on almost any topic. For some, an additional benefit is the relative anonymity of the process. Other participants know as much or as little as the person wishes. A posting can be responded to quickly or ignored. One's personal reactions to what others say can be hidden. Thus an on-line community provides the access to the insights and understandings of others who share the experience of living with aphasia, while placing control for the sharing of personal information and reactions in the hands of the person living with aphasia. On-line self-help communities support interactive communication in socially validated ways that reduce the requirements for flexibility, timing, and fine tuning in conversation.

On-line discussion groups are not available to all, since many persons living with aphasia are not comfortable with computers and the Internet, in part because of generational differences in exposures to technology. In addition, support groups in general are resisted by some individuals, for a variety of reasons. Some individuals do not wish to adopt a new identity as a person with aphasia or a person with stroke. They are working to overcome that part of their altered self, and the support group encourages them to do the opposite, to embrace this new part of their life story. Others feel the need for community but find it elsewhere, such as church involvement. One person whose husband has experienced multiple strokes steadfastly refused to consider attending a stroke support group, indicating that such programs "are not for me." Ironically, she was willing to attend a support group for caregivers of persons with Alzheimer's disease, noting that she felt she "could be of some use" to participants.

Why are support groups so important to some persons living with aphasia? That question is answered, in part, in Chapter 4, particularly through Rappaport's (1993) theoretical perspective on support group processes. Personal narratives are somewhat private, linked with identity and self development, maintenance and change. In contrast, support groups provide a kind of community narrative. Thus by joining a group, individuals living with aphasia can explore opportunities for reframing narrative self, a process that occurs through communication of individual and shared stories. It is the merging of private and public stories that is so important. For example, in the presence of new participants in a support group, existing members often introduce themselves by sharing their stroke experience. In such setting, this telling and retelling serve vital functions (Holland, 2007), including validating the person's membership in the stroke or aphasia community and welcoming others to share their experiences as well. Further, one's choice of illness narrative provides others with insight into member perceptions and can reveal critical matches or mismatches between the perceptions and expectations of the person with aphasia and her loved one.

Marie Putman (personal communication, May 12, 2007) has been quoted elsewhere describing her experience in a stroke support group. One additional comment is included here:

> The most wonderful help for survivors of stroke and their caregivers are support groups. In a support group, the

survivor along with the caregiver receive hope as they are able to tell their story and be heard. They are listened to and verified with understanding and compassion. At a support group the caregiver is able to voice their concerns and frustrations and begin to grasp what the stroke victim has experienced during and after their stroke.

Over and over again in this particular group, caregivers comment on what they have learned from other stroke survivors (not their loved ones).

The comments of a new member after her first session capture the need to be with others who can understand and validate one's experiences. She described her lack of success of finding such a group in the city where she lived previously, indicating, "I just wanted to be with people who understand." She then commented at length about her husband's inability to talk about her stroke, even though he was by her side constantly in the hospital. Dennis's comments about the group are also relevant. During his first session, he explained that he had come to the group to learn, ask questions, and see if there was anyone like him. As the meeting progressed, he began to realize that all strokes are very different, but there is a common thread or bond that can be shared. Thus at the end of the first session, he indicated:

> That's what I have missed the last 3 years —having a family, someplace where I belong . . . Finding out there are others like me—I can't believe it—it's like a dream come true. I'm comfortable with these people. They understand. They look at me and don't see a freak.

Most importantly, Dennis stated: "I'm not the same . . . Okay, so I have to accept that

I can't be the same, but *we* sure want it." Notice the powerful transition to the term "we," an indicator of steps in embracing membership in this community.

On most occasions, support groups provide exactly what Rappaport (1993) suggests, a place where the communication of stories helps give meaning to the experience and provides opportunities for others to validate each other. It is hard to imagine a more important experience for those struggling to move forward with life with aphasia. Thus it is best to close with an e-mail from the family who drove so far to attend the support group:

> Thank you for talking with us before the stroke support group meeting yesterday. After the meeting, Daddy was laughing and talking up a storm. Not sure what all he was saying, but we didn't care if he was happy. Driving back today, he started to get mad when he couldn't say something right, then just sort of shrugged as if to say, "oh, well." I think Mom got the best night sleep she has had in all this time, maybe because she felt a little hope. The people in your group are wonderful. We don't know what went on when the family members went to another room, but the fact that Daddy didn't want to end the "conversation" says a lot. We'll be back next month for sure.

Communication Treatment and Tools

One interesting part of the process of storying of self is the relative contribution of treatment (in this case, speech-language therapy) to moving on with one's life story. In today's treatment climate, life participation receives considerable focus, so treatment goals are being framed to emphasize restoring a sense of agency and competence in some settings. However, availability of extended treatment past the first few months post-stroke is limited, and many turn to on-line forums for support and suggestions for ongoing improvement.

Persons with aphasia share tales of success and failure in speech-language therapy. For example, Harry reflects on his interactions with all of his therapists, including their centrality to his positive feelings and his sense of abandonment when he went home. In the following quote, he notes the fact that his therapists had apparently been very validating of him and his efforts while he was in treatment. So the obvious pain he felt at the lack of contact after discharge was related to feeling that the previous interactions had not been authentic.

And the therapist would work very patiently for that 90 minutes or whatever it was, not scolding or anything like that, but just encouraging and pointing out successes that I made at small points. I began to feel that my therapists were proud of me and they were friends of mine. And when that therapy ended, I was very very hurt to realize that that was not candid—I became more and more aware that that was a job they were doing and that the friendship part ended pretty abruptly. I remember expecting to have a social life having dinner with a therapist or something. And one therapist did have lunch between me and her husband or boyfriend and expecting that to happen more and then gradually finding out that I was pretty much back alone again except for you caring about me and spending time with me. And that was very important during that period of time.

When asked to reflect on what could have been done differently to reduce his sense of abandonment, Harry suggests:

There may be something that needs to be done in terms of that transition period, because I went from being interested in the therapy and eager for the next session of whatever it was, male or female therapists, to that leaving the hospital and the feeling of abruptness. The contrast was unsettling. Maybe having the therapist do some follow-up more—either coming by or calling. At the time when I could at least understand, I couldn't dial a phone to call somebody but maybe a call from the therapist just saying "Harry I'm missing you" or "How ya doing" and being authentic about that . . . a phone call, a card not necessarily a greeting card, a letter a brief statement some connections there from going to successful to no process the feeling of no process, even though I may have been making progress at the time.

While these suggestions may not be realistic or even possible, they underscore the importance of professionals in the lives of persons with aphasia. More importantly, they highlight the fact that, at least for persons living with aphasia, clinical interactions and treatment efficacy are often measured in terms of support for the narrative self. As Hinckley (2007) suggests, the speech-language pathologist is a partner in a clinical discourse process that may be at least as important as any impairment-based therapy activities.

In Section IV, the implications of a clinical perspective on narrative self will be discussed in greater detail. Our discussion of the four dimensions of self, and our focus on life stories, interfaces seamlessly with current practices and models. For some persons with aphasia, treatment may involve facilitation of the use of communicative tools. In discussing ALS, communicative tools were featured prominently at the end of Chapter 6. Questions raised related primarily to why some persons embrace augmentative and alternative communication (AAC), and others reject it completely. Issues of fluidity, spontaneity, timing, and personal style were described as influencing willingness to use AAC. These issues are equally important for persons with aphasia, but the challenges are very different (Hux, Manasse, Weiss, & Beukelman, 2001). Since the onset of aphasia is abrupt, there is no opportunity to gradually acquire the skills needed in using AAC. Further, aphasia is essentially an impairment of the ability to use language symbols, and AAC systems rely on some degree of symbolic representation to convey meanings. Thus, traditional AAC devices may not be effective with some persons with aphasia.

Use of computers and Internet technologies was described earlier as opening up opportunities for communication and life storying. In addition, the Internet is one vast information resource. In fact, the National Aphasia Association Web site addresses the possibilities inherent in technological tools, noting that technology can change lives and that computers do not demand responses (unlike some people). The need for portability of devices and independence in using them is highlighted on this Web site. However, persons with aphasia cannot immediately use such tools without careful, individualized training.

This point is well illustrated by an experience years ago in a hospital. A speech-language consult was requested and the clinician was informed at the nursing station that the patient was uncooperative and resistant to intervention. Immediately after she entered the patient's room, he looked up and threw a handheld communication device at her. The device required the user to spell out messages using a small alphabetical keyboard. Sadly, no one at the hospital had realized that this patient's aphasia had left him unable to spell as well as talk. Whenever a new staff member entered the room and urged him to use his device, his frustration mounted.

Throughout this text, reference has been made to other types of animate and inanimate tools that may be available in one's cultural tool kit to support communication and the presentation of the narrative self. Such tools include significant others who can be used to coconstruct one's story, as well as artifacts (pictures, personal items), simple notebooks, and vehicles for sharing basic information. Technology may enhance personal sharing in others ways, such as exchanges of pictures and personal information. Clearly, those with aphasia need other people in their lives to help them communicate (Liechty, 2006). There are no quick communicative fixes, just as there are no immediate cures for the language deficit that has set up roadblocks to the process of moving forward with one's life story. Tools must be used to address the challenges to self found with respect to one's cultural status, roles, interactions, and biography. A primary goal must be restorying of self over time. Part of restorying of narrative self involves reassertion of a sense of control or agency with respect to one's life.

Moving Forward

In Chapter 4, life story, illness narrative, and biographical accommodation were presented in a circular schematic. For persons with aphasia, illness narratives are a step toward biographical accommodation, toward moving forward with one's life. For some, it may be something as simple as rediscovering ways to engage in former hobbies such as woodworking. As a spouse living with a husband with aphasia, Rene has taken up painting, a lifelong desire, and is filling her time productively with classes and producing art. For others, it is finding meaning in helping new stroke survivors, exemplified in Wayne's simple statement, "We are still here so . . . we do what we can . . . we give back . . . people stroke people need help." For yet others, it may be finding a way to return to work, perhaps in a different capacity.

It can be difficult to identify when illness narrative ends and the biographical accommodation necessary to reweaving this narrative into the larger life story begins. Harry speaks about the months and years post-stroke, picking up the threads of his life story defined almost exclusively in terms of the impact of the stroke and communication impairments:

> I began aware . . . became aware that I was spending time alone and I did care about that. So it was somewhere about that period of time of being back from the hospital and the therapy to being back home. . . . Anyway, this growing understanding of how different my life was going to be became an issue and depression began to set in and despair and anger all of those things combined. I'm still angry about how people interact with me since I can't speak at full speed or understand what they are saying full speed. I for a long time have made myself go out into public and go to the store and go to a restaurant and interact with people. I have gradually been able to understand sentences and then paragraphs after I went over them a number of times and could . . . now concepts in general.
>
> [In projects at home] For example trying to work on a simple project working with tools something that could have taken me 10 or 15 minutes to accomplish maybe take most of a day and still do it incorrectly. An example would be just trying to make a frame for a map turned out to take many hours and my measurements were off even though . . . I measured things over and over. And I have still made sometimes a difference of two inches off in measuring something. But there is a growing sense of being less impatient with myself increasing the frustrations and at some point I need to talk about things I've done to what I call getting around the stumps ways of functioning in daily life.

For Harry, life continues to be exhausting. Each day is defined in terms of challenges that arise from the consequences of his stroke, and each day raises questions of competence and value, and each challenge becomes a proving ground. While this may be a part of the process of biographical accommodation, he still seems more oriented towards the past—what he used to be and do—than to a present and future living with his altered abilities. However, he actively shares his new life particulars with others, in an effort to present a capable self. He also seeks new challenges that may help him define the way forward.

At the beginning of this chapter, it was suggested that narrative self construction is uniquely challenging in the context of aphasia. Part of the challenge evolves from multiple associated impairments and life changes. More important is the unknown status of self and personhood when communication is abruptly disrupted overnight in seemingly incomprehensible ways. However, the very fact of the unknown, coupled with the promise of some degree of recovery, provides tremendous possibilities of moving forward with life and a self associated with aphasia. In contrast, varying forms of dementia are distinguished from other disorders in this text by the very fact that it is indeed selfhood that is perceived as being steadily erased by the disorder. In the final life stories chapter, we turn to dementia and explore the status of self construction through the course of the disease process for one woman and her children.

CHAPTER 9

Life Stories in Dementia

Nuland (1994) reminds us that diseases are medically described in terms of patterns of physical cause and effect that are traceable to specific pathological changes in cells, tissues, organs, and biochemical processes. When describing death from Alzheimer's disease (AD), he goes on to state that a description of such physical change does little to " . . . chronicle the emotional carnage visited on the families of victims" (p. 92).

Surely the story of AD is one of the most feared of all the neurogenic communication disorders in this section. Why? Kitwood (1997) suggests that early social psychology focused on dependence, mental instability, and the un-being of the individual to such an extent that these became fears that dominated responses to the disease. More basically, the question "Why?" can be answered in terms of selfhood. We fear loss of the person—to themselves and to others. These two aspects of fear are emotional responses that shift from the individual during early stages to that of family and friends as interpersonal life disintegrates. Powell (1988) has said that we remain persons to each other in our memories, shared interpersonally or relived alone yet populated by those others in our lives. As the ability to remember or construct memories with others falls into the abyss of AD, an increasingly fragmented self emerges.

The Present Clinical Context for the Dementias

Several trends in recent years have been responsible for increased attention to the impact of AD on identity and self, for both the person with dementia and loved ones. First, probable AD is being diagnosed earlier in the progression of the disease (Beard, 2004). Thus we are able to communicate directly with those with AD, raising questions about making sense of changes, identity and meaning construction (Beard, 2004; Beck, 2005; Kitwood, 1997), as well as perceptions of self. It is also possible to explore how persons with AD feel others respond to them. Second, the focus on biomedical models of illness in the 20th century has yielded to broader biopsychosocial models (Charon, 2001, 2006; Kitwood, 1997; Langdon, Eagle, & Warner, 2007; Sabat, 2001). These newer models have given rise to intervention approaches, such as Kitwood's person-centered treatment, that emphasize support for the changing personhood of people with dementia. Finally, there is a burgeoning body of research literature on the experiences and needs of caregivers and loved ones in all illnesses, and specifically in the context of dementia. In addition to understanding caregiver stress and burden, it has become important to recognize and understand the impact of disorders such as AD on the life stories and illness narratives of these caregivers (Hinton & Levkoff, 1999; Karner & Bobbitt-Zeher, 2005).

In this chapter, we will first outline the changes in communication and self associated with progressive dementia. We will then introduce Flo Watkins, whose 13-year longitudinal case study material will be used to elaborate changes to the narrative self that can accompany dementia. We talk next about the cultural, role, interactional, and biographical tools for self construction and how these change as Flo progresses through the stages of the disease. As we turn to a consideration of Flo's narrative self, three themes will be highlighted that emerge from her story. The presence of these themes in the life stories of two other aging individuals, living with and without dementia, will be discussed briefly. The chapter will close with a discussion of this question: If the person with progressive dementia can no longer use any of his tools of self construction, does the self remain? We will respond by claiming that something about the self remains until the very end of dementia, but that much of the final story is written by others. We will argue that this differs only in degree from the storying we all do and that all of our stories are cowritten with others. Thus, we return at the end of the chapter to issues of agency and relationships that hinder or facilitate the storying of self. We shall return to the question, is the storying of self inherent in the individual even as tools are lost, or is this a product of the relationships that one has developed?

Communication Impairment Associated with Dementia

In Chapter 2 the dementias, particularly AD, were described as degenerative neurological disorders with a gradual onset and a decline that eventually ends in death from related causes. Cognitive impairments, specifically memory loss, are the most recognized and reported early features of dementia. Thus the cognitive dimension (see Figure 2–1) most specifically characterizes deficits in dementia. However, as dementia deepens, symbolic skills in general become impaired. As a result, all aspects of language can be affected including reading, writing, and other symbol-specific knowledge such as that involved in music and art. Over time, therefore, the impact of dementia broadens to include the linguistic domain and may begin to involve the motor speech systems. Sabat (1991) provided an example of the changes in conversational skills of a 74-year-old female diagnosed with dementia. Her word-finding problems were of major concern to her. Indeed, in the transcript of her conversation, time lapses and circumlocutions were the predominant speech-language disruptions. This individual experienced losses of speech (as motor output), language (as a symbolic system), and cognition (including focused attention and remembering). These domains can be affected singly or in combination, with the profile of deficits reflecting the specific underlying pathology of the dementia.

Within ongoing communication events, difficulty in one domain can influence other aspects of communication. For example, the person with dementia (PWD) may appear to have greater difficulties with memory or attending to the particulars of conversation when apraxia (motor planning) disrupts speech flow. In the attempt to get something said, what the person wanted to say (content) may be lost or abbreviated. The same can be said for Sabat's patient with word-finding problems, reflecting her deficits associated with symbolic language functions. Her combination of language and cognitive issues together decreased her communicative functionality. As a very general statement regarding the course of deterioration in the communication of PWD, the cognitive aspects are first noticeably affected, followed by changes in language organization and content, and perhaps in some but not all cases, speech production issues. If the individual lives long enough, the most common end communicative result is silence with only the occasional meaningful word or phrase.

As has been said in earlier chapters, we refer to narrative as the telling of stories. Changes in narrative processes can be addressed along a hypothetical timeline that involves both the PWD and social others. Time is an element in most stories. Things about distant as well as immediate past events are talked about in typical conversations. During the telling of personal stories, PWD tend to first lose (or not be able to construct) immediate past events but can construct stories about events that happened in the distant past. With time, even this skill is lost so only immediate happenings are talked about. Thus, storytelling is gradually replaced by exchanges of information in the present. Contextualizing this pattern of loss within families can shed light on communication changes that extend beyond the individual. If we accept Sabat's (1991) criterion for successful communication as the fulfillment of purposes negotiated between two or more speakers, as the PWD experiences decreases in storying skills, family and friends may provide the necessary shared elements during communication episodes. In other words, when narratives are viewed as shared constructions of loved ones and PWD, there is a kind of reverse continuum. Initially in joint storying conversational activities, the family member would supply the immediate past elements and would gradually have to add distant elements over time. Finally, during conversational episodes in the later stages of the disease process, family members would be required to provide all aspects of the "joint" storytelling, simply hoping for a glance, nod, or some recognition of the PWD being an interlocutor.

As noted earlier, many persons with AD are being diagnosed earlier in the disease progression. Thus it is possible to examine the perceived impact of communication loss from the perspective of such individuals. One of the most complete and revealing documents of the impact of living with AD can be found in Richard Taylor's (2007) recent book. He reflects frequently on his fears and concerns about loss of language and communication, explaining, "If I don't have words, if I don't have access to words, will I be thinking? How can I know and understand what I'm feeling if I have no words to describe it?" (p. 26). And elsewhere, in describing how others react to him, he notes: "I'm not sure what family and friends expect to hear when they begin a conversation with me. But I do know that somewhere near the end of the conversation many of them say to me 'I just can't believe you have Alzheimer's'" (p. 172). The thoughts and reflections of persons with dementia, particularly early-onset versions of the disorder, can also be found on many on-line forums for persons with AD and their significant others.

The loss of symbolic skills extends beyond the speech and language output features of communication. As is well documented (Gardner, 1975; Vygotsky, 1971), other symbolic forms, such as music and art, are regularly used for communication. These include written versions of language and nonverbal modalities such as music and art. The latter two would both meet the definition of communication suggested above in that the individual is purposefully intertwined with two or more others. A significant difference may be that those others may not all be involved in the immediate action of communication. In the production of music and art, the "other" can be imagined. This is in part what makes art forms symbolic. They constitute a dialogue with unseen but understood others (Bakhtin, 1990). The individual engaged in artistic communication is employing dimensions of self (Chapter 3) to dialogue with and through these same dimensions projected onto imaginary others. The artistic product conveys to others (in the immediate time) what the person who produced the artwork experienced and understood about his subject. Because each product from this point of view is a "telling" it is a story that is being nonverbally communicated. These tellings, such as in the case of verbal-linguistic storytelling, will change and be gradually lost over the course of dementia.

William Utermohlen's chronicling of his progressive dementia through self-portrait is an example of this (Grady, 2006). An artist known for his detailed figurative paintings, his drawings over a 5-year period document the loss of spatial awareness, geometric form, and in the end even the ability to work with color. In the beginning, he reportedly used his paintings to express emotions such as anger and fear. By the end of the series, he had lost all verbal communication and could no longer use any materials associated with his art to create nonverbal symbols. This same progressive loss of symbolic communicative products can occur with any medium from the arranging of food on plates to arranging flowers in vases. The message here is that even the small things in life that become symbolic means of storying are lost in the course of progressive dementia.

Self for Self and for Others in Progressive Dementia

To keep the self alive (metaphorically) is to maintain storying. For PWD and their families, the status of self as the disease pro-

gresses is of paramount concern. Guendouzi and Müller (2006) consider the major theme associated with dementia in Western culture to be loss of self. This same position was earlier stated by Albert and Mildworf (1989) who suggested that it may be more meaningful to conceptualize progressive dementia as a progressive diminution of personhood rather than a cluster of medical symptoms, since this provides a basis for understanding and addressing what is experienced by patients and those with whom they interact. For Kitwood (1997), the issue of self is highlighted when he writes, "So, how do you relate to a Thou who does not act or think like Thou?" (p. 23).

The fact that dementia is indeed a progressive disorder presents unique challenges to all persons living with dementia. Harman and Clare (2006) note that the two dominant themes in interviews with PWD are: "it is going to get worse" and "I want to be me" (p. 484). In the beginning, the patient struggles with obvious disruptions in everyday living routines as schemes, time, space, and objects that depend on remembering where, when, and how to do things are lost. These changes in daily functioning can be frightening for the individual and lead to fears about a possible diagnosis of dementia. A primary concern may be that the person will no longer be himself for himself or for others. In this context, Tappen and Williams (1998) looked for persistence of self in conversational analyses with PWD. While noting that self preservation does continue through the disease progression, they also acknowledged that a failure of others to recognize that selfhood can lead to dehumanizing of dementia patients. Thus, like the other neurogenic communication disorders considered in this book, AD takes away tools that have been used to construct the self. However, unlike the other diseases we have considered, the question is how self might be sustained if none of the tools remain. Thus, rather than considering, at the beginning of the chapter, the cultural, role, interactional, and biographic tools for self construction, as we have done in previous chapters, we will delay that discussion until later. Instead, we turn first to the case of Flo.

The Story of Flo Watkins

Flo Watkins was the oldest of three daughters born during the Great American Depression to a stay-at-home mother married to a father who worked as an assembly plant mechanic. The stories she shared as her earliest memories were of life during the Depression: little food to eat, gathering scraps from garbage cans in the alleys of city restaurants, taking care of her sisters, loving her grandmother. Flo and her family lived in a large Midwestern city and then its suburbs until she was married. She finished high school and wanted to go to college. Instead she married the young man who first claimed her as "his" wife-to-be in the third grade. Like her father, he worked in an assembly plant. Together he and Flo created a family that consisted of seven children. Flo, like her mother, was a stay-at-home wife. She balanced the budget, took care of the elderly in the family, and mothered her children. She was a friendly, open person who talked to everyone and anyone. Her passion was painting and seeing all she could of the United States. In essence, Flo Watkins was no different from many women of her generation, no different from her high school chums, buddies, and TV personalities who would today be in their 80th decade.

Flo was in good health throughout her life. There were no major illnesses or injuries. She was hospitalized only twice, when delivering two of her seven children. Her family health history was remarkable for

dementia. Flo described her beloved grandmother as becoming increasingly childish in her old age, to the point of wandering away and finally not being able to take care of any of her personal needs. The same fate was replayed with her mother, diagnosed as "senile" in her early 70s. All were healthy women whom Flo described as having "lost their minds."

Prior to Alzheimer's Disease

Flo's Children

Flo had her first child, a girl named Bea, at the age of 19. This was followed by a second girl child 2 years later, and then a boy. Four years passed before the second son, and then a third son, a third daughter, and a final son entered the family. Flo always explained her desire for a large family by saying they kept her happy and comfortable because she was never alone and always busy. This is an important point within Flo's historical construction of narrative self because it establishes why loneness may have been an early feature of her dementia. What she most relied on was being surrounded by and a part of the lives of others. This old and established way of being was part of her essential construction of self as a mother and as someone who was loved by others.

As adults, all of Flo's children lived a distance from her, but two remained in the same state. These children, the middle boys, visited her on a regular basis and made sure Mom was all right. Her three daughters lived in three different states, and the oldest (Buzz) and youngest (Bart) sons lived in the same area as the oldest daughter (Bea). Flo visited each child yearly after the death of her husband. From the perspective of the children, Flo was doing well after adjusting to this death. She had an active life. She immersed herself in the much-loved hobby of painting, did needlework, and worked word puzzles when just sitting or visiting in order to keep, in her words, "the mind alive."

Flo's Life

Flo's children grew, married, and left home, but until her husband's death at the age of 57, she had never lived alone. This was a major change in Flo's life reflected by her often stated claim that she always wanted a big family to keep her company. Now in midlife no one else lived in the house. There was no one depending on her, no one to look after, no one to work with to frame everyday life situations. Frequently during the first 5 years of this study, Flo would talk about her relationship with her husband saying, "He always gave me a long leash, but if I got out there too far he was always there to pull me back." She described herself as the energizer while her husband was the rock. He remained a viable part of her life in the stories told and as a mental partner to whom she attributed roles in continued decision making.

During this time, Flo was an active church member with a variety of friends in the community. A weekly correspondent with her daughter, in a letter dated approximately 5 years after her husband's death and before any signs of dementia were noticeable, she chronicles the small activities that were part of her everyday life.

> Page 1. I've been painting and finishing my Christmas presents up. I should get the box off UPS this week. The only excitement in my life is budgeting.
>
> Page 2. Well, I'm going to clean house today and repair Linda's booties. She asked me to do that two years ago. I just found them in my work basket, on the

bottom of course. I have my home study Bible lesson to do. So my day is full.

> Page 4. I've got presents all wrapped and I'll get box off Monday UPS.
>
> Page 5. Well, this is Monday. / [the slash indicates a change in time before the letter was continued] This morning is Tuesday. I got to cleaning the living room and today is Tuesday. I'll listen to news, drink coffee and get ready to write "Happy Birthday."
>
> Page 6. Today I clean another room. I've retired the paint brushes to get this done. I'll take the lower storm window from the door to the lumber yard to get it repaired. I've got to get tape for the box and UPS to pick it up on Friday. Time gets shorter and shorter.
>
> Page 8. This is Friday [a week gone by]. I baby sitted a dog yesterday and all today it looks like. I went to the farm yesterday, checked the house out and read the electric meter. Well, that's about all going on here. It's a beautiful sunny 52 degrees. I'm putting off cleaning the kitchen until afternoon when the sun is back there. Well, that's the news. UPS picked up the box.

Each of Flo's letters from that time period was similar. Rather than being written in one sitting they were a journal of her days, often spanning a week, that served as a conversation with the missing family member. When asked about her habitual letter writing, Flo said they were better than a phone call because you could read them again and again, making you feel that the person was really with you.

Hallmarks of Flo's letters to her family were reminiscences that she included as well as her observations on life. These are particularly salient with regard to narrative self since they communicate "who" Flo is to her self and how this is situated in her worldview. The following samples were taken from the same 10-page letter from which the daily routine was abstracted.

> Page 2. I'm beginning to realize my paintings are reflecting my saving too much. Cluttered paintings are not good.

> Page 5. (Your father) swore you talked by three months. I used to tell him he just understood baby language as you and your sister had your own language for years, even after you spoke our language . . . I believe babies have a language of their own.

> Page 6. One doesn't place furniture. The space rules.

> Page 9. Babies need love no matter who or what the parents are or do or not do. I don't believe the world's doings, human wise, have changed since creation.

> Page 10. It's a wonderful life out there as long as one doesn't get caught in the riptide of life.

Flo's letters tell how she organized her life: cleaning one room of the house each day to make the week flow, painting and sewing, visits friends and relatives, and going around the small town in which she lived. They also reflect the values and beliefs that she regularly shared with others, in a sense her storying of who she was as a person. And finally, from Flo's letters, we know about the roles she filled in life. Flo was primarily a mother and someone who had been a wife. She planned her days, managed her finances, communicated with friends and relatives, took care of herself, and was dedicated to her hobby, painting.

The preceding details of Flo's life pre-AD capture the self she presented to the world and the self that was to be altered with the beginning of dementia. Certainly, the picture presented conveys a wealth of biographical particulars that were part of her self at all times.

First Years of the Slow Descent

The moments when things begin to change in small ways can be some of the most critical times in the lives of persons falling into dementia and their families. It is difficult to know when such changes are the results of normal aging processes associated with shifts in relationship patterns and living conditions as contrasted with neurological impairment (see Chapter 5). Indeed, the critical incidents that mark the onset of perceived change are highly individualized.

Perhaps because of changes associated with widowhood, Flo's slide into dementia was not dramatic or even particularly noticeable to those outside the family. She was still friendly, funny Flo to those who conversed with her in casual contacts. Changes first became noticeable to her children in letters. These had more ramblings and disconnected ideas. The day-by-day chronicle of small activities was lost, and the letters became briefer as well as emptier. Verbal communication also changed. As telephone calls replaced letters, she would no longer simply report what she was going to do, but rather ask questions about what to do. This shift itself represented a marked transition from independence and agency to growing dependence on the input of others in daily activities. While she continued to laugh and make commentary on the quirkiness of life, other emotions were just as potent. She frequently talked of being lonely, wanting to live with her children, and missing her husband. There were tears and silences with each good-bye. Those children who lived near Flo began to say that, "Mom has lost her touch with housekeeping. The place is really a mess though she is always cleaning. She needs to throw some stuff out." And, "Mom just can't finish a painting before starting another one! Her paint room is full of half finished stuff."

The incident that signaled change beyond just loneliness or aging was a Saturday call to her oldest daughter, Bea, from a very irate Flo. The grocer had moved crackers to another shelf and she couldn't find them. On the visit that followed this call, and based on an accumulation of changes over months, it became apparent that Flo was relying on routines to maneuver through everyday life. Shopping was one example of this. Any product that was moved could not be found even with verbal directions from others. The grocer said they always knew to help, so it was no problem for them. But for Flo all the little "lost" things contributed to insecurity that was becoming a part of everyday living.

Following Bea's visit, Flo's children were called together for a discussion of Mom. Thoughts on Mom varied between daughters and sons, and between oldest and youngest. All agreed that she was lonely, but all also agreed that she could still live alone. The youngest son claimed that all Flo needed was to paint more. The middle son's solution was marriage, which he had been working on with no success in changing Mom's mind. The youngest daughter thought Mom just needed more visits and more love. The middle daughter thought it was hypochondria, and the oldest daughter suggested that all wait and see but in the meantime, visit more and make sure friends and neighbors could keep an eye out for Mom.

In the months after this meeting Flo began to report changes in memory and in her sense of space. In the excerpt below Flo talks about this:

My neighbor drives me to church. I could find it (the church), but not the room. She lets me out at the door, but I can never find the room where my ladies' group meets. Now they leave the door open for me, or come looking if I don't show up.

Shortly after this, Bea and her husband decided to have Flo move in with them. They felt that Flo, like her mother and grandmother, was beginning to experience dementia. Therefore, they wanted Flo to feel comfortable in and know her way around their home before she could no longer function. This point of transition marks an important shift in Flo's story. Up to this point, she was the acknowledged definer of herself. Now, for the first time, the perspective of others not only intersected but also began to control aspects of Flo's personhood.

The Middle Years

The middle years of dementia are considered that time after a diagnosis has been made and accepted by others, and during which cognitive functions noticeably decline. Numerous accounts written by professionals, family members, and even persons with dementia depict these changes. For example, in the chronicling of his own dementia, Taylor (2007) speaks of it in this way:

I am starting to fear the coming of the end of me. Not the death of me, but the end of me as I know myself and as others have know me. . . . The consequence of this creeping fear is that I have noticed I have started to pull more into myself. . . . Even before we must withdraw because of the failure of our cognitive processes, we begin to pull into ourselves. (p. 69)

Taylor's wife, who wrote the introduction to his book, says this:

I wish you knew Richard before Alzheimer's disease changed his life and my life. I am so glad you will at least have the chance to get to know him as he was several years ago through the essays that are collected in this book. (pp. xx–xxi)

Flo's children had all accepted the diagnosis of dementia during the early years of her move to Bea's home. Two other children lived in the immediate area. The goal was to have a support system in place for Flo and for Bea during the years in which care would be needed. Changes in Flo during this time period mirror those presented in the research and clinical literature. What will receive focus here is the identity assigned to Flo by her children. Space and routines are two socially shared identity parameters (Hagstrom, 2004; Sarbin, 2005) that are reflective of the cultural self. Both of these will be used to discuss Flo's identity as reflected in the actions of her children.

Buzz, the oldest son, and his wife brought Flo to their house regularly for the first few years of her stay with Bea. As Flo's dementia deepened, these visits became more problematic. Flo could no longer sew, work word puzzles, or paint. Her inability to paint had the greatest repercussions for one son's perceptions of her self and identity. Buzz had never known a time when his mother was not consumed with or preparing for a painting project. He constantly provided materials and topics for painting while Flo visited, but little came of this. At last, 3 years into Flo's dementia, Buzz let her go.

Mom used to paint all the time. We kids always talked about her painting, She always talked about it, smelled like it, heck, even her food tasted like it. I was sure if she would just keep painting she could beat this and finish life okay. I knew she had trouble thinking of something to paint; I could see that. And she didn't use any of the books or pictures I got for her. Well, this past Christmas I got a idea. That was to ask Mom to do a chalk drawing of Santa and his sleigh, like she did when we were kids. The books all say to use familiar things to keep the mind going. I was going to hang that picture on the wall, make it a center piece for the holidays. It was terrible, really terrible. Mom kinda got a sleigh with almost a stick figure for Santa standing next to it. The reindeer were no better. The whole thing looked like something a first grader could do better. It was just terrible . . . and I mean not just the picture but that I finally realized Mom was gone. My mom, the mom I remembered and wanted her to still be was gone.

Shortly after the picture incident, Buzz stopped having Flo over to his house. His visits with her were limited to a short drive once or twice a month. As she lost other skills and her speech became so dysfluent that conversation was difficult, he stopped coming at all. Buzz did not see or talk to his mother for the last 2 years of her life.

Bart, the youngest son, and his wife also had Flo to their house for regular visits. These became increasingly difficult to manage because of Flo's constant movement, even at night, and her inability to orient herself in his house. This resulted in night terrors and agitation that only stopped or lessened when she returned "home" to

Bea's house. Even with all this Bart and his wife remained in Flo's life.

> She's not the Mom I grew up with, but hey, I'm not the son she raised all those years. I've got lost a time or two myself. Like Buzz, I thought Mom just needed to paint. Said that from the get-go when we all started talking about this thing. I don't know. She isn't Mom the way Mom was, but she is still my Mom and will be until the day either she or I die. So, I make the best of each visit. A visiting nurse helped us rearrange the bedroom in our house that Mom uses. We learned to change the way light comes in, stay on the same routine that Bea uses at home, same foods presented in the same way, and we talk to Mom. She jabbers a lot . . . sometimes it is pretty clear and makes sense, but other times she just can't get those darn words out. She'll just say, "mumble, mumble . . . Damn!" And then she laughs. She laughs at herself, at us, with us. That's Mom.

Ending

While the middle years of dementia bring with them shifts in identity, the ending period of time is a focus on self from the perspective of the family as well as, we will argue, the individual. A key question and concern is where the person with dementia spends his final months, weeks, or days. When the person with dementia becomes a danger to himself or to the family, placement in an assisted care facility is considered. Those are the "facts," but the narrative that goes with this choice is about the identity and self of the person. If the person no longer knows family members or himself, the narrative of care changes. An excerpt from Flo's daughter reflects this time.

Mom doesn't know who she is. We couldn't figure out for the longest time what she was talking about . . . her talk doesn't make much sense these days and sometimes she just stumbles over words. Any how, she kept asking who that lady was in her room. We thought she was talking about the new weather-girl on TV. We keep the TV on in her room during the day and in the evening so she is not alone. While that seemed to be the answer, at least for us, after a while that just wasn't right. Mom would wake up in the middle of the night, screaming and afraid of "that woman." She would be terrified and run out of the bedroom some mornings almost as soon as her eyes were open, again terrified of "that woman." No matter how smoothing we were, how we talked about there not being any strange women in the house, it just didn't help. Of course, she . . . I don't think . . . was getting much of what we said because she was so distracted within herself. Anyhow, one morning when I came running into the room at her shriek and ask her to show me the woman, Mom pointed to the TV, which wasn't on. For the first time, I noticed that the morning sun coming in the window made the TV screen look like a mirror and that Mom could see herself reflected in it. I asked if that was the woman. Of course, Mom couldn't answer, but she did point and shriek and kept pointing, crying and rocking. After that, we noticed that she had the same reaction if she unexpectedly saw herself in a mirror.

As can be seen, in the eyes of her daughter, Flo no longer knew herself. Rather than dealing with identity issues (e.g., who am I, who are you, who are we), which were paramount to the narratives of the middle years, the change in perception of self was the clarion call of the endgame. A few months later Bea again talked about Flo's "other woman":

> There has been another change in Mom. Remember how she used to shriek and be afraid of that "other woman" who was really her? Now she's not afraid, thank god . . . no more shrieking. She spends hours, it seems like, talking to "the woman" now. Of course the talk is really just a bunch of gibberish, but you would swear it is conversation of some kind. Mom just stands at the mirror or in front of a dark TV screen mumbling and laughing. She sure looks and acts crazy. But I guess it is like the doctor said. She just has Alzheimer's.

Bea saw this as another step toward the end of her mother being a self-perceiving person. In fact, Bea felt that her mother needed her company less and less as a shell formed around Flo's personhood that excluded real others.

Just prior to an assisted living placement Flo was for the most part nonverbal. Attempts at speaking were extremely dysfluent as well as disorganized. Flo still made eye contact, would respond to changes in the tone of voice, and matched laughter. During one joking episode Bea stated that Flo looked directly at her and said, "Won't be long now." Those words were the last clearly spoken ones in her home according to Bea. One week later Flo was moved to an assisted living placement, and 3 weeks later to a nursing home. Within a week of that placement, she lost the ability to swallow and was moved to hospice care. Bea and Bart regularly visited for hours with Flo during this series of moves. Flo's other children, including Buzz, came to see her in the hospice. They brought small paintings or

pictures to share with each other and with Flo, just in case she could hear them. Bea, the firstborn child, did needlework at Flo's bedside as she died. The journey was over, but as Bea said, "She was not alone. Like Dad said, she wouldn't be alone."

Dementia and Self Construction

In previous chapters, we have argued that people have cultural, role, interactional, and biographical tools that they use to create a self. In this chapter, we delayed this discussion until after the introduction of Flo's life story, because it is important to consider whether the person suffering from deep dementia retains any tools for self construction. In the following, we discuss this issue.

Cultural Tools and the Person with Dementia

Predementia, Flo's roles were consistent with cultural expectations for women in her generation, as we have discussed previously and will continue in the next section. This was validating for her sense of self. When it became initially apparent that Flo had progressive dementia, the members of her family responded to this with knowledge of the disease conveyed by our culture. This cultural story of dementia contributed to the roles assigned to Flo within the homes of her children, shaped interactional content and form, and was a part of the ongoing biography of Flo's life . . . now with dementia. As Taylor (2007) says:

> I have become keenly aware of a patterned response from some individuals as soon as they find out I have Alzheimer's disease. They switch their eye

contact and attention to whomever I am with. It is as if knowledge of the disease immediately cloaks me in invisibility. (p. 152)

In the middle years of Flo's journey with dementia, much of what occurred is being discussed theoretically about the impact of this disease. Kitwood (1997) notes that "Often personhood has been disregarded, particularly when the 'patients' cannot easily speak in support of their own interests" (p. 43). For example, Flo's son, Buzz, could not move past his sense of his mother's lost personhood.

Finally, in the late stages of the disease, the person with Alzheimer's has essentially lost the tools of self construction and some would argue the very self, which is part of what is feared when a person is first diagnosed. In all ways from social interaction through life's pleasures and self-care (discussed below), however, others are the key to continuously being oneself in the moment. Persons with Alzheimer's do need the assistance of others in storying themselves, and unfortunately, as communication is lost, the actions of the PWD are interpreted through the cultural stories of dementia as a disease, what Sabat (2003) called the malignant positioning of the person. When the individual becomes the disease, all their words, actions, fears, health concerns, upsets become interpreted from that frame of meaning. In a sense, when this happens the disease as a societal construction swallows them. In the story of Flo, we see that some of her children, for example, Bart, kept their mother's self alive. In the end, Flo's move out of the home of her children to a strange place, even though she no longer spoke or seemed to know them, was perhaps the final life impact because those around her could only construct her self from their perceptions of the disease.

Roles and the Person with Dementia

Flo's predementia self was characterized by multiple validating roles—wife, mother, homemaker, churchgoer, friend and neighbor, and painter, among others. She was also very much a creation of the social and cultural times in which she grew up during the Depression. It is interesting to note that the centrality of many of her roles was a direct product of the larger culture in which she was raised. In the pre-World War II Depression years, women's roles were clearly defined, particularly in terms of being a wife and mother, and Flo's sense of self in these roles was important throughout her lifetime, even when dementia intervened.

Flo often spoke about important defining relationships, particularly with her husband, who remained part of her narrative life even after his death. He had been a support to her during her grandmother's and mother's disease process, and would reportedly always tell Flo, "I won't let you lose your mind and I won't put you away." Through Flo's own stories about his role in caring for her relatives with dementia, he was part of her personal journey into dementia. From her letters, after her husband's death and in a house devoid of children, it was not so much the habitual self that changed, but rather her identity as defined by her roles in the lives of others. In other words, the ways that life roles structured self changed. The loneliness of daily living in a house without children or a spouse was real. So, this woman whose life revolved around the busyness of a large household was, even in the midst of a well-managed everyday life, no longer the person she thought of as herself. Life was not "right" for her. However, for a while, letters with her children maintained her previous relationships and roles, and also shared who she was. By writing letters instead of making phone calls, she said that others could reread and constantly recreate her presence in their lives, just as she could think of them constantly being with her.

Interactions and the Person with Dementia

Kitwood (1997) discusses how important social interactions are in the maintenance of a self, emphasizing and associating the I-Thou with personal recognition and intimacy. Taylor (2007) underscores the centrality of intimacy issues when stating, "Alzheimer's disease shuffles the intimacy deck! It upsets the apple cart. It's a whole new ballgame" (p. 169).

The importance of intimacy to Flo is apparent in the following telephone conversation about her move into the home of her married daughter. As Flo discusses the move, her focus is on the fact that she was wanted, and that it was the son-in-law as well as her daughter who wanted her.

Flo: Well, is anything going on important?

Int: Well, not a thing that I know of.

Flo: Well, I'm still here.

Int: You haven't moved yet?

Flo: No (laughter) obviously! I'm moving up to Bea and Larry's.

Int: Uhuh, I know that.

Flo: You know, Larry he asked me to live there.

Int: That's great.

Flo: Didn't you know that?

Int: Well, I didn't know exactly who asked you.

Flo: Larry called and said he wanted me to move in with them. And, well, I tried not to bawl.

Int: M-m-m.

Flo: You know, I'm not happy about packing things up. I don't know why I haven't painted. And forgot the paint room!

Interactions are also illustrated by the different responses of Flo's sons, Buzz and Bart, to her progressive inability to actively construct a self with them. During the middle years of Flo's dementia, her son, Buzz, found it increasingly difficult to interact with her, because he could find no evidence of her previous self, nor could he find any new self with whom to interact. However, Bart continued to find his mother within the interactions that they shared:

That's Mom. Always has been and I think it always will be. Her mind might be going, but that humor, the way she joins in with us sometimes, that's Mom and I'm real glad she is still with us.

This illustrates how important interactions are to constructing the self. Because Buzz highlighted the structural role-governed aspects of self, particularly how painting defined his mother for him, her violation of this role negated her selfhood for him. On the other hand, Bart gave priority to his mother's instances of humor as points of interpersonal contact. As a result, Bart perceived his mother as still some version of the person he had always known. While it is unknown whether Flo was able to participate in the construction of her self, she either was lost or remained in the selves constructed by her children.

In the later stages of her dementia, Flo was still displaying some interactional aspects of self when "the woman" (her reflection) frightened her. Her shrieks were a call to social others who responded in some way, anchoring her to a shared social world. When that world narrowed so only Flo and her unknown reflected image shared social space, she stopped asking for the intervention of others. In fact, Bea felt that her mother needed her company less and less as a shell formed around Flo's personhood that excluded real others.

Biography and the Self

It is perhaps the biographical particulars which are the most affected by progressive dementia, so that by the end of the disease, Flo did not even remember her own face. When she saw her reflection, that reflection was someone foreign and alien to her. Then, as an intermittent companion, the reflection came to be accepted by Flo, but as separate from her. Flo's body continued, but her biography of self ceased, except in the interactions during which other people assigned meaning. Her narrative was, by this point, being written entirely by others. This brings us to a discussion of the narrative self and the illness narrative.

Storying and the Illness Narrative in Dementia

Throughout this text, claims have been made about the role of communication in the construction of the narrative self. As neurogenic disorders of communication were discussed in Chapter 2 the various "costs" of impairment on the communication system were presented in a Venn diagram. ALS and Parkinson's disease exact the greatest toll on the speech output aspect of communication. Aphasia exacts the greatest toll on the language system. And dementia exacts the greatest toll on the cognitive system. Of course, none of these disorders is

that simple, and all aspects of communication can be affected. What is of importance here is that in dementia, communication as a key to the construction of narrative self is lost. Taylor (2007) clarifies this importance as follows: "Words not only describe my world, they create my world. What happens when the meaning of words changes from one day to the other, from one hour to the other, when words sometimes lose their meaning? This is where I and my world are right now (p. 258).

Reeve Lindbergh (2001) described her mother, Anne Morrow Lindberg, in the last years of her dementia, as becoming silent; this was a woman who had had a love of words and whose professional career was based on words. She did not talk. She appeared unaware of others except for the rare and unexpected word(s).

The concept of storying is useful in understanding the ways in which communication framed in narrative and delivered in social contexts contributes to the ongoing construction of narrative self. Although all of the disorders discussed in this text can be considered from a storying perspective, a question of particular interest with dementia is, "Who is doing the storying?" (Wertsch, Tulviste, & Hagstrom, 1993). If, as we have claimed, communication is essential for the construction of self, can we logically conclude that the individual with deep dementia continues to have a self for self, or is what lingers as self only the construction of others (Gubrium, 1986)? Within the context of this book and the way that we have discussed aspects of self, the following is suggested: It is the actions of others, the world of symbolic meaning that is no longer expressed by the person experiencing dementia but supplied by the interpretative stories of others, that survives for this person even in the final stages of the disease. Gubrium (1986) posed the question, does AD steal the mind or the capacity to express it? This is a fundamental question for the storying of self for the person with dementia. Gubrium vividly describes the ways in which families from the support groups he observed gave meaning to actions, glances, and even the moans of loved ones with AD and in the end reached the conclusion that mind is a social, not individual, preserve. In the case of Flo, she had lost the need for identities. Each had dropped away as she no longer functioned as a mother, an artist, a friend, a correspondent. The storying that surrounded Flo supplied the means for those around her to maintain the identities they had for her, or to lose sight of those identities, in the case of Buzz.

Dimensions of the Self

Throughout the story of Flo, her perspective on herself and the perspectives of her children flow across the four dimensions of self that we have used in this text. Flo was a mother, a wife, and a homemaker, roles that were considered especially appropriate for women, so Flo was always in tune with her culture. She was a storyteller, and that role especially as a correspondent and a painter gives priority to the self that is constituted by roles. This aspect of her personhood is what became so violated by dementia that her oldest son no longer saw Flo as a person. Flo's story of herself, shared with her husband and children was not only about her life experiences, that is, biographical, but included interactional dimensions reflected in her relationships with her grandmother and mother during their living with dementia. As such, health and illness narratives about the experience of dementia were part of Flo's biographical self.

Relationships were fundamental to Flo's life story. Her own assertion that hav-ing a large family kept her from being lonely and her need to be with family as she perceived changes in her ability to manage everyday life reflect the priority given to the interactional aspects of self. Flo was not alone in giving priority to this aspect of self in that her youngest son's assertion of Flo's essential self was based on construed interactions. Each of these storied dimensions of self allowed Flo to construct her self, but they also provided tools for the family to use when Flo no longer participated.

Narratives of Age and Illness

Every person's life has major thematic elements, consistent with the idea of narrative. These themes are unique to each individual, and they are typically critical in understanding the construction of self in dementia. Three major themes frame the storying associated with Flo's life: (a) social living, (b) life's pleasures, and (c) self-care including home management. Each of these also frames biographical, interactional, structural, and cultural aspects of selfhood. These themes will be described in the following sections, with two additional examples of adults aging with and without dementia, in order to illustrate how narratives of age and illness frame stories of dementia.

Social Living

McAdams (1993) made the case that our identities are composed of stories throughout the life span. These stories are about ourselves, others known and unknown to us, things, happenings, and the many multilayered aspects of daily life. Everyday stories among friends, relatives, and neighbors are part of the ritual of daily life that reveal the social processes that surround and involve each of us, and are instrumental in forming and reforming what is remembered (Sarbin, 2005).

Gibson (2004) suggested that telling stories about oneself and one's life as it relates to others is in actuality a quest for relationships. This is such a powerful force in the lives of humans that Bruner (1999) claimed the willingness to story one's life is tantamount to the desire to live. Thus, seeking and maintaining relationships in storied form, as well as in actual acts of living, may be essential for the preservation of self. Changes in the desire or ability to story are observable actions. Following changes in Flo's storying provides insight into the dropping of identities and her struggle for self as her dementia deepened.

It is clear that a major task for individuals as they age is finding ways to maintain self despite declining health and mental functioning (Kitwood, 1993a, b; Tobin, 1988) and in the face of the loss of relational ties and family members through distance or death (Powell, 1988). We see from Flo's life story that she, indeed, had to deal with the loss of her husband through death and of her children through distance. Her health declined as did her mental functioning. Still, in social situation after social situation until almost the end of her life, she maintained connection. Her sense of humor remained recognizable even when speech was basically lost, and when Flo could no longer inject humor, her children told stories of her humor. In these ways Flo's self was maintained.

Family was an important point within Flo's historical construction of narrative. What she most relied on was being surrounded by and a part of the lives of others, especially her children. The retelling of the biographical self becomes a tool used by the person to question, answer, make sense of, or reformulate tasks that become diffi-

cult with the onset of dementia. This old and established way of being was a main theme in her biographical self. What is suggested here is that the rituals of everyday life (Sarbin, 2005), when revealed in stories, bring into focus the social processes upon which maintenance of self depends.

Because some of these same issues are part of the normal aging process, storying of life skills being lost conveys the concerns of the individual who experiences changes in memory. Jessica, age 88 at the time of her interview, provides a contrast to Flo in several ways: she was older, the mother of only one child, and lived in a retirement community rather than with this child. The following excerpt was a response to questions about her physical and mental well-being.

Age has affected parts of my brain—mainly the parts of the brain dealing with mathematics. I always took care of the financial part of marriage. Richard (Jessica's deceased husband) worked out the details of money. Then I took over keeping the records—checkbook—account book—bank statements. After he died I had to take over the task of making decisions about finding which bank had the best CD interest rates. As I got older I found it was harder to make such decisions. Recently I began to realize that getting higher interest also meant I was getting more income which led to being in a higher bracket for income tax. I never actually sat down to see what the difference was. Maybe not much—not enough to make me uneasy. Here is where I realized I was becoming more incompetent to keep my records accurate. Writing checks and entering them accurately in my check book and then account book—I began to make mistakes—small ones—foolish ones like writing amount in my account book like 9.097

instead of 907.00. Remembering that if I had written checks but they hadn't been cashed which meant the bank account didn't agree with my account book. The part I always have to go back to other months to see if I added the uncashed checks to the bank statement or subtracted the amounts.

Jessica answers the question, "Who am I?" by telling us about one of her valued family roles. Because of the value placed on this role, her story about problems with maintaining financial records is a pivotal miniature drama (Sarbin, 2005) about self. Is she the person she always believed herself to be? Jessica is not certain. She also speaks about her social world. People are important to her, but she finds herself dissatisfied with those she sees on a regular basis, for example, in meals in the central dining room.

You know I eat with these same people twice a week . . . I mean each one is different . . . and we just don't discuss anything that's going on. It's so boring . . . and uh you can't get out of going there any more you're sort of stuck because you're here but really they may mention in passing something and oh isn't that too bad but they don't discuss it. Now whether they always were like that or they were getting old . . . that's their reaction.

[Int: Do you feel trapped?]

Oh God yes. I more and more don't try to eat with people if I don't have a date.

In Flo's early stories, she talked about the role of others in her life. However, as the dementia progressed, while everyday life continued to affirm the centrality of interactional self for Flo, she was no longer able to reflect on relationships. In contrast,

Jessica struggles with issues of closeness in friendships, issues that would not have been present 20 years earlier when most of her core friends and her husband were still alive.

I find I've met people that I like and go along with them and all that and then after a while I get what's the word I want—critical of them for no reason and I withdraw. I don't like that. I don't know why.

Thus, it can be seen that the two women juxtaposed themselves differently in social space. Social others had different roles in their lives, different affordances allotted to them. Jessica's search for social grounding for her interactional self also reflects a sense of isolation from those who would have been important in her younger years. Such people would be intelligent, interesting, diverse, and passionate about liberal issues. In her current, somewhat isolated situation, she states:

I just haven't . . . somehow gotten involved with them . . . and when you read their backgrounds they really are of an intelligent type. We've got professors and doctors and business . . . lots of military . . . I always have to be careful. I read the background that they send us so that I avoid those people. Which is safer. No, we've got 'em . . . the people . . . I guess I haven't latched on to them.

Flo and Jessica are both dealing with aspects of aging, including personal losses. Swidler (1986) talked about how individuals select goals that are aligned with their symbolic tools. In Jessica's case, mathematics was a symbolic tool that she was used to having the power and skill to use. When those skills began to erode through normal aging processes, she worked to maintain them, almost testing herself on a daily basis, as seen in the following interview excerpt:

> Along this problem (with mathematics) I was doing something stupid like counting. For example, my bras have 6 hooks and eyes to close. I find myself counting as I hook them. So totally unnecessary. When putting clothes into or taking them out of the washing machine/dryer, counting things like underwear or socks. What difference does it make!!!

Flo, prior to the onset of dementia, kept track of her financial accounts as did Jessica. However, even in the early stages of dementia, once she had moved in with her daughter, Flo gave away this everyday ritual of living. For her, it would seem, understanding one's financial assets were not pivotal to who she considered herself to be. Like Jessica, keeping her mind alive was important. So what was in her tool kit, with what did she identify?

Life's Pleasures—Keeping the Mind Alive

In this section on keeping the mind alive, we will address life's pleasures since those things that give us pleasure do become habitual parts of our lives, things that we become skilled at through doing. Even in the face of progressive dementia, these skilled activities may remain useable for keeping the mind alive and maintaining self. This was exemplified by Maria, who became increasingly forgetful in her 80s and remembered few new and many old things in the years before her death at the age of 91. Her story is told from the perspective of a colleague.

Maria was a Swiss immigrant who came to America just before the beginning of World War II. She had a Ph.D. in philosophy and had been participating in research in her home country until the impending war resulted in her relocation. Between the ages of 30 and 70 Maria taught at American universities, with her last appointment spanning more than 20 years.

I met Maria, then retired, during my Ph.D. studies. This amazing little woman would regularly attend faculty meetings and social gathering in "her" department. She greeted all, new acquaintances and old friends alike, with the opening sentence, "I won't remember your name, but tell me about your research." Maria would listen carefully, ask penetrating questions testifying to habitualized skill as a researcher, and provide suggestions for furthering her interlocular's research or writing. One could walk away, come back 10 minutes later, and Maria would again greet you with, "I won't remember your name, but tell me about your research," and the sequence of telling, listening, advising would again unfold. This was a staple in her life, and even at the time of her death, Maria was writing a book, one she had been writing and rewriting for over 10 years. With regard to keeping the mind alive, it is important to note that Maria's advice was not simply a repetition of what she had said before, but was novel to the current discussion. Even when she did not grasp the content, she demonstrated skill in the dissection and refinement of research organization.

We can ask, how did Maria keep her mind alive, and what does this say about her self? Maria's pleasure was her work, and most of all she identified herself as an academic. She did not sew, paint, cook, or take on household tasks for others. As a person who never married, she maintained her household as needed, but most of all, she read, wrote, and taught. The department faculty, many of whom had never worked with Maria, maintained her identity as the grand dame of the department, and were instructed by senior faculty members in how to honor and care for Maria's sense of self as a productive department member. Therefore, Maria's social unit cooperated with the ways she worked to continue to story her life in the department. Maria used the habitual skills of her long life and social others within the academic community to keep her self intact, to keep her mind alive.

Jessica, our normally aging interviewee, found pleasure in life by taking on new challenges, by challenging her mind. Over many years, she had attended courses to learn to do many creative things, such as stained glass and weaving. These were true delights for her, and her physical inability to continue these pleasures was discouraging. Jessica also prided herself on being willing to try new technological challenges. She obtained her first computer (an Apple II-c) at the age of 72, purchased WebTv for Internet access several years later, and transitioned to a Windows-based computer with full Internet access at the age of 87. Instead of feeling good about these newer challenges, she has felt defeated as she states:

> The body is being defeated, the brain is being defeated, and most people over . . . they just . . . go with the flow . . .

She elaborates further on the relative ease she experienced in adding Internet access to her TV, as contrasted with more recent computer challenges:

> Such as adding Internet to TV. Lately I don't do this easily. The new computer and the Internet has been very difficult for me to remember. I have to continually check back to Barbara's notes. I have been so slow at this that I haven't been able to do things on the Internet—like working with pictures, playing games,

working with spreadsheets (whatever that is). I have become so frustrated with this lack of understanding how to do these that I wish I had never decided to buy a new computer and connecting to the Internet. I was satisfied with my old Apple which of course couldn't do all the things of the new set-up. So I more and more wonder why I get involved with more advanced technology. If I can't learn to do the "fun" things why have I wasted the money and hours sitting in front of the computer/internet and not progressing.

And she goes even further in stating:

> It seems like the brain is not responding quickly to the new mechanics and this bothers me, you know. You know there are lots of women here who are really into this computer bit, it's very interesting, even the 98 year old woman I love dearly. Well she only uses it to e-mail a large family and she doesn't get into the good . . . and somehow, the computers don't go off like mine has gone off.

For Flo, the pleasures that she indulged in were few—sewing, reading, and painting. The last was her passion that spilled over and intruded on housekeeping, cooking, and managing her time. In other words, Flo's story of self was most of all connected with the pursuit of self via the symbolic forms associated with painting. Her children saw her as a painter even when she could no longer paint. Hence, paintings and pictures of her paintings were shared with her even in the hospice. Bruner's (1999) conjecture that the willingness to story one's life is tantamount to the desire to live places Flo's pleasure, especially painting, in the realm of storying. Painting is more than putting brush to canvas. It is the telling of a story where the painter as "I" is telling a story. Each painting as a story also tells something of the storyteller, that is, the "me," in the way it is structured and used as a communication tool.

In the case of Flo, early on her sons thought she just needed to paint to be well. Flo in her own words began to see unwanted changes in her paintings, calling them "cluttered." Before she lost speech, before she lost the ability to write and correspond, Flo lost the ability to take perspective, to communicate to others via this vital symbolic form who she was. She dropped the identity of being a painter even though her children maintained this as a core aspect of her self (via stories and in the exchange of pictures on holidays and visits back and forth). Flo replaced painting with things she could do, most notably sewing, which became gift items to her children and others, and in her own words, "kept the mind alive." When Flo's eyesight was lost due to macular degeneration and she could no longer sew, when she had lost the ability to link thoughts and words in writing, and when she could no longer articulate fluent words, her storying of life depended on others. She had no way to tell the story, in Bruner's sense, no way to live.

The stories of these three women tell much the same narrative. They *were* the habitual actions of their lives. For all three, aspects of their identities were heavily connected to life's pleasures (as uniquely defined for each). In all three cases, they and others in their living sphere continued to story their selves through these fading images of who they were, stories now spoken and transferred by others rather than by their own telling. The stories and habitual skills of Maria and Jessica can be contrasted with those of Flo. Maria's focus and identity was linked to academia; Jessica's focus was on domestic competence and independence in taking on new challenges; and Flo's habitual skills were in linked to being a mother, wife, and painter. Our normally aging respondent Jessica has become particularly despondent over her inability to find pleasure and stimulation in the challenges she used to enjoy, an emotion not experienced by either Maria or Flo as they progressed into dementia.

Self-Care

The experience of living is filled with wants and needs that give rise to goals, planning, and just doing what we want at the time we want to do it. The needs in our lives are mundane actions and activities that in this chapter have been grouped loosely under the section heading of Self-Care.

A large part of the experience of living is the care we have to take of ourselves. Our bodies demand food, liquid, evacuation, and cleansing. As we master these skills as children, we become independent; we become "little people" to others and to ourselves. Illness and age systematically rob us of self-care skills. And with each robbery, each care that must be transferred to others for personal maintenance, a little of our sense of self is impinged upon. Others see us differently. The content of communication changes as does the focus. Tobin, among others, has suggested that the task of old age "is to be 'oneself' until the last breath of life" (1988, p. 550). Changes in self-care are a significant challenge for this task.

Self-care is on a continuum as the individual moves through the life span, whether or not this progression is altered or accelerated by dementia. For normally aging persons, self-care involves considerable independence in activities of daily living (ADLs) and independent activities of daily living

(IADLs). For persons in situations like Jessica's, progressive loss of physical independence to motor problems associated with severe arthritis raises the specter of institutional placement. In reflecting on people who have been moved into one of the care units at her retirement community, she states:

> . . . but you know I've found that people who felt that way [afraid of placement] and then again mentally you accept it they don't seem to mind once they get in there. I could cope with Laurel house but Holly House. . . . I couldn't—I'd become another Mildred Simon . . . I probably would. And that's again not what I used to be . . . I would accept . . . not accepting . . .

For persons living with dementia, self-care prior to and early on involves taking care of one's own life in everyday ways such as maintaining the house, shopping, and being fiscally responsible. These everyday activities change in various ways and degrees as dementia progresses with others taking a more active role in their management. In the later stages of the disease, self-care is restricted to tasks and routines such as maintaining simple cleanliness, nutrition, and safety. This progressive change of self-care was seen in the story of Flo. In the beginning phase, the local grocer assisted her when shopping and the lady's group at church left the door open. During the middle phase her youngest son rearranged his house and routines to make visits easier. In the last stages of the disease, Flo's basic physical needs were taken care of first by her daughter and then by strangers in assisted living and hospice care. Flo's earlier stories of washing her grandmother in order to keep her clean as dementia claimed her mind became Flo's own story.

Narrative Self in Progressive Dementia: Who Writes the Story?

Situating self in relation to others is a lifelong endeavor (Haight et al., 2003; Sullivan, 1953), one that is fundamental to conversation (Bakhtin, 1986), and one that becomes more difficult as individuals experience forgetting (Obler, 1980). Gubrium (1986) when writing about AD claims that the mind, while a state embodied by the individual person, is in reality not something possessed by the individual but rather a dialogical social preserve that is a product of its own discourse. Part of that discourse for Flo was the family history with progressive dementia.

As seen in her story, both Flo's grandmother and mother were described as having "lost their minds." With modern technology we know they are losing brain cells, brain connections. We know that the higher mental functions, such as remembering, attending and self-directed and regulated action, decreases. Therefore, 'mind' as a subset of body is constantly being lost. However, self is also fragmenting in that the ability to construct memories and the social interactiveness that builds and supports mindfulness becomes diminished in the disease process. This is not to say that "self" is lost, but rather that the form of communication associated with self and shared intersubjectively with others including family members, changes.

Armstrong (2005) suggests that when an individual's use of language regularly fails or is compromised during the negotiation of meaning in a social context that it be considered disordered. Certainly, language changes occurred over a ten year period for Flo as she progressed through dementia. An avid correspondent, she lost the skill to convey her thoughts in writing. An engaging conservationist, she lost the power to sequence and organize speech production. A companionable listener, she lost the skill to follow conversation or make sense of questions ask of her. A life-long reader, she lost the ability to derive meaning from print. These kinds of language changes are typical with progressive dementia. The disorientation that results from changes in memory in conjunction with progressive dementia impinges on how well " . . . physical and social settings and abstract frames and premises for communication" (Linell, 1991, p. 1), that are so necessary for the maintenance of personhood, can be socially negotiated. Aspects of conversation are subsumed within the goal of maintaining and communicating a self perspective.

We opened this chapter with this question, "Thus, shall we consider the agency involved in the storying of the self to be something inherent in the individual or a product of the relationships that one has developed?" As we have claimed throughout this book, narrative self accumulates from persistent acts of storying. As we have seen from the story of Flo, vebal-linguistic and other symbolic means of storying were lost to her over a ten year period of time. Was Flo lost? As Flo gave up the roles that mattered to her, and as her story was replaced with the stories of others, did Flo remain? This is essentially a question about agency, and the question highlights critical aspects of agency, in ways not possible with the other diseases we have considered in this book. If Flo no longer uses the tools of her culture, of her roles, of her interactions, and of her biography, and if these tools are picked up by others or simply lost, who retains agency? Who writes her narrative self, her illness narrative, her story? Current research on dementia suggests that the agency is retained by others, who create

the demented individual as they wish. So, whether these others privilege the cultural expectations of someone with Alzheimer's ("as the doctor says, she has Alzheimer's") or the role expectations (she no longer paints anything of value), or the interactions (she still has her humor), or her biography (she is the mother of her children), these are not necessarily the tools that would be used by Flo, if her self continued to matter to her. As the dementia deepens, Flo progressively abdicates self construction to others.

However, this may not be fundamentally different from how we all story ourselves, differing only in degree. Powell (1988) claims that life is created through relationships, and that the inter-human "we" that emerges from these provides possibilities of existence. As a result, individuals need to establish and maintain relationships, even if these are in remembered form, throughout life. He states, "Memories of our relationships linger with us as we age (p. 550) . . . (and) are the currency that makes life's transactions and transitions possible" (p. 562). Self is constantly being created and renewed by means of interactions and through relationships. We have argued, with Gubrium and Holstein (2001), that each self is constructed anew in each situation.

As long as Flo had her family around her, even though she may have lost both receptive and expressive language, the routines, the rhythms of the daily life in the home were a means of interaction. It was hardly interaction on the symbolic level. However, at the level of a "sensory self," which we can say is part of the biographic dimension, her family was renewing memories of something. This would be an example, perhaps, of how self is sustained over the course of the dementing process through others who are socially engaged with the person experiencing dementia (Kitwood, 1993b). Others replenish the personhood of PWD when that individual remains somebody to someone, and is treated as someone rather than some body in need of medical treatment and assistive care. Thus, the essential task of dementia care is to maintain personhood even as mental powers fail (Kitwood, 1993a). We can argue that this is the essential task of any self creation, to create self when previously used tools become lost or we forget how to use them. Agency is not made evident when one is able to create a self entirely alone, but when one is able to create a self in interaction with others. The life story is a shared story, a story of how someone "remains somebody to someone." And even though Flo no longer used recognizable tools to preserve herself for self or others, it was her narrative bequests to her children that allowed her to live on as a person until her death.

SECTION IV

In today's outcomes-driven health care environment, at least in the Western world, the demand is for product. Theory without practice implications is devalued. Instead, clinicians are constantly exhorted to do more with less. They are often driven by the need for quick, simple answers to questions such as: what can I do, with what tools, with whom, in what contexts. Because of these concerns, Section IV of this text was originally intended to be the obligatory clinical implications portion of this text. It soon became apparent that we each had our own unique perspectives about what the implications of a narrative self perspective might be for clinicians, researchers, and those living with neurogenic communication disorders. We also began to realize that the primary contribution of this text may indeed be the development of and support for a strong theoretical foundation for considering narrative self in future dialogue about the life impact of neurogenic communication disorders.

At the heart of our work is the premise that everyday communicative acts and interactions are powerfully linked to who we are, as we see ourselves and as others see us. If we accept this premise, it alters our perception of what is "broken" and what needs to be "fixed" for those living with acquired communication disorders. The focus shifts to self, as narrated through everyday actions and communications. This shift then demands different clinical roles, broader intervention environments, modified intervention targets, and greater involvement with those important social others with whom our clients interact.

However, if our conceptual work is solid, there can and should be many ways to understand this work in the context of the real people who populate the lives of clinicians in multiple disciplines. Consequently, what follows are our personal "take-home" messages to the reader, our initial efforts to translate theory into today's clinical practices.

In Chapter 10, Koski places our premises in a broader postmodern context, challenging practitioners to respond to the implications of our exploration of narrative self. Hagstrom uses Chapter 11 to explain how the constructs of this text fit within a sociocultural perspective, with particular attention to clinical action and to provision of tools for the necessary storying of self in the clinical interaction. Finally, Shadden's Chapter 12 provides a summary of key text premises that hold greatest promise in guiding future theoretical development, research, and most importantly, clinical practice. A common theme is the role of the clinician and clinical interactions in providing a social context for ongoing construction and renegotiation of self for persons with neurogenic communication disorders.

No chapter pretends to have all the answers clinically, since there is much more work to be done. In fact, one person who reviewed a draft of this text suggested that we have actually laid the conceptual foundation for relatively uncharted territory in clinical work. We agree, and we hope that this will be the beginning of an important theoretical and clinical dialogue about how we can address narrative self in our interventions.

If we do manage to move towards a focus on narrative self, new interventions that emerge will not succeed unless we can also help the public appreciate the fact that communication is so much more than simple acts of listening and talking. This is a tremendous challenge, and it is one that varies depending on the specific neurogenic disorder. Most people living with adult-onset communication disorders want communication impairments to be "fixed," focusing on the outward manifestation of communication in language forms and intelligible utterances. We need to find ways to reorient these persons to a better understanding of the role communication serves in supporting self construction in everyday life, so they can become partners with us in activities designed to sustain and reframe self in the context of a communication impairment.

CHAPTER 10

Postmodernism and the Story of the Self: A Call to Action

by Patricia R. Koski

This is a postmodern book. It is unlikely that it would be written, much less published, in a modern world. We have spoken of the creation of the self in the face of debilitating illnesses; we have not spoken of cures. We have talked about storying the self, creating narratives that allow people to continue to create selves even when they have lost many of the most critical tools for doing so. We have not talked about restoring those tools. We have talked about accepting people with disabilities and fully integrating them into a social world. We have not talked about treatment modalities and plans. We have extended the person-centered treatment concept of "late modernity" (Giddens, 1991) beyond its original boundaries to argue that every self is a social construction created at four levels (at least), and that the differences between those who are "well" and those who are not is only a matter of degree. Thus, we have not spoken of deficits and differ-

ences, but of similarities and common challenges. We have spoken of agency and hope, not the hope that someone will be restored to a former self, but that she will find or be given new tools and will interact in affirming ways with others, so that "storying" of the self continues.

I write this chapter as a sociologist to reflect on the implications of our theory for practice. Because I will never be called upon to actually implement the theory "on the ground," I have the luxury of extending a call to action that ignores the complexities of actual practice. However, what I say here is the result of listening to my colleagues throughout this project—because it is not my field, my perspective comes largely from them. In the two chapters that follow, as speech-language professionals, they will be able to speak to those who understand the full implications of this perspective. Here, I take the prerogative to offer a few personal reflections.

When an Illness Narrative Becomes a Life Story

One major theme in this book has been that people use a cultural tool box that contains tools at the cultural, role, interactional, and biographical levels, to create a self, which has agency to create a story. This story or life narrative is the way in which people present their selves to others, and the way they move through and build a life. We have argued that this is the case for all of us, but that those with neurogenic communication disorders have lost some of their most cherished tools at a time when they most need them to make sense of their altered selves. If they are able to respond to this crisis by finding and learning to use other tools (and if such tools exist), and if they thereby are able to create a changed life story, they will create a new self that will take them into the future. For all of the neurogenic communication disorders we have discussed in this book, that new story will be, for a time, an illness narrative, where the fact of the illness is given priority in the plot. For those with ALS, the illness narrative is likely to last until the person's death. For those with Alzheimer's, as the narrative comes to be written by others, the fact of the illness may only explain why others have become the authors of the story. For those with aphasia and Parkinson's, the degree to which the illness narrative remains central or gives way to a new life story, which takes the illness into account but does not privilege it as the plot of the story, will depend on those tools that the person and her social others are able to recapture or find.

However, whether an illness narrative or new life story, it is important that people be allowed to move on with their lives in ways that affirm the person apart from the disease. For this to happen, it is essential that new tools be made available. In the pre-

vious chapters, we talked about how SLPs may help clients obtain and use tools at each of the levels of culture, roles, interactions, and biography. In this section, I wish to emphasize the role of the SLP in helping the client find and use cultural tools, because this is where our charge is most radical.

Cultural tools provide the individual with a way to adeptly use cultural values and norms to present an appropriate self. People who have lost the ability to talk effectively, whether because of motor, linguistic, and/or cognitive impairment, have lost these tools. As a consequence, they find it difficult to negotiate interpersonal interactions. We have seen several examples of this: Harry, with aphasia, is angered because people will not give him time to process information and thus truly engage in a conversation; Jerry, with Parkinson's, fears that he will lose authority in his classroom if he cannot talk without the self-described stuttering that disrupts his lectures. For persons with ALS, there are powerful computerized tools that can be substituted for deteriorating communication skills. However, some persons, such as Penny's mother, emphatically refuse to use any type of communication device, effectively isolating her from family members at considerable emotional cost to everyone concerned and with associated losses of self, at least in the interactional domain. SLPs have always attempted to assist these interactions, whether through specific therapies addressing the actual impairment or through facilitating use of other animate and inanimate tools to support communication.

In this book, though, we make a more radical charge. Our culture must create new tools for everyone, so that well people interact with "diseased" people in ways that affirm the personhood of those with disease, not requiring them to be hidden, *and* that also contribute to the personhood of those who are well, as Frank (1995) suggests.

Certainly, such a charge goes beyond the current expectations for the SLP, but these professionals are in a primary location to facilitate the process of interaction, creating these tools at least at the micro level. After all, as we have suggested, all selves are created situationally. This charge is certainly consistent with some of the new directions in the field, but in our theory, SLPs must interact with their clients, not as professional and client, but as two people cocreating a story. Social approaches to intervention (such as those found in the management of aphasia) have gained prominence, an important start in the right direction. However, these approaches often maintain the professional power and distance between the therapist and client. Concepts of personhood in understanding and working with those with dementia are more consistent with the theory presented in this text. What is central is an understanding that, in order to create the tools of which we speak, the speech-language professional must actually empower the individual to write her life narrative, by doing so himself in the same setting.

This is why we began this chapter with the statement that this book would not be written, much less published in a modern world. This charge to the professional would be outrageous in such a world, and certainly frightening even in a postmodern world. An understanding of the differences between modernism and postmodernism is necessary for this point to be understood.

Modernism and Postmodernism: The Creation of the Self

A postmodern world is fundamentally different, in basic assumptions, worldview, and expectations, from a modern world. In a modern world, we believe in the "project of the enlightenment" (Giddens, Personal communication, December 4, 1991): that it is possible to build knowledge upon knowledge, and that knowledge ultimately leads to increases in the common good. In a modern world, there are experts—medical doctors, university professors, SLPs whose word is uncontested and who have the ultimate power in interactions with subordinates. In a modern world, there is an emphasis on self construction and self identity, almost a fascination, but the acceptable self must conform to fairly narrow prescripts. An acceptance of diversity is typically one of assimilation—we welcome new groups to this country, to a social situation, to a new social structural level, but expect them to accommodate themselves to the existing culture and language (or jargon) as quickly as possible. In a modern world, there is a sense of linearity in many ways, including an optimistic belief that the development of society is always positive.

In contrast, a postmodern world is messy and chaotic. There is no privileged set of assumptions; diversity is valued because it brings together people who think and see and believe and talk differently, and none of them is considered to be superior to the others. In fact, it is assumed that we can learn from each other. Instead of knowledge building upon knowledge, there is contested knowledge between different interest groups. To build knowledge is to take what we know, from many perspectives, and create an amalgam. Power is more diffuse and more explicit. A person in a powerful structural role may be challenged by those with less power. A postmodern world is likely to be more pessimistic, not assuming that progress equals the betterment of society, and on many dimensions, progress will not be linear.

We argue that we are now in a time where we retain some of the assumptions and features of the modern world, but have moved into a postmodern world as well.

The implications for the construction of and narratives of the self are profound. Gubrium and Holstein (2001) and Holstein and Gubrium (2000) have provided an extensive discussion of the concept of the postmodern self. While I do not repeat their arguments here, much of this chapter is based on their ideas.

Modernism and Postmodernism: The Self and Illness Narratives

As Frank (1995) argues, in a modern world, the medical narrative is one of restitution. From this follows the assumption that a patient must submit completely to the power and knowledge of the superior medical professional, allowing herself to be categorized and diagnosed, in order to be returned to her former state of well-being. In modernism, the emphasis is on perfectability: the claim that science can cure the ill is a central belief (Frank, 1995). This is part of the "grand narrative" (Lyotard, 1979) of modernity, the cultural belief that nature must succumb to science.

The promise of postmodernism is that there is no longer a grand narrative, no longer an expectation that science will overcome nature, no longer the expectation that the only possible cultural outcomes of an illness are either a return to "normal" or death (Frank, 1995). The promise of postmodernism is that people will be seen as ill and accepted as ill and that their illness will spark real communication between them and others. For example, in Chapter 7, we heard the story of Jerry Patnoe, who went into his classroom without having taken his medicine to control the symptoms of Parkinson's disease, to make a deliberate point about his condition. We heard him say, "It, it's for me, it was the strongest statement I could make that they—simply, I'm

here, deal with it. There are other people like me here, deal with it . . . "

This is an example of what Frank (1995, p. 137) calls testimony: "Becoming a witness assumes a responsibility for telling what happened. The witness offers testimony to a truth that is generally unrecognized or suppressed. People who tell stories of illness are witnesses, turning illness into moral responsibility." This is not a modern concept, but it is an example of the moral imperative that Frank discusses: "The moral imperative of narrative ethics is perpetual self reflection on the sort of person that one's story is shaping one into, entailing the requirement to change that self-story if the wrong self is being shaped" (p. 158). Again, unlike the modern "restitution" narrative, which is a story of becoming well, of returning to normal, a postmodern story of illness is the "intrusion of the ill body," (p. 158) itself, into self presentation. If it is true that one no longer has the same tools, and the same abilities to use those tools when one is ill, then Frank would have us believe that in a conducive social environment, one has an immensely more important, overriding tool, the ability to teach normal people about the importance of living on the edge of acceptance. And in a completely postmodern society, one would not even need to live on the edge, but would be accepted into the community as a person with a unique and important story to tell.

Thus, the promise of postmodernism is that the construction of the self will require fewer specialized tools, as the tasks themselves will become less burdensome. Whereas modernity wants the predictability of bodily control, a postmodern society may accept that control is not always possible or even desirable, certainly that the energy it takes to maintain control may not be worth the effort. If society does not require that we use the tool of language or the tool of bodily control within a narrowly allowed range, then the possibilities for agency multiply many-fold. What if having a chronic illness marked the boundaries of society as a way to highlight the potentialities of all humans?

For the SLP, such a world would be one in which he worked with a client in several ways: (a) to help the client find, refurbish, recreate, and learn how to use tools at the cultural, role, interactional, and biographical levels to write a new narrative and create an ongoing story of the self; (b) to facilitate the writing of an illness narrative or to help the client move beyond the illness into a new life story; (c) to work with others to reduce the stigma of a neurogenic communication disorder and to reposition the ill as an important example of diversity; (d) to refuse to collaborate in any project that lessens the agency and power of the individual; and (e) to actively participate in the writing of the new life story by coconstructing the narrative. A more specific discussion of these challenges will be found in the following chapters, 11 and 12. The major point here, however, is that we have now come to a time in our history when the assumptions of modernism no longer hold, and it is possible for SLPs to actually engage in these activities as part of their professional role.

We have presented a hopeful view of postmodernism, but a more negative view is also possible. The fracture of society may lead to competing groups of "experts" who do not build on either previous knowledge or the experience of others unlike themselves. Lack of authority may result in competition for power, including the power to label the sick as deviant. Postmodernism may bring together all of the worst features of modernism along with lack of control. This future is in the hands of those who respond to people with neurogenic communication disorders and, ultimately, in the hands of us all.

As those at the forefront of interacting with people with neurogenic communication disorders, and as those often given the primary responsibility for helping them story their new selves, SLPs have both the challenge of deciding how best to assist with that storying and the responsibility to set the future course of the story. We have suggested that these professionals may assist their clients not only by cowriting narratives, but by also helping our culture provide more tools. The charge is both awesome and exhilarating, and we hope that our colleagues join us in this challenge.

CHAPTER 11

A Sociocultural Approach to Clinical Action

by Fran Hagstrom

A Sociocultural Approach

The horns of my personal dilemma as a clinician and scholar in the field of communication sciences and disorders have been theory and clinical action. While both theoretical and empirical evidence are recognized as important to the field of communication disorders, the ways they are differently valued stratifies the profession. On the one hand, the long tradition of empirical measurement of individuals has translated into empirical measurement of clinical outcomes. In a sense, it is no longer about the individual, the client, but about the outcome that is directly linked to the plans and activities of the clinician. Both the patient and the clinician become invisible in churned data points. This empirical accountability is of questionable value if clinical action, as is the case with narrative self, is conceptualized as dynamic and coconstructed. As can be seen, embedded in the above argument is the "touch" of theory, that is, "conceptual-

ized as dynamic and coconstructed." All clinical action, even the seemingly most objective and measurable, is based on theory whether this is the formal stuff printed in books and memorized for tests in graduate school or informal beliefs that have resulted from personal experiences or hand-me-down routines and procedures.

I bring up this point, this dilemma of theory and clinical action, because this is essentially a book about theory, the theory of narrative self. Grounded in the work and theorizing of others about self, identity, and personhood, it branches out in ways particular to the clients and practices that are the concerns of those working in the field of communication sciences and disorders. In so doing this book presents a position statement where the individual as a person is the key to better practices. My goal in this chapter is to address particulars of clinical action using theory about self, identity, and personhood, and to then ask and suggest some answers to the question, "What is a clinician?"

Theory about Self, Identities, and Personhood

Each of the authors of this book has written individually and collaboratively about self, identities, and personhood. The perspectives that we each take on these concepts have resulted in a healthy tension for this final product, a book on narrative self. As a developmental psychologist, I am intensely interested in what it means to be a human being across the life span. As a speech-language pathologist, I am intensely interested in how individuals and families deal with being human when faced with the disruption of something so central to humanness: the ability to communicate ideas, dreams, and just plain needs of the moment to others. All these things, the stuff of communication, create the richness of social-emotional life. Having said this, I now want to apply what I've just said to the concepts of self, identities, and personhood in order to illustrate how these terms have came together in the cowriting of this book and how the resulting matrix of ideas can be woven into patient care.

Thought in action consists of the things we say and do in everyday life. It is these actions, all the little ones that are habitual to me as well as the large tasks that result from a myriad of actions, that give me a sense of who I am to me. This results in a sense of self that centers me in the good times as well as at those times when life is disrupted by change, illness, or loss. My sense of self is intricately woven into my ongoing autobiographical storying. Others look at or are mutually involved in these actions. They identify me by these very same actions, as well as the roles I play in conjunction with them. This is social identity, in other words, the identities that others see as me (Sarbin, 2005). This social identity is part of my ongoing biography that is cowritten through

social action and roles. Some colleagues identify me as a psychologist, some as a speech-language pathologist, some as a mentor, and others as a friend. My own sense of self is threaded through these identities but is also shaped by these others in my communicative life. The persistent sense of self that becomes predicable in modes of action and reaction that shift even as they remain the same constitutes my personhood.

I would claim that when I am functioning well, in optimal flow (Csikszentmihalyi, 1990), the predictable gradients across self and social identities are woven into health narratives. Imbalance of the gradients when I am ill shifts the self-social balance (and personhood) so illness narratives rather than health narratives become central aspects of storied action. This same kind of thing happens when life-changing events disrupt the ability to communicatively construct self or contribute to how others are constructing any or all of my social identities. Each of the disorders used to illustrate narrative self in this book represents this kind of shift. The gradient between self and social identities in the stories of ALS is shifted toward preserved self with lost identities as the roles the client can take on in life shifts. Persons with ALS use self as a strength to preserve personhood as the roles they fill are dropped as a result of impaired communication and motoric loss. For many, the strong sense of self is maintained. This can be contrasted with the experience of those with other disorders, as can be seen in dementia, where the self can become invisible to others as social roles and identities aligned with these are dropped.

In summary self, identity, and personhood are constructions that are at the same time individual and socially shared. They become stable (i.e., predictable) over time even as they remain dynamic.

From Theory to Therapy

Bridging theory and practice requires analysis and synthesis of two or more bodies of knowledge, in this case theory about narrative self and the mundane as well as interactive aspects of therapeutic intervention. One of the tasks that we have set for ourselves in this book is to provide clinicians with tools and perspectives through which they can include narrative self work in their practices. Several key terms drawn from discussions of theory throughout this book will now be reviewed and recast for clinical purposes. These include the cultural tool kit, cultural tools, and storying.

Cultural Tool Kit

The concept of tools was introduced and linked to our theoretical position on self in Chapter 3, and elaborated throughout Section III of this book. We used Swidler's (1986) conceptual cultural tool kit as the basis for addressing narrative as a tool and linking tools to the four dimensions of self (i.e., cultural aspects, roles, situational interactions, biography). Working with the tool kit is doing clinical work in the area of narrative self. Culture viewed as the collection of ways that people live, work, and play together, using the things they have made to control and function in their environmental settings (Leeds-Hurwitz, 1993) provides the "job'"space in which the cultural tool kit becomes a resource or a source of frustration.

Cultural Tools

Socially Shared Cultural Tools. Clinicians also need to work with (and as) tools if the kit is to be functional for communicative purposes. Like any good kit, tools should be interchangeable and with a little creativity be used in ways beyond their original intent. Culture and cognition "create each other" (Cole, 1985, p. 146) as individuals use signs as tools to communicate, and as a result, these become the means by which individuals think and act (Wertsch, 1998). Thus the stories that generate narrative self become the means by which individuals think and act. They are the stories that are retold by family members and received as part of storying when the individual can no longer do so herself.

Wertsch (2002) focused on a particular kind of storying, narrative accounts based on remembered historical events, to illustrate how individuals use texts as a resource for thinking and talking about their national identity. He could have easily used an illustration from neurogenic communication disorders where the power of the medical label impinges on the biography of the individual and on the roles that the person is allowed to regulate in various situations. Of note is the fact that the reciprocal creation of culture and cognition is replicated continuously over a person's lifetime and is central to narrative self. The stories told by others about us (i.e., biography) that are filtered through social and cultural norms and expectations (cultural dimensions of self) as they relate the roles we've played (situational interactions) become part of self presentation and a tool for remembering and reconstructing that self in future situations.

Tools for the Person. When explaining cultural tools for the mental functioning of the individual, Wertsch draws on the writings of Luria (1981), who used examples from patients who had suffered brain damage, and Vygotsky (1987), who provided examples from children with sensory deficits, as well as Bakhtin (1986) who examined texts. Wertsch's (2002) unit of analysis is mediated action. He states,

...from this perspective, to be human is to use the cultural tools, or mediational means, that are provided by a particular sociocultural setting. The concrete use of these cultural tools involves an "irreducible tension" between active agents, on the one hand, and items such as computers, maps, and narratives, on the other. (p. 11)

Wertsch (1998) used societal examples to demonstrate how tools, not just as physical objects but as mental objects derived from their use, become the means by which individuals regulate their attending, problem-solving, and remembering. Clinically, these are kinds of actions that are as salient for thinking about the analysis of narrative self as they were for establishing a position on mental functions. In the act of storying, individuals are giving priority to what is attended to and remembered and how these things (within the story) address (solve) life situations (problems).

Because tools are vital to the ways we each negotiate everyday life, culture as reflected in and through the use of tools is fundamental to the narrative self. In addition, considering cultural tools as the means by which individuals move through everyday life helps us to better understand the needs and challenges of persons with communication disorders. First, understanding the tools used (i.e., physical, symbolic, animate) allows for the adjustment of communication. Second, describing a person's use of the tools for storying reveals the network of meanings (i.e., cultural dimension) that are being deployed during self construction. And lastly, the selection, manipulation, and social negotiation of communication via tools allow the clinician to "see" the person as an agent of narrative self in action.

Along with others who take a social and cultural constructive approach to self,

identity, and action, I propose that the unit of analysis, in other words what is actually observable, is an individual who is completing an action by means of tools. Taylor (2007), for example, used valued cultural creations (e.g., blogs and book writing) as tools to maintain self in the face of dementia. Some individuals with motor speech disorders adopt augmentative communication devices that begin with clinicians acting as animate tools (they provide a selection, work with programming, and write reports that support choices) while other individuals experiencing these problems rely on themselves to find cultural resources that allow them to maintain interactions. This is what we mean by agency, and as indicated above, the agency of narrative self in action is our analytical target. This stands in stark contrast to a biological position on neurogenic communication disorders where the focus is on the description of the disordered communication or on the physical differences associated with the disease process.

Storying: Cultural Tools and Agentive Action

The concept of storying was introduced in Chapter 1 and has been used as a fundamental form of action throughout this book. This notion of storying as action was derived from Wertsch's (1991) discussion of mediation. Specifically, the question that frames all action via cultural tools is that of who is doing the acting (Wertsch, 1998, 2002; Wertsch, Tulviste, & Hagstrom, 1993). With regard to the storying of narrative self, the question is who is doing the storying. If communication is indeed essential for the construction of self, can we logically conclude that the individual (regardless of the kind or degree or communication impairment) engages with family and friends, therapists and self-help groups, and even the government to do the work of storying? In other words, all those dimensions of self laid out in Chapter 3 are aspects of storying as a cultural tool that is involved in agentive action of individuals at all levels of social strata. The job of the clinician as well as the patient and family is to be aware of the cultural roots of their agentive action and, if it undermines the respective relationship upon which care and treatment rest, facilitate restorying.

Restorying would not be possible without cultural tools because only reconstruction, often partial, would result from tools that cannot handle new and enlarged roles in the individual's life now lived with a neurogenic disorder. Therefore, it is important to keep in mind that Wertsch (1998) claims that an individual's mental functioning is made observable by the use of cultural tools, a claim that is just as pertinent for narrative self. Previously in this book, we talk about agency as power, a postmodern perspective that has demonstrated the legacy of doctrines, laws, procedures, and other shared semiotic vehicles of ideology. Now I will situate this agency in the actions of the individual or families as agentive action. Specifically, I am talking about the expression of agency on the part of the individual that is observable by others in what is seen, heard, and touched in everyday life as well as during therapeutic intervention.

Through various forms of communication that can extend from insurance forms and service codes to the words used for diagnosis by a physician, the sociopolitical agentive narrative becomes part of public discourse, which in turn becomes part of situated personal storying. This personal storying is an agentive action and as such an analytical target that can be used during clinician-client communication. This stands in stark contrast to a biological position on neurogenic communication disorders where the focus is on the description of the disordered communication or on the physical differences associated with the disease process.

Putting Tools to Use

Self Construction and Sense of Self as Part of Clinical Action

In this text we refer to the personal self as the distilled construction of the sense of who one is in private and public communicative space. We claim that this sense of self is a composite that results from the use of tools (mainly symbolic across dimensions of self) used for social interchange. Thus, the unavoidable clinician question for this volume is, how can one engage in the ongoing process of self construction if a tool goes missing or is damaged? What other resources, replacement tools, can be employed to serve the communicative personhood function?

The main role of theory in clinical action is to provide a window for viewing and informing practices. While saying that one constructs one's self and that this construction is a moment–by–moment endeavor may have theoretical integrity, this premise lacks everyday sense. Few clinicians want to say to themselves or family members or patients that they are really having to recreate themselves all the time, in each interaction. As clinicians we want to treat patients who are someone to us, a self. For many clients there would simply be no logic at all to telling them or inferring or planning treatment based on a transient self. Each person knows who he is to himself and who he is to others. At face value then, the theory would even seem to violate a major purpose of this text: to include issues of self and personhood in clinical practice. Yet the claim that self is constructed in the moment adds to rather than violates the belief that therapy can include narrative self work. Why? Because this claim actually offers the possibility for analysis, and analysis is critical to clinical action.

As already noted, the action of narrative self put forth in this book is storying, a communicative act encompassing telling a story or having a story told about you. Each story is a narrative. Therefore these self stories are narratives about self that are recognizable and available for analyses. As clinicians, we hear each day self stories from our clients. They tell us about their self-care, their work or leisure activities, their families, their concerns, their jokes, and their beliefs. They are telling us about themselves in these stories. Within the narrative self theory outlined in this book, they are in the instance of that telling, in conjunction with the listener(s), constructing self. The act of storying is the means by which self in constructed in the moment.

This storying depends on semiotics, which refers to signs and symbols that convey recognizable meaning (Leeds-Hurwitz, 1993) rather than simply language or speech production. In everyday life, habitual routines such as getting breakfast can become symbolic when the routine is taken over by another for communication purposes. When the routines are used symbolically, because these come with prior contexts of use, they are considered scripts (Nelson, 1986), which can be found in the literature as part of narrative. So the action of storying can take place by means of gestures, vocalization, or verbalization to semiotically convey routines and scripts where the self as teller functions as the "I" at the same time that he is the "me" of the story. Since the semiotic communication is not a solitary act (even if the physical other is not present; in other words you are having a conversation in your mind with someone else), the other as well as the roles of I and me are part of a continuous action within the storying cycle (Bakhtin, 1986).

Clinical Action in the Moment

The clinical moment(s) are those times that you as the clinician are engaged in communicating with your client. Respect for the self of the other (Gladwell, 2005) is either present in this construction, making the therapeutic interaction one of care, or it is absent and the storying is a clinician/cultural imposed construction. As we all know, each minute we are with the client, from the time we pick him up in the hospital room for transport, or in the case of outpatients, when he enters our clinic and then therapy room, we are engaged in clinical moments. Episodes of storytelling on the part of the clinician as well as on the part of the client occur throughout. Narrative self analysis can be used to examine one particular episode or the entire clinical session. The questions that might be asked regarding self construction for each episode of storying are: (a) how am I (the patient) saying who I am; (b) who am I saying I am (four aspects of self from Chapter 3); (c) what is the listener hearing about me; (d) who are we jointly in this action of storying? Because storytelling can be recorded, it can be analyzed. The framework for this analysis is guided by the questions being asked, which in this case are about narrative self (Hagstrom, 2004).

Synthesis

The Sense of Self

The forest is always more than the trees, which is also true for personhood. While the case has just been made for how examining storying yields information about self construction, this does not in itself provide the solution to the notion that self is not constant, at least in the way we live our lives and treat those we serve in clinical situations. Personhood is the forest. It denotes the persistent sense of self that we have of ourselves and that others have about us even if the actual construction/reconstruction is in the moment. Therefore, it can be said that one's sense of self emerges out of situational and role consistencies woven together in storying over time. This results in a persistent sense of self for the individual as well as for those around him. This sense of self is an expectation frame for how a person will act with others or in a given situation. It provides the sense of what can be depended upon. The point here is that while self may be an ongoing construction, the sense of self that the individual has guides what he expects of himself even as these expectations are challenged and revised within everyday interactions. So it is important to both theoretically recognize self as construction and at the same time accept that individuals achieve a pervasive sense of self that guides actions and participation with others in everyday life.

Clinical Action

Having recognized and acknowledged the vital role that sense of self plays in daily living, we will now revisit the notion of self as construction and outline how this can inform clinical action. Theory in general (Hagstrom, 2001) and certainly about self construction provides analytical units that allow scholars to recognize and think through personhood. Theory does the same thing for the clinician. We treat/habilitate/ rehabilitate what we identify as the disease or disease characteristics that fall within the purview of speech-language pathology.

What about this concept of self construction allows for improved services to patients during narrative self work? Cultural tool kits and tools.

People and Communities of People as Tools

People are another tool. All people in all cultures have other people. This is not to say that they have intimate relations or friendships with all or any people (especially with age and illness, etc.). At the beginning of our lives people care for us or we die, and as we mature and age our lives and the lives of people in all cultures become embedded in communities of people. Therefore, socially organized as well as personally organized others are a constant in human life.

People are a constant in our lives even as the roles they take on in our lives change. Knowledge is common to all cultures and is also a product of culture, which preserves as well as creates it. This knowledge may differ. Some will remain personal, some will be shared within family units, while some will be organized within schools, companies, communities, agencies, and so forth. The point being made is that moments of actions—the very moments that constitute self-in-construction—are made possible by the individual's use of other people as animate tools.

Communication is an action made possible by tools that will be employed between people as they are involved in problem-solving life's dilemmas. One particular communication action is telling a story. When the story is about the life or actions of the teller, in this text we refer to that as storying, and in particular the storying of self. The language used, the content, the knowledge, the social others are all present in the act of storying. And in the very construction of the story, the sense of self is reflected.

Our long told and often repeated stories framed by contexts and situations with others over days, weeks, months, and years become *the* story of our lives. In the retelling of the episodes, we are in that moment reconstructing the self. With time as others tell the same stories about us, tell different versions of the same story, make up plausible stories with us, a sense or feeling of who we are as a person to ourselves and others emerges.

Clinical Action for Narrative Self Work

Clinicians are medical professionals as well as communication specialists. As such, they are unavoidably immersed in and conveyors of public discourse on health and illness, and in danger of "malignantly positioning" (Charon, 2006) their clients. If, as has been asserted throughout this book, SLPs are in the position of uniquely meeting the personhood needs of patients, they must move beyond this positioning to see and participate in the moment-by-moment construction of narrative self. Patients and families may come to therapy with discourses that revolve around the loss of self or changes in identity, their helplessness in the face of disease progression, and fear about the future (Guendouzi & Müller, 2006). None of these issues is amenable solely to standard clinical practices, for example, practicing decontextualized tasks such as telling the names of presidents, stating their own name and age, or completing story forms.

Self is not an issue of biological or neurological sciences. If, as we have claimed, self is a narrative construction that is socially shared, the clinician working with patients and their families must deal with the action involved in narrative construction, the ac-

tion of storying. This storying must include any and all modalities of interaction that can represent (i.e., be semiotic) no matter how unstandard. This might include repetitive routines or uses of space, light, or touch. Self resides in these socially shared aspects of living as surely as in the words and ideas exchanged between family members. Most importantly, the role of the clinician is to not " . . . overlook the individual in front of us and address the stereotype" (Guendouzi & Müller, 2006, p. 166).

To Be a Clinician

We have defined the patient at some length in this book, focusing on four dimensions of self. We have said that the patient, family members, and socially significant others are part of the same constructive process with regard to self. Now we must redefine the clinician within a narrative self approach to the therapeutic practice. To answer the title question of this section, one must first perhaps define what a clinician is. And perhaps that definition is one thing this book is actually about. What is a clinician, as defined by her actions with individuals whose means to story themselves have been impaired? Is she the person who works with their mouth, the person who works with their brain and retrains the parts, or (and in addition) is she the person who enters into at least a small part of their lives, becomes a role giver and receiver, and a part of their story?

Gladwell (2005) reported on a variety of studies that focused on doctor-patient communication. Each of these reported that the quality of the interpersonal interaction influenced how satisfied individuals were with their medical treatment. In fact, one study found the most vital aspect of the interaction was respect for the individual conveyed through tone of voice rather than facts or specific content (Ambady, 2005). While it may be of little surprise that respect is an essential aspect of care and caring, it is of note how much of this is communicated by subtle aspects of the mutual (or not) engagement. Part of our definition of the clinician, then, must be that the interaction communicated in touch, voice, and glance as well as word and deed is respectful of the person and family. At various points in this book we have addressed self, identities, and personhood, themes returned to in this chapter. Of note here is that respect clearly relates to self. If the latter aspects of clinician-hood are pivotal to the work, the job, does this get planned as part of the service delivery or it is both more basic to as well as more globally organizing of therapeutic interaction?

There is always the desire to find or put into place simple solutions to complex problems. Simple solutions in the case of therapy are to use a straightforward hierarchical approach as if life and life-related tasks really do unfold on a sequential time line. After all, speech-language pathologists (SLPs) are trained to write goals and objectives that unfold in just this way. Still, we would say that issues of self and personhood and our role in this as clinicians are not simple. They are messy. Therefore, it must be asked, can we write goals and objectives for clinical action around a messy issue like narrative self without reducing something this complex to a formulaic approach to remediation? In fact, are we even interested, should we be interested in remediation of narrative self?

Writing Goals and Objectives for Narrative Self

As has been stated, self is predicable. That is why we can identify the self of others even in the sea of identities. Actions in everyday life are the material of this predictability. Perhaps after neurogenic disruption to the biographical self we are seeking (within our own stories of self and the others in our lives in the stories they tell about us) pieces of predictability that may be evidenced in roles, situational interactions, or culture. If this is the case, clinical actions that pertain to narrative self should assist clients and their families in finding or rebuilding predictability among or across the four dimensions of self.

Therapists are accountable for the services they provide. This accountability is fundamentally about ethical practices rather than empirical measurement. Yet demonstrating results of services provided is common to both. Good clinicians think about what they are treating, why they are treating particular behaviors, and how they are going to illustrate that their treatment is making a difference in the life of the individual and family with neurogenic communication impairment. Simmons-Mackie, Elman, Holland, and Damico (2007) wrote about layered clinical skills that extend from activities and tasks, which are highly visible, to how clinicians actually carry out therapy, which is an implicit level of action, to why clinicians do what they do, which involves cultural biases, tacit knowledge, and other invisible ingredients. Therapy plans as textual discourse reflects all these layers. However, that very accessible layer of activities and tasks is often the only layer clinicians subject to accountability. In a sense, this reduces the vitality of the other two layers by collapsing them into an empirical set that is not of the same category. The "how" of therapy often becomes a comparison of amount or accuracy of responses by a client during individual treatment versus group therapy sessions. The documented how is seldom about the dynamics of therapy that is by necessity negotiated between the clinician and client or, in the case of group therapy, between members, one of whom is the clinician. As Nelson and Butler (2007) state, there is a science of using mediational discourse to establish supportive contexts for success. This is the how of therapy that needs documentation above and beyond Simmons-Mackie et al.'s (2007) highly visible and easily described layer of client responses to tasks. And beyond this, there must be recognition of the beliefs, values, and concerns (Kovarsky, 2007) associated with ethical practices that each clinician negotiates during clinical action with individuals and groups, which constitutes the layer of "why" (Simmons-Mackie et al., 2007).

In this book we are calling for clinicians to go beyond simply recognizing that clients have a narrative self to actually working with narrative self as an accountable practice. Our task is to now put this "new wine" into the old practices associated with but not limited to formulating goals and documentable objectives. We use the term documentable instead of measureable only because to measure assumes a predetermined endpoint, while to document allows for dynamic and open-ended change.

Goals are written to indicate what the clinician plans to achieve in a particular domain within a specified period of treatment. As such, goals are broad and reflect the scope of a treatment plan. We, as well as others (see Nelson & Butler, 2007), see therapy as dynamic and coconstructed activity on the part of both the clinician and client. Clinician self-awareness of this coconstruction is vital to the identifying process. Hagstrom (2004) used Sarbin's (1986a) approach to narrative analysis of person to address identity in clinical action. Three questions are constantly a part of this process: who am I, who are you, and who are we? These are contextualized by two broader questions when working with narrative self: is this making my client's life better, and does this make sense of the ongoing storying? A value held by the clinician is evident in the first of these questions in that what constitutes a better life is a matter of opinion that will vary between clinicians, clients, and even clients' families. For example, in a PBS broadcast about adults who were thalidomide children, inherent in each of their stories was a statement about how they perceived their own functional needs versus the goals of their fully bodied parents and therapists. Prosthetic limbs were attached to legs and arms so the children could walk as we do and write as we do. These adults made the point that prior to ever being fitted with these prostheses they had mastered rolling across the floor to get where they wanted to be and using their mouth or whatever partially formed appendage was available to hold objects such as spoons, cups, or pencils. As adults, they have jobs and spouses and raise children without the use of prosthetics. The value behind the interventions with these children was to make it possible for them to have a better life. The judgments that guided the goals for treatment were cultural biases (Simmons-Mackie et al., 2007) about the physicality necessary for this.

Person-Centered Goals and Objectives

Worrell (2006) calls for person-centered treatment. She reminds us within evidence-based medicine (as contrasted with EBP) there is a place for and the need to situate services in the will of the patient. Rather than writing specific goals and objectives the discussion of tools as presented in this text can provide a nexus for person-centered practices.

In planning treatment, whether individual, family, or group, if Worrell's position is combined with sociocultural theory and narrative self work, the three kinds of tools discussed above can be used to determine goals. In other words, regardless of the deficits that the clinician identifies, the patient would work with the clinician or intervention team to decide what forms of assistance would be most useful for gaining functionality for specific everyday actions. Family members would also decide what forms of assistance they think would best serve their family member in order to make functional gains. Negotiations about getting things done from both perspectives as well as shifts in the forms or amounts of this assistance would reflect change, what we commonly associate with objectives.

For example, does the patient want to complete specific tasks (such as taking a bath) with the assistance of another person? What aspects of this task does the patient want assistance with? Then from the perspective of the family with regard to the same specific task, what level of assistance do they think their family member needs in order to reach functionality (with bathing)? While all concerned might want bathing to be more personal, perceptions about levels and amounts of assistance might be quite different for family members and patients. Perhaps the family was smothering the patient with care when that individual wanted less animate tool assistance but increased tangible tools to work on the activity himself. These differences would be negotiated points and points of communication. As a result, therapy may be considered more meaningful for the patient and family because it is focused on activities that impact everyday life for all of them. This approach is person-centered because patients and families are communicating about how they will get tasks done rather than accepting what we as clinicians think they need to achieve. Since self and social identity are about the storying of life and this storying is about everyday actions, the negotiation of personhood, maintenance of self, and construction of identity remain central to therapy. In other words, these three issues contextualize the treatment rather than treatment being contextualized by the disease process.

Final Thoughts

The ending to any project that has consumed one's life for well over a year is mixed with the sweet sense of accomplishment and a deep feeling of loss. The "baby" must grow with others now, and if we, the authors, have done our work well enough the readers of this text will have the foundation necessary to begin their own journey with narrative self. We don't have the answers, but perhaps the people whose stories have been told and our work with these stories will provide the readers of this text with touchstones for their own journeys into issues of self, identity, and personhood as they work with those who live with neurogenic communication disorders.

CHAPTER 12

Supporting the Narrative Self

by Barbara B. Shadden

There are some clinical moments you never forget. The following is one such moment.

Franklin Ruston suffered a severe stroke at the age of 61. His receptive and expressive aphasia, coupled with a severe apraxia of speech, left him incapable of communicating through verbal channels. He was referred for an AAC evaluation by his current speech-language pathologist (SLP), who acknowledged that the aphasia might interfere with his ability to use symbolic communication on such a device but indicated that the family was desperate to find a "cure" for his problems. During the evaluation, Franklin was unexpectedly successful in dealing with symbols as representations and grasping the categorical framework of the system as set up. While exploring one screen, he selected the icon of a heart, and heard it say, "I love you." He immediately went back to a previous screen, found his wife's name, and selected it, then touched the message window to say, "I love you, Connie." With a big smile, he held up a finger ("just wait") and pointed to the door leading to the waiting room where his wife was sitting.

At the end of the evaluation, his wife returned to the room and the SLP described briefly the outcomes of the evaluation, ending by saying, "I believe Franklin has something to say." He looked his wife straight in the eyes, selected the message window, and the device said, "I love you, Connie." And the wife, looking at the SLP with an annoyed expression, said, "That's a weird voice. I'd hate to have to listen to that all the time." After a pause she added, "He never felt comfortable with computers anyway."

Why does almost everyone gasp after hearing that story? What is it that strikes at some basic level of humanity, even without knowing the people or the specific circumstances? Franklin Ruston had just rediscovered the gift of communication in letting his wife know he was still there, still loving her. He had found one small way to affirm his narrative self in relationship, in interaction. His wife totally ignored this expression of self, focusing instead on the altered message quality and the fact that it was not socially acceptable. In that one moment, one of those many small moments of self construction, the wife rejected his communicative offering and the person behind that offering. His wife was not necessarily uncaring or cruel; she simply did not know who either of them was in a world with aphasia.

Or what about the following?

Harry and his wife were having lunch in a restaurant on his first outing from a rehab facility. At the next table was a well-known coach of a university athletics team. Despite his wife's attempts to dissuade him, Harry immediately got up and went over to the coach, trying to introduce himself and explain when they had met before. After months of hospitalization, it was clear that he needed to validate himself in the world outside of the medical system.

Unfortunately, Harry's receptive aphasia was extremely severe at that time, and his expressive jargon made little sense. The coach mumbled a few words, said "Good to see you, buddy," and turned back to his table companion, even though Harry was still trying to talk with him. Harry's wife helped him return to their table. Before they had even sat down, the coach loudly said, "Boy, how pathetic can you get." Fortunately, Harry did not understand, but his wife did.

Again, most readers will shudder when reading this story. Harry's strong need to obtain recognition from a high status individual, the coach, was treated dismissively. Further, the coach's use of the term "pathetic" when it could be overheard makes clear just how devalued Harry was because of his inability to communicate effectively. And his wife was humiliated for both of them. I was that wife, and thus my summary of the essence of this book is necessarily colored by personal, as well as professional, experiences.

Why begin this chapter with these two stories? Because it is critical to return to the original premises that led to writing this text, particularly the centrality of communication in the construction and reconstruction of self. For me, the following are the key recurring themes in our theoretical and life stories chapters:

1. Life and one's sense of self are storied.
2. Self is socially constructed in the domains of culture, roles, interactions, and biography.
3. Communication is at the core of life storying, with impaired communication discrediting us with others and disrupting our ability to use narrative as a meaning-making tool.

Each of these themes will be elaborated further in terms of the clinical implications of the need for continuing one's life story and renegotiating one's identity or narrative self.

In Chapter 1 of this text, we described a number of existing models and frameworks that have expanded our understanding of living with neurogenic disorders. A focus on narrative self is supported by such models but also raises additional questions about the nature of assessment and treatment when self takes center stage in the intervention process. Throughout the text, we have also acknowledged that we have not provided a comprehensive literature review, one that would target those master clinicians, researchers, and best practices that characterize the clinical landscape of the early 21st century. That has been particularly difficult for me, since I feel a sense of unpaid debt—to those who came before, to today's visionary leaders, thinkers, and clinicians, and to the passion of those who work with people with neurogenic communication disorders. In this text, however, we have endeavored to focus on the extraordinary commitment to narrative self of those whose stories we have shared.

This final chapter is my attempt to articulate my "bottom line." What would I like readers to remember when they finish reading this text? Where would I like to see clinicians and researchers investing time and effort if our concepts of narrative self do indeed illuminate our understanding of the impact of neurogenic communication disorders? Are the insights suggested here applicable beyond the discipline of communication sciences and disorders? The remainder of this chapter provides a summary of key themes, with reflections on the clinical implications of a focus on narrative self.

Key Themes Revisited

Life as Storied

We have stated that narrative, the storying of one's life, is fundamental to human existence, a position readily accepted in many disciplines today. We communicate about who and what we are through moments of storying. Kovarsky and Curran (2007) recently cited Ray Kent's (1990) discussion of the need for a science of the person in the following quote:

And thus we now return to our starting point, the assertion that each client is a

biography, a narrative of life history. . . . To appreciate the individual histories of clients or patients, we need to go beyond the traditional scope of science. The unity of personhood is beyond any approach or quantification. (p. 57)

Almost two decades ago, Kent acknowledged the centrality of narrative and of personhood expressed through narrative. He also acknowledged that personhood as a construct is so complex as to be almost impossible to grasp with our existing research methodologies.

The idea of narrative self is grounded in an understanding of storying across the life span. Thus it is not surprising that some of the clearest statements about the centrality of narrative can be found in publications about aging. For example, Bruner (1999) suggests that "[l]ife is a work of art . . . the art is in the telling" (p. 7), acknowledging elsewhere that "[t]here is no way to describe lived time except in the form of narrative" (Bruner, 2004, p. 692). In this text, we have suggested that neurogenic communication disorders disrupt the presentation and ongoing renegotiation of narrative self, in part because communication is a primary tool in the storying of self. Our basic premise is that one cannot understand the impact of these disorders without considering the changes in self.

Bruner (2004, p. 692) would suggest that the telling of one's life, in any format, can be considered a "cognitive achievement," in that a series of decisions must be made as to what to convey in what format to whom. He has used the term *dysnarrativia* (Bruner, 1990, p. 222) to describe an "inability to tell or understand stories," one associated with various neuropathies. He further suggests that dysnarrativia is "deadly for selfhood" (p. 223), a premise consistent with the theory and life stories we have presented in this text. While the use of this term may not be relevant for all of the conditions we have described here, the premise of an impairment of narrative is central to our theoretical work. It is important to note that we are not using narrative here in the sense of the grand life story, although that is indeed one form of life narrative. Instead, we are referring to the fact that every communicative encounter with others contains elements of narrative and associated identity construction. As Hagstrom indicates in Chapter 11, it is the many small actions and interactions of each day that build the story of our life, our self. These narrative and interactive building blocks depend on cultural conventions and linguistic processes, with the narrator consciously or unconsciously structuring perceptions and memories to convey a message about his life.

Singer (2004) notes that each person's narrative is a "fluid and evolving work in progress" (p. 445). At any given point in time, depending on context and circumstances, our narrative exchanges create local spheres of meaning that allow us to present ourselves in a specific manner and to know others in that moment. Examination of narrative at these moments is much like taking a snapshot of the interaction in order to frame a transitory understanding of the identities of the parties who are interacting.

Self as Socially Constructed

Throughout, we have asserted that self is socially constructed and negotiated in each social interaction. Hagstrom (Chapter 11, this text) highlights the paradox in such statements, emphasizing that we also have a persistent and personalized sense of self that allows us to move through each day with some confidence. Some of that sense of unified self exists because of those narrative processes that allow us to create and modify the many identities that define who

and what we are in social contexts. The idea of socially-mediated narrative self is not a new one (Bauer, 2005). For our purposes, we have proposed that narrative construction of self occurs in at least four dimensions, including culture, role, interaction, and biography.

Our taxonomy of dimensions of self emerged naturally as we began to recognize that our original concept of identity was potentially too simplistic. When we listened closely to the life stories of those with ALS, PD, aphasia, and dementia, we recognized just how diverse individual experiences were. Our dimensions of self reflect the different social ways and contexts in which life stories are exchanged and narrative plays out. Further, any personal narrative or life story must "mesh . . . within a community of life stories" (Bruner, 2004, p. 699). Being "different" is only acceptable to a certain degree. Beyond some invisible boundary, being different in one's life story sets the individual apart from others. When our differences cross the threshold of acceptability, we no longer receive recognition and affirmation from others. Further, at moments of change or life "trouble" (Bruner, 1999), the need for acceptance and recognition increases at the same time as the risks of rejection also increase. Thus, the gradual or abrupt onset of a neurogenic communication disorder potentially disrupts this critical process of self presentation and recognition.

Communication at the Core of Life Storying

Communication, often in the form of narrative, is a primary mechanism through which we both ascribe meaning to our lives and life events and also convey to others who and what we are as persons. In the context of life-changing events such as the onset or diagnosis of a neurogenic communication disorder, it is the sharing of narrative, specifically illness narrative, that provides opportunities for renegotiating an identity that incorporates aspects of the illness as a part of self (Frank, 1995). The inability to share such narratives, as well as elements of the larger life story, can discredit us with others, making us difficult to know. Thus we are at risk for losing agency in the creation of personhood, while also losing tools needed to attribute meaning to life events.

Discrediting the Narrator

Loss of communication makes us difficult to know. Further, it has been suggested that illness and disability may create a kind of spoiled identity (Goffman, 1963). In part, this risk for acquiring a spoiled identity is at the heart of our focus on narrative self; disability is known to be a socially constructed process. Numerous authors have spoken of the need to use unflawed communicative tools in the life storying processes that help us maintain selfhood. For example, Holstein and Gubrium (2001) emphasize the need to present "reasonably familiar identities" (p. 13). Without such identities we risk not being taken seriously or being attributed personhood that is eccentric or inadequate. Goffman (1967) notes that the study of self can only be grounded in a study of the "traffic rules of social interaction." Others have written of the importance of using acceptable social tools in identity negotiations, particularly language codes that are familiar and culturally validated (Beard, 2004; Becker, 1999; McFadden, 2005). Beck (2005) suggests that the act of telling one's narrative allows "my story" to be transformed into "our story." Use of a flawed communication tool can lead to loss of agency in social contexts. We must justify any violation of conventions of normal communication, or we will be discredited.

In many instances, what may be impaired in the communicative interchange with persons with neurogenic communication disorders can be as subtle as small shifts in timing, in speed of responsiveness in interactions. Pasupathi (2006) suggests that much of the small talk found in everyday life is at the heart of social validation of narrative self. Small talk is critical in maintaining the interpersonal contacts that are the foundation for negotiation of self (Malinowski, 1923). All of the neurogenic communication disorders described in this text are characterized, at the very least, by a slower rate of conversation than found in unimpaired interaction, by some breakdown in how well each person understands or is understood. Given the spontaneous and evanescent nature of acts of creating meaning through communication (Charon, 2002), time pressure alone may undermine the process of self construction in daily exchanges.

In the medical ethics literature, a great deal has been written about narrative processes that occur between health professionals (particularly physicians) and patients. Carson (2002) has discussed the "hyphenated space"—the silence that occurs in the absence of narrative, and the common turning away from the patient, rendering her voiceless. In many instances, the absence of narrative is construed as evidence of mental incompetence. Thus, the challenge to medical practitioners is to develop stronger narrative competence, which implies interpreting and acting on the stories of patients. The same challenge applies to other health care providers, as well as family, friends, and society in general.

Loss of Mechanism for Filtering Life Experiences

Impaired ability to tell one's life story also affects sense-making processes for those experiencing the communication disorder.

In much of the literature, there is discussion about the ways in which individuals cope with or adapt to life change. Regardless of the label for this process, humans deal with change by modifying their narratives or stories. Guendouzi and Müller (2006) describe this as a homeostatic mechanism for maintaining a sense of stable self, with language as a major system for constructing meaningful culture. Loss of communication and the meaning-making processes of narrative disrupts our ability to understand our experiences and make choices about what must be added to our storied self. In particular, narrating illness can create openings for other kinds of narratives critical to renegotiating identity. If our life story has been temporarily derailed by some form of trouble (Bruner, 1999), and that trouble cannot be eliminated or overcome, a new narrative must be created, one that incorporates the trouble and restores meaning to the narrative self.

Nakano, Hinckley, and Paul (2007) raise questions about how one can reflect on self and the life changes created by any disabling condition when one is devoid of words. It is a question well worth pondering. Most of us have experienced moments of insight that occurred only because we were sharing some piece of our life story with another person. Narrative does more than present some version of our perceived self to others. It also allows us to filter our experience through the narrative lens (Singer, 2004, p. 442), to craft causal, temporal, and thematic coherence in order to revise our sense of self. In part, this occurs through illness narratives, although sense-making takes place in other narrative contexts as well. Illness and other life-altering experiences open the door to considering both lost and new possible selves.

Individuals with neurogenic communication disorders may struggle to maintain aspects of their previous narrative self. They may not be able to use communication to accommodate flexibly any newly emerging sense of self and life story. They may experience challenges in presenting themselves as competent in the context of impairment, advanced age, or both. They may struggle to convince others that they are not incompetent, and they may have problems sharing the vast spectrum of human reactions, including those evaluative and judgmental responses that define who they are (Armstrong, 2005a). Bauer (2005) and McAdams (1993) write about transition stories, those narratives that address life changes by either focusing on personal mastery and status in the face of these changes (in the agency domain) or by highlighting themes of personal growth and relationship (in the communion domain).

Narrative Self and Clinical Practice: Clinicians as Facilitators of Narrative Self Reconstruction

The key premises summarized here provide the rationale for claiming that challenges to narrative self must be addressed in interventions with those living with ALS, PD, stroke-related aphasia, dementia, and other neurogenic communication disorders. Speech-language clinicians must be in the front lines of the battle to restore and renegotiate a sense of viable narrative self for these persons, including their significant others whose life stories have also been affected. Part of the challenge for clinicians may be finding ways to enhance an understanding that the loss of communication goes beyond loss of words in daily interactions. Part of the challenge may also be finding ways to support and nurture other actions in daily life that are self-enhancing.

In the following sections, suggestions are made about how an understanding of narrative self might be incorporated into present day intervention practices. There are no "cookbook" treatments when dealing with issues as complex as those associated with self and narrative. However, speech-language clinicians are uniquely positioned to probe the impact of neurological conditions on a person's sense of identity and self, guide persons through a process of narrative self renegotiation, and participate as coconstructor of self through acts of clinical discourse. Some readers may be uncomfortable with these roles; that is perfectly understandable. But none of us can afford to blatantly disregard issues of identity and self, since they are fundamental to the outcomes of good quality of life and full life participation despite the constraints of communication impairment. Implicit in these statements is recognition of the importance of taking the time and exerting the effort required to truly understand the person's life story and narrative self as affected by neurogenic communication disorders and to assess the impact of communication impairment over time.

Targeting Dimensions of Self

Fundamental to this text is the question of how changes in one's perceived sense of self affect recovery and reintegration into life and society. Self needs to be considered in the overlapping domains of biography, interaction, roles, and cultural contexts. Targeting narrative self requires unique and comprehensive forms of assessment that probe multiple life domains (see Assessment of Living with Aphasia, Kagan et al., 2007, discussed later in this chapter). If our conceptual framework has merit, targeting narrative self also involves helping clients

and significant others identify resources in their tool kits (see Chapter 3) and facilitating use of these tools in all domains in order to support ongoing storying of self. In the following chapter sections, each of these levels is discussed. Examples from Harry's life story (Chapter 8) are used to illustrate successful and unsuccessful intervention approaches to narrative self in the face of aphasia.

Biographical Self

The idea of biography or autobiography is perhaps easiest to understand. In fact, if you imagine being asked, "Tell me about yourself," you can begin to understand the diverse elements that may be associated with any one individual's biographical self. Information about biographical self can be somewhat easier to gather than about aspects of self in other domains (Faircloth, Rittman, Boylstein, Young, & Van Puymbroeck, 2004). Biographical self is closely aligned to who we think we are in relationship to others. On the surface, many elements of biographical self remain in place after diagnosis of a neurogenic communication disorder. One is still a woman, a wife, a person of a certain age, a daughter, and a churchgoer, and that history remains unchanged. Other aspects of biographical self (such as employment) may be more challenged by the communication impairment.

The biography of the client may be a fertile area for rediscovering tools for self negotiation. In a sense, the SLP may act as a kind of biographical detective, identifying biographic priorities, past and present. By truly listening to what the individual and her family say, the SLP may identify or highlight tools that even the client has overlooked or forgotten. For example, for a client who privileged her previous work activities, discussions with the SLP may help identify other priorities and move the focus to a biographic characteristic that remains within reach. In current clinical practices, support for sharing of biographical self is particularly evident in work with persons with Alzheimer's disease (cf. Hepburn et al., 1997). In aphasia management, biographical self is also being targeted in work assisting such persons to create their own Web sites. Various on-line posts and forums also provide support for sharing of life information with all of the disorders discussed in this text.

Of course, it is possible to gather most of the information needed to describe the biographical particulars of a person's life story and still not know which of those is most important. In the case of Harry, although he had already retired prior to his stroke, the idea of returning to work became a priority during his months of rehabilitation. He needed the sense of validation he had experienced previously in his work as a case manager for the chronically mentally ill. Tied in with that priority was a need to feel useful, competent, and contributing. The relative privileging of employment as a priority had to be understood in working with Harry, even though its importance would not have been predicted based solely on the facts of his life. In this case, the SLP would need to listen even more carefully to what Harry had to say about his past and understand that some previous tools were essential for Harry to move forward with revising his life story.

Interactions and Relationships

In most neurogenic communication disorders, interactions and relationships receive primary focus. After all, most people grasp the fact that communication is central to relationships. From an intervention perspective, it is relatively easy to target daily interactions. As with other dimensions of self, we must identify premorbid interactional styles, important relationships, and the value placed on these relationships by the other party.

However, the role of interactions and relationships in the ongoing storying of self must not be neglected. It is this aspect of interaction that is less readily understood by those living with neurogenic disorders. While it is certainly important to be able to express one's preference for dinner to one's spouse, it is equally important to move forward with life, to be able to discuss and express responses to the changes that have occurred in all life spheres, to tell one's own illness narrative and discuss life since diagnosis.

Thus SLPs must explore the impact of the communication impairment on the storying of self within important relationships and must facilitate storying processes. This requires working with clients and families to develop an understanding of how communication operates within previous and existing interactions and relationships. Sometimes, even when old and new communicative tools for interaction are identified, too much attention is paid to refurbishing these tools, with insufficient attention to the underlying changes in perceived self that will continue to impair relationships. Shadden and Koski (2007) have discussed how a stroke support group and a communication treatment program helped one client strengthen his sense of self post-stroke and thus begin to use existing tools for moving forward with his life story. Interactions between the SLP and the client may be important elements in intervention, not only because of the tools that are created in such interactions, but also because they provide the client with opportunities for success in negotiating relationships.

For Harry, interactions with others had been a primary tool for validation of self. He defined himself in relational terms, both professionally and personally. When his communication impairments disrupted those interactions, he was both depressed and angered. His response was to take others to task for failing to provide the communicative responses and attention he expected. A kind of vicious cycle of communication and self breakdown evolved. Harry needed the self validation that derives from everyday conversational interactions. Instead of validation, however, he was forced to confront his deficits in virtually all interactive encounters. His "lecturing" of others sometimes changed communicative interactions but also tended to limit interpersonal exchanges. He sensed others' altered response to him and tried harder to obtain validation, and the cycle continued. These issues would have been excellent targets in intervention if they had been identified early or if treatment had extended over time. As Harry stated frequently, when he was alone, he did not feel impaired or incompetent. When he turned towards interactions for validation, however, his experience was typically one of failure of narrative self.

Roles and Situations

Roles, particularly tied to specific situations, are most closely associated with what many think of as identity and with more measurable aspects of disability. Our roles are associated with characteristic interactions, communicative modes, communication partners, and settings. The impact of communication disorders on roles is highly variable. For example, the role of employee may be altered as a consequence of stroke, or ALS, or PD, or dementia. For some, this loss of work role would be relatively insignificant. As discussed in Chapter 6,

while Jim valued his university position, once he was diagnosed with ALS, he was relatively content to retire early and expressed no sense of regret for the lost role and status. In contrast, Steve's work was strongly linked to his sense of self and value. He independently pursued all technological options to ensure that he could continue to contribute in his job for as long as possible.

Speech-language clinicians and other professionals must probe the importance of life roles to the individual client. What is at stake is developing an understanding of which roles are critical to self construction and validation. If a critical role can be maintained with some accommodations, then these accommodations can be facilitated. If the role cannot be maintained, the SLP must work with the client and significant others to adapt to that loss and to seek out other validating roles and opportunities. Again, the focus of the SLP is on identifying tools that are still in the tool kit despite the communication disorder, that can be added to the tool kit, that can be reworked and used, or that can be reanimated with a different power source.

Harry's desire to return to work reflected his need for self validation or recognition in his previous role as professional. Because the SLP was the first professional who spent much time talking with him after his stroke, she became a pivotal social figure. For Harry, success in therapy related directly to his perception of how he was treated in the therapy room. Success was also measured in terms of how he was treated when he went out into community social environments such as restaurants. He was impatient with worksheets and other impairment-level activities that did not appear to directly address his role needs.

Harry's focus on work included a preoccupation with another role, that of wage earner, of "bringing in" income, a rather surprising priority given his limited concern about financial issues earlier in his life. His SLPs and I understood his need for recognition in his previous employment role but missed early cues that there had been such a dramatic shift in his priorities with respect to income generation. Only after several weeks of escalating frustration was the problem identified. At this point, a plan was developed to allow Harry to return to work part-time, with therapy targeting his interactions with clients and an analysis of factors contributing to success or communication breakdown. I was able to work with him to create an aphasia-friendly report format that would allow him to complete case management forms. He carefully reported his earnings every 2 weeks.

Self in Culture

For persons with neurogenic communication disorders, there are many cultural stigmas that must be dealt with on a daily basis. An inability to communicate effectively is perceived as an indication of a more fundamental social incompetence. The SLP can be particularly effective at helping people to understand that there are strategies for dealing with such stigmas. Some individuals choose to become active in local or national organizations that provide advocacy and public information. Examples might include the Amyotrophic Lateral Sclerosis Association (ALSA), the National Aphasia Association (NAA), the Parkinson's Disease Association (PDA), and the Alzheimer's Association. Similarly, some clinicians choose to take an active role in such organizations, attempting to create change at the cultural as well as the individual level. Other persons living with neurogenic communication disorders choose to educate society one person at a time. This can be a daunting task, but it is an important one.

Typically, those who choose a more active role in addressing cultural stigmas and social lack of understanding are validated by their involvement. While we do not argue that the SLP is obligated to take an activist role, clinicians must support the client by providing tools for dealing with negative interactions based on cultural beliefs.

Harry had been involved with a stroke support group for many years prior to his stroke. As might be expected, it was difficult for him to switch from visibility and prominence as professional facilitator of the group to his new status as group member. This issue of position within the support group culture has not been resolved. However, Harry independently decided to start a new stroke support group closer to home. In doing so, he set himself up as group leader and thus a person with power and social status. While this example is at the interactional level, it is also cultural because status is a valued cultural goal (Huberman, Loch, & Onculer, 2004).

Using Intervention Tools and Processes More Effectively

If clinicians make a commitment to support life storying, there are numerous aspects of the intervention process that can be manipulated. These include, but are not limited to, goal setting, optimal treatment contexts, timelines for restorying of self, mechanisms for eliciting narratives, and tools in the life storying process. Each of these is discussed briefly.

Goal Setting

Clinicians must engage in active collaborative and functional goal setting with clients and significant others (Worrall, 2007). Goals should be established within a framework that considers the need for ongoing storying of self, of moving on with life with neurological impairment. Goal setting can be facilitated by use of tools such as the Assessment of Living with Aphasia, which is currently under development (Kagan, 2007; Kagan et al., 2007) and which visually depicts aphasia and living with aphasia as a potential barrier to life participation. This assessment tool was built on the premise that the client is the most important agent in judging meaningful life challenges and changes.

If narrative self plays out in multiple domains, we might expect different clients to have different priorities. So . . . who sets those goals? Worrall (2006) has expressed concern about our failure to meet the true needs of our clients. She traces practice patterns in speech-language pathology, noting that we have moved from clinician-driven goals to client-driven goals and hopefully to a new perspective on person-centered goals. Person-centered goal setting acknowledges the social grounding of our work and the fact that more than one individual is living with challenges to narrative self. For Harry, it is doubtful that he could initially have expressed his needs for self-validation. However, as his wife, I was able to share information about Harry the person, including personality and style of interaction. Based on this information, "functional" therapy activities were developed to provide him with success in social validation.

In goal setting, we must consider the question of whose value system is guiding the process. While person-centered goals will be more personally relevant and better linked to life participation and quality of life (Simmons-Mackie & Kagan, 2007; Worrall, 2007), there are always potential discrepancies between client and clinician values in the goal-setting process. For example, many clinicians presume that talking better is a universal goal, but there is no evidence to support this presumption. Sometimes, the clinician may recognize that a client can benefit from use of AAC. Without probing how that use of AAC affects the client's sense of narrative self, the AAC recommendation may be made, only to find the device gathering dust in a closet because we failed to ask the right questions about client priorities and life story needs.

The challenge is to determine how we move towards interventions that use treatment goals that privilege narrative self. To do so, we must learn to ask the right people the right questions. We have to learn to listen better, to identify the voice of the client and significant others as they attempt to express their needs and share who they are. We need to learn more about the life stories of our clients so we can facilitate their expression (Gubrium, 1986; Randall, Prior, & Sarborn, 2006; Shotter, 2003, 2005; Stanley, 2004).

Working Directly with Life Stories and Illness Narrative

We have been cautious about suggesting that every client with a neurogenic communication disorder should be provided with opportunities to tell her life story in a formal manner. Telling one's story is a powerful exercise in self-reflection, and one that can be fraught with emotion at times of crisis. Active storying may be uncomfortable to some, maybe to many. In addition, the life story continues to evolve as those living with neurogenic communication disorders continue to reconstruct who they are in the various life domains they occupy.

Having said that, clinicians should encourage sharing of pieces of the life story whenever possible. These pieces may reflect perceptions of self in the larger culture, in roles, in relationships, and in the lifetime of amassed biographical particulars. The more clients feel they can share about who they are, the more successful the therapeutic intervention will be. In addition, illness narratives occur much more readily in therapeutic contexts, since the reason client and clinician are in the room together relates to a specific disorder or disease process. Significant others also have illness narratives to share and may be struggling to understand who they are in relationship to the pronounced changes in their life stories. If the clinician truly listens to these bits and pieces of narrative, it is possible to develop a much clearer understanding of the valued identities of clients and family, and goal setting is facilitated.

In the context of encouraging sharing of life stories, it is appropriate for the clinician to share personal information as well. This sharing creates more parity in the communicative exchange and shifts the locus of power from the clinician. Sharing of self is an intimate experience, even if the details of the shared self are as simple as love for a cherished dog. In everyday relationships, the volunteering of such personal information is almost always matched by the communication partner, if indeed there is a desire to continue the interaction. Failure to share in the clinical exchange may result in the client feeling devalued.

There are times when the exchange of life stories can be formalized in treatment. At the University of Arkansas, there have been ongoing communication groups that often focus on life stories (Shadden & Koski, 2007). Our life stories groups began as a relatively straightforward conversation group and evolved into the life stories format after a spontaneous decision in one session to create a chronological time line for key life events for both clinicians and clients. Ironically, when a new group started up, it was formally called the Life Stories Group. However, drawing attention to the process made

some members uncomfortable. Since that time, we have used elements of this process in the context of a variety of group formats.

What is truly remarkable is the transformation of our clients (and student clinicians) when they become involved in such a group. By creating a therapeutic environment in which storying of self is explicitly encouraged, we see many facets of our clients that do not emerge in more traditional one-on-one therapy. One outcome that is particularly important is a desire to share with others the experience of the stroke—the illness narrative. This desire emerges spontaneously, without clinician prompting, and is explicitly oriented to other persons with aphasia.

Optimal Treatment Contexts

No single treatment program can possibly address the need to recreate a narrative self in the multiple social contexts experienced by each person living with a communication disorder. The challenge to the clinician is to be aware of all treatment options within the community and proactive in developing alternatives to those treatments typically funded through insurance. A needs assessment may be part of this process. If so, needs to be considered should also include issues of access and participation in community-based activities. In fact, the terms *treatment* and *assessment* may be the biggest barriers to meeting needs for storying of self. Invariably, for both clinicians and clients, these terms suggest deficits or impairment to be fixed. Narrative self does not fare well in this context. As asserted by Koski in Chapter 10, health care professionals need to engage with broader community-level initiatives that address issues of participation. It is difficult to imagine doing the required work of storying of self if one is cut off from the many social and community activities that supported that self prior to illness diagnosis.

Throughout this text, groups have been highlighted as contexts that provide a community for validating the self of persons with various neurogenic communication disorders and their significant others. Groups serve a variety of functions. In Chapter 4, for example, it was noted that personal and community narratives sometimes merge to affirm the ongoing life story in support groups. Communication and conversation groups are also widely accepted as powerful environments for improving interactions and validating self (Elman, 2006). Groups underscore the essentially social nature of our presentation of narrative self and thus provide a more natural environment for moving forward with one's life story. Stanley (2004) has said that one fundamental characteristic of an illness experience is a sense of profound isolation in multiple arenas. Isolation in turn contributes to a sense of having lost one's way in one's own life story. In a group environment, the isolation is lifted somewhat.

If we wish to use groups to support the narrative self of persons living with neurogenic communication disorders, care must be taken to avoid assigning the person with aphasia the role of patient who then automatically cedes control to the professional (Horton, 2007). Group processes can be complex. Simmons-Mackie, Elman, Holland, and Damico (2007) recently identified core attributes of successful groups, including discourse equality/symmetry, engagement in everyday communicative events, use of silence and gaze solicitation to promote participation, genuine respect for other group members, and clinician adherence to her own personal style. All of these also support the presentation of self.

Opportunities for facilitating the storying of self occur in other contexts as well.

As suggested above, the dyadic clinical interaction provides opportunities for recognition of self, for letting one's voice be heard and understood. In addition, as previously noted, some persons find self validation by participating in groups or organizations designed to serve advocacy and political action functions. By affiliating with a local chapter of the ALS Association (ALSA), for example, persons with ALS and their families acquire a new identity, find meaning, and feel empowered by the commitment to action, even when the family member with ALS dies. Those who have lived with Alzheimer's disease often find meaning in advocacy for funding for this disorder.

There will always be clients or significant others who vehemently oppose any form of group involvement. However, some who are reluctant to participate in face-to-face groups find comfort in the distance and anonymity of the on-line support groups and discussion communities that have emerged in recent years. For the neurogenic communication disorders discussed in this text, there are numerous such communities. Health care providers should respectfully visit one or more on-line groups. There you will often read painfully honest postings about what the experience of loss of communication means to each individual. Invariably, the tone is one of support, acceptance, and understanding. The work of the narrative self, of storying of life, occurs here on a daily basis. When appropriate, clients and family should be referred to such sites for support and self expression.

Time Lines for Intervention

Creating and sharing one's life story occurs over time, indeed over the life span, assuming no disruptions in the normal allotment of years. We have discussed the centrality of time in understanding the distinctive challenges to narrative self associated with living with each of the neurogenic disorders described in this text. Intervention needs are constantly evolving for all persons touched by the communication disorder. There are also stages in meaning-making that occur through life storying at different times, as there are stages in readiness to deal with information and to take on different treatment challenges.

Communication is rarely a priority early when medical issues take precedence or when initial communicative changes are slight. Thus client and family awareness of changes in narrative self will probably not emerge until later in the timeline of recovery or decline. Clinicians need to monitor evolving needs and concerns over time, despite the fact that the health care system in America is not designed to support extended monitoring and assessment. If our premise about the centrality of storying of self is valid, the challenge to practitioners is to find ways to maintain involvement with persons living with neurogenic communication disorders for months and even years. The solution may be something as simple as a telephone check-up at fixed intervals (depending on the disorder), or a group gathering to touch base about issues of living with the specific disorder. These activities allow monitoring of the evolution of narrative self and typically do not take inordinate amounts of time.

The life stories chapters in this text hint at unique timeline issues associated with each disease. For example, several persons living with ALS have stressed the importance of not having to deal with the full medical picture at the outset. Thus, clinicians must be sensitive to this need and must offer new information with care. Since the primary involvement of SLPs with persons with ALS tends to be in the AAC domain, there is some time pressure to make decisions about AAC

early on, while intelligible speech and motor skills remain functional. However, the process of considering AAC cannot be pushed upon the client and her family. SLPs need to remain in contact with families, ready to provide support and information when needed. Similar examples of unique timeline challenges apply to each of the other disorders addressed in this text. What is clear is the fact that little is known about the maintenance, evolution, and/or decline of narrative self and about the factors that influence these processes. Research and trial clinical interventions are needed.

Tools for Supporting Narrative Self

Throughout this text, we have underscored the idea that we all have tools for supporting our narrative self, and it is the communication tool that is jeopardized in neurogenic communication disorders. In Chapter 10, Koski describes the challenge to clinicians as one of helping those living with communication disorders to use existing tools better, or to acquire new tools, in the ongoing storying of self. In Chapter 11, Hagstrom also focuses on the types of tools available to support efforts to create and share an illness narrative and to move forward with the reconstruction of narrative self. Both animate and inanimate tools can facilitate these processes.

Inanimate tools include a variety of objects—notebooks, AAC devices, a card explaining the communication impairment, artifacts. When used appropriately, these tools can indeed support communication, particularly in the biographical domain of self. Every clinician should explore with clients and family members those tools that are available and acceptable in the context of *client-* or *person-centered* goals. Creativity is encouraged. For example, when Harry was first moved to a geriatric psychiatric unit due to unmanageable behaviors, I was concerned about the patronizing and dismissive behaviors of the staff in interacting with him. I typed up a one-page life history, giving many specific and hopefully interesting biographic particulars so that staff would see Harry as a person, not just a behavioral problem. By the end of the first 24 hours, several nursing assistants had asked me additional questions. The change in interactions was remarkable. Staff now approached him with good eye contact, using his last name, mentioning items on his life history. One nursing assistant in particular talked repeatedly with Harry about fishing. Although he had little understanding and nothing but jargon output, his behavior became less agitated when he was approached as a person first. It is this type of creativity that we are encouraging, and the SLP may be one of the few professionals in a position to facilitate information gathering and brainstorming.

There is at least one major caveat with respect to use of tools. What appears to the SLP to be the most appropriate and effective tool in supporting communication may not be acceptable to the client or significant others. Any attempt to force a particular choice is doomed to failure. Only the client can determine what alternative or augmentative communication tool she is willing to use. For some, no artificial tool is sufficient as a substitute for speech.

Each clinician is or can be an animate tool whose actions and responses can provide a voice for those whose communication is impaired due to a neurogenic disorder. Our ways of interacting and facilitating the communication of our clients should support their presentation of self to social others. We can also train significant others to support communication in order to empower the client in presenting a self to others. Once again, the tool is critical but we must first understand what aspects of narrative self need to be supported.

Narrative Self and Clinical Practice: Clinician as Coconstructor and Character in Restorying of Self

While clinicians can be animate tools, they can also adopt an important role as communication partner. As communication partners, we can help persons living with these communication disorders to recreate a narrative that provides meaning to their experiences, facilitates coping and adaptation, and promotes a sense of agency and healing, as well as a perception of being recognized and valued for who they are (Caplan, Haslett, & Burleson, 2005).

One important part of the role of communication partner is listening. Menninger (n.d.) has written, "Listening is a magnetic and strange thing, a creative force. The friends who listen to us are the ones we move toward. When we are listened to, it creates us, makes us unfold and expand." Repeatedly, clinicians are encouraged to listen, truly listen, to the stories shared by their clients (Gubrium 1986; Usita, Hyman, & Herman, 1998; Worrall, 2006). Listening to life stories is described by Rappaport (1993) as an antidote for professional centrism. Ganzer and England (1994) note that the challenge for social workers is to attend to the client's story in a highly privileged manner, but not to reauthor. Instead, they suggest that professionals can serve as coauthors of a new story. In other words, health care providers must recognize that we are indeed characters in the client's illness narrative (cf. Haidet, Kroll, & Sharf, 2006). Finally, Shotter (2003, 2005) repeatedly emphasizes the importance of the health care provider's focus on the client's perspective, as narrative self plays out in stories. He highlights the importance of respect, attunement, acknowledgement, and mutual obligations.

It is fitting to close this chapter and this text with consideration of the clinician as member of a clinical interaction, as a person who also has a storied life that can be shared, and as cocreator of the narrative self that emerges in treatment contexts. In a 2007 issue of *Topics in Language Disorders*, Kovarsky took on the challenge of considering the role of discourse processes in our clinical interactions in order to provide a rich narrative environment. It is up to the clinician to recognize the opportunities and to use them to support expression and validation of narrative self. Quite possibly, those who are referred to as master clinicians are simply clinicians who understand and use discourse possibilities.

How many times have we said (or heard others say), "We didn't get much done today. He just wanted to talk." Implicit in this statement is a kind of apology for time wasted, time that could have been used for impairment-based tasks. I would suggest that it is indeed those times when the work of narrative self is most in evidence. Because of the outcomes-driven health care environment in which we operate, we are somehow embarrassed by our inability to record numbers to characterize the success of such moments.

Hagstrom (Chapter 11) suggests that, in the clinical interaction, we should ask questions about our own identity or self, as well as about the client's self. In asking "Who am I?" the clinician is really asking what aspects of his self or personhood are being brought to this conversation. Is it the role of health care provider that will dominate the clinician's presentation of self? Is there a willingness to bring into play some biographic particulars of self (e.g., dog lover, football fan)? Is there a need to control the interaction, or a contrasting willingness to allow more balance and less control? Cohen-Schneider (2007) suggests these are questions that are "underexamined." In asking, "Who are *we*?" the clinician is acknowledging that the dyad exists as a social, interactional unit and can potentially function in ways that go beyond the administration and monitoring of therapy tasks.

Thus beyond techniques and specific tools, the clinical interaction provides opportunities for facilitating the recreation of narrative self. Part of the process includes conveying multiple verbal and nonverbal cues that suggest we are ready to interact in the sociorelational domain, not just in the "business of everyday" therapy talk (Walsh, 2007). Penn (personal communication, October 11, 2007) refers to magic moments of interaction that characterize the best of therapy sessions. In those moments, two or more people are united in the experience of sharing some dimension of self and identity, and that sharing is a vital piece of the life story. Such moments cannot, indeed will not, occur if the clinical interaction is characterized primarily by roles of client and clinician, with associated power imbalances, interactive rules and constraints, formalized discourse, and constructed incompetence (Kovarsky, Duchan, Mastergeorge, & Nichols, 2003; Nelson & Butler, 2007).

Kitwood (1997) has written at length about the distinction between *I-It* and *I-Thou* perspectives on the clinical relationship in dementia care. In an I-It framework, the other person is viewed more as an entity or label, rather than as a viable human partner. This I-It perspective is cool, detached, distanced. In contrast, an I-Thou perspective carries implications of self recognition, disclosure, and reaching out. The clinical discourse approach we are recommending is one that adopts the I-Thou perspective, in which clinicians assume responsibility for acting as agents in the ongoing storying of self.

In Closing

In Chapter 10, Koski challenged SLPs and other professionals to confront the broader implications of an understanding of the impact of neurogenic communication disorders on narrative self. Her challenge is remarkably similar to the moral imperative identified by Audrey Holland and Martha Taylor Sarno at the 2007 conference, Living Successfully with Aphasia: Intervention, Evaluation and Evidence. Their moral imperative was defined as a willingness to take on responsibility for more than management of linguistic deficits, to engage fully in quality of life issues.

The concept of narrative self as constructed in multiple domains and as threatened by a communication disorder appears to resonate with many. During the final months of writing this text, we were surprised at how responsive other professionals, friends, clients, and their families were to the ideas we were developing and how rich the ensuing dialogues were. Thus one of our goals in writing this text appears to be within reach. We had hoped to provide a foundation for further dialogue about narrative self, and that dialogue is already in progress. An example of one such dialogue emerged in a series of e-mails with colleague and friend Jon Lyon (personal communication, November 23, 2007). Years ago, Jon took the courageous step of walking away from the medical model of aphasia treatment, deciding instead to engage in the difficult work of understanding life as seen from the perspective of those living with the problem. He chose to focus on facilitating life reengagement. Despite the success of his work, Jon indicates that he "came to see, first hand, the magnitude and complexity of the life issues these individuals face." He became

concerned that he was playing with the fringes and not the core components. "What I was doing 'helped' . . . usually . . . but the bigger and more essential issues in life needed much, much more. We'd need a cadre of folk and resources [not available today]."

Jon's concern was that his work still did not reach to the core of "a profound sense of isolation from that community of folk who [the person with aphasia] most wished most to be united with." In this text, we acknowledge his concerns. Indeed, they have been at the heart of our exploration of the life stories. We have learned about the similarities and differences in narrative self challenges across four diverse disorders. We believe that it is possible to do a better job of supporting and maintaining narrative self if issues of engagement in life storying receive greater focus in our interventions.

Jon and his life partner Marge also raised the following important question:

> . . . isn't it often that survivors of traumatic occurrences in life . . . when they and their lives have been altered inexorably . . . first seek guidance, therapy and ultimately solutions for their changes in life from the "outside" (experts who "treat" this disorder) . . . [and] few seem to know or understand, at these very initial moments of despair, that their truest and greatest asset lies "within," and it is their common commitment and values to each other and their long-term preservation that will serve them best over time.

In other words, in our desire to help persons improve speech-language skills, we may run the risk of failing to help them recognize the resources within, the core personal and interpersonal strengths and commitments that can sustain them over time. Jon suggests,

"It's critical that readers grasp that 'hidden' within these very 'inner' realms of selfdom (shared respect, honor, trust, caring, mutuality, touching, giving) are greatest promise and reward for recovery and are not destined, necessarily, to change or decline." Jon and Marge both underscore the importance of personal bonds, since "they're the strongest predictor of whether you (the affected parties) emerge from this reformation process whole, partial or forever disabled." They suggest that as therapists, we can be most effective " . . . in keeping loved ones together and united through all of these identities shifts. The real core key is staying together . . . in heart, respect, honor and understanding (of what's happened and what's possible)."

That goal is at the heart of this text. We believe more can be done to support the core life issues Jon has described, and our hope stems from those whose lives we shared briefly. And while we have repeatedly underscored the importance of communication in moving on with the storying of life, we do not mean to imply that it is the sole determining factor in sustaining narrative self. Most of us know individuals who, despite loss of communication, have maintained what Jon calls "vibrant, strong and good" identities or selves. We need to understand these stories of successful living as well as the broken narratives.

Hagstrom (Chapter 11) notes that the concept of narrative self is not analytically tidy and is instead somewhat "muddy." Similarly, Koski (Chapter 10) warns us that this postmodern world will be messy and chaotic. Years ago, in grappling with the complexities of human relationships and self, Prather (1970, p. 143) wrote:

> Ideas are clean. They soar in the serene supernal. I can take them out and look at them, they fit in books, they lead me down that narrow way. And in the morning they are there. Ideas are straight— But the world is round, and a messy mortal is my friend.
>
> Come walk with me in the mud . . .

We encourage you, the readers, to join us in exploring the messy but powerful relationships between communication impairment and maintenance of a viable sense of self.

References

Aarsland, D., Larsen, J. P., Karlsen, K., Lim, N. G., & Tandberg, E. (1999). Mental symptoms in Parkinson's disease are important contributors to caregiver distress. *International Journal of Geriatric Psychiatry, 14,* 866–874.

Abudi, S., Bar-Tal, Y., Ziv, L., & Fish, M. (1997). Parkinson's disease symptoms: Patients' perceptions. *Journal of Advanced Nursing, 25,* 54–59.

Albert, M. L., & Mildworf, B. (1989). The concept of dementia. *Journal of Neurolinguistics, 4,* 301–308.

Allard, D. D. (n.d.). Tools of the thoughts. Retrieved October 15, 2007, from http://www.aphasiahope.org/experience.jsp?id=41

Alter, H. (2006, June). *Presenting NAA bill of rights: A call to action.* Presentation at the National Aphasia Association Speaking Out Conference, Boston, MA. Retrieved October 7, 2007, from http://www.wingoglobal.com/transcripts/0606-Harvey-Alter.doc

Alzheimer's Association. (n.d.). Alzheimer's disease. Retrieved October 15, 2007, from http://www.alz.org/

Alzheimer's Foundation of America. (n.d.). Alzheimer's disease. Retrieved October 15, 2007, from http://alzfdn.org/

Ambady, N. (2005). In M. Gladwell (Ed.), *Blink* (pp. 42–43). New York: Little, Brown and Company.

American Heart Assocation. (n.d.). Aphasia. Retrieved October 15, 2007, from http://www.americanheart.org

American Speech-Language-Hearing Association (ASHA). (2007). Amyotrophic lateral sclerosis (ALS). Retrieved October 7, 2007, from http://www.asha.org/public/speech/disorders/ALSCauses.htm

American Speech-Language-Hearing Association (ASHA). (2007). Apraxia of speech. Retrieved October 7, 2007, from http://www.asha.org/public/speech/disorders/ApraxiaAdults.htm?print=1

American Speech-Language-Hearing Association (ASHA). (2007). Dementia. Retrieved October 7, 2007, from http://www.asha.org/public/speech/disorders/dementia.htm?print=1

American Speech-Language-Hearing Association (ASHA). (2007). Dysarthria. Retrieved from http://www.asha.org/public/speech/disorders/dysarthria.htm?print=)

American Stroke Association. (2006). Stroke support groups. Retrieved September 21, 2007, from http://www.americanheart.org

American Stroke Foundation. (n.d.). About aphasia. Retrieved October 15, 2007, from http://www.americanstroke.org/

American Stroke Association. (n.d.). Aphasia. Retrieved October 15, 2007, from http://www.strokeassociation.org

Amyotrophic Lateral Sclerosis Association. (n.d.). What is ALS? Retrieved October 15, 2007, from http://www.alsa.org/

Andersson, S., & Fridlund, B. (2002). The aphasic person's views of the encounter with other people: A grounded theory analysis. *Journal of Psychiatric & Mental Health Nursing, 9*(3), 285–292.

Armstrong, E. (2005). Expressing opinions and feelings in aphasia: Linguistic options. *Aphasiology, 19,* 285–295.

Armstrong, E. (2005). Language disorder: A functional linguistic perspective. *Clinical Linguistics & Phonetics, 19*(3), 137-153.

Armstrong, E., & Mortensen, L. (2006). Everyday talk: Its role in assessment and treatment for individuals with aphasia. *Brain Injury, 7,* 175-189.

Armstrong, E., & Ulatowska, H. K. (2007). Stroke stories: Conveying emotive experiences in aphasia. In M. J. Ball & J. S. Damico (Eds.), *Clinical aphasiology: Future directions* (pp. 195-210). London: Routledge.

Armstrong, E., & Ulatowska, H. K. (2007). Stroke stories: The aphasia experience. *Aphasiology, 21,* 763-774.

Baars, J. (1997). Concepts of time and narrative temporality in the study of aging. *Journal of Aging Studies, 11*(4), 283-296.

Bakhtin, M. M. (1986). *Speech genres and other late essays.* Austin, TX: University of Texas Press.

Bakhtin, M. M. (1990). *Art and answerability* (M. Holquist & V. Liapunov, Eds.) (V. Liapunov, Trans.). Austin, TX: University of Texas Press.

Ball, L. J., Beukelman, D. R., & Pattee, G. L. (2004). Communication effectiveness of individuals with amyotrophic lateral sclerosis. *Journal of Communication Disorders, 37,* 197-215.

Barker, K. (2002). Self-help literature and the making of an illness: The case of fibromyalgia syndrome (FMS). *Social Problems, 49,* 279-300.

Barrett, A. E. (2005). Gendered experiences in midlife: Implications for age identity. *Journal of Aging Studies, 19,* 163-183.

Bauer, J. J. (2005). Review: Narrative self and cultural influences. *Infant and Child Development, 14,* 103-105.

Beard, R. L. (2004). In their voices: Identity preservation and experiences of Alzheimer's disease. *Journal of Aging Studies, 18,* 415-428.

Beck, C. S. (2005). Becoming the story: Narratives as collaborative, social enactments of individuals, relational, and public identities. In L. M. Harter, P. M. Japp, & C. S. Beck (Eds.), *Narratives, health, and healing: Communication theory, research, and practice* (pp. 61-82). Mahwah, NJ: Lawrence Erlbaum.

Becker, B. (1999). Narratives of pain in later life and conventions of storytelling. *Journal of Aging Studies, 13,* 73-88.

Ben Yishay, Y. (2000). A holistic perspective. In A. Christensen & B. P. Uzzell (Eds.), *International handbook of neuropsychological rehabilitation* (pp. 127-136). New York: Kluwer.

Berger, J., Fisek, M. H., Norman, R. Z., & Zelditch, M., Jr. (1977). *Status characteristics and social interaction: An expectation-states approach.* New York: Elsevier.

Berger, P., & Mensh, S. (1999). *How to conquer the world with one hand . . . and an attitude* (2nd ed.). Merrifield, NJ: Positive Power.

Beukelman, D. R., Ball, L. J., & Pattee, G. L. (2004, December 14). Intervention decision-making for persons with amyotrophic lateral sclerosis. *The ASHA Leader,* 4-5.

Bhatia, S., & Gupta, A. (2003). Impairments in activitirs of daily living in Parkinson's disease: Implications for management. *NeuroRehabilitation, 18,* 209-214.

Biemans, M. A. J. E., Dekker, J., & Van der Woude, L. H. V. (2001). The internal consistency and validity of the Self-Assessment Parkinson's Disease Disability Scale. *Clinical Rehabilitation, 15,* 221-228.

Birgersson, A. M. B., & Edberg, A. K. (2004). Being in the light or in the shade: Persons with Parkinson's and their partners' experience of support. *International Journal of Nursing Studies, 41,* 621-630.

Birren, J. E., & Cochran, K. N. (2001). *Telling the stories of life through guided autobiography groups* (3rd ed.). Baltimore: Johns Hopkins.

Birren, J. E., Kenyon, G. M., Ruth J.-E., Schroots, J. J. F., & Svensson, T. (Eds.). (1996). *Aging and biography: Explorations in adult development.* New York: Springer.

Blustein, J. (1999). Choosing for others as continuing a life story: The problem of personal identity revisited. *Journal of Law, Medicine & Ethics, 27,* 20-31.

Bogdan, R., & Taylor, S. (1989). Relationships with severely disabled people: The social construction of humanness. *Social Problems, 36,* 135-148.

Borkowski, D. (2004). Not too late to take the sanitation test: Notes of a non-gifted academic from the working-class. *College Composition and Communication, 56*, 94-123.

Bourdieu, P. (1991). *Language and symbolic power.* Cambridge, UK: Cambridge University Press. (Original work published 1972)

Bramley, N., & Eatough, V. (2005). The experience of living with Parkinson's disease: An interpretive phenomenological analysis case study. *Psychology and Health, 20*, 223-235.

Bremer, B. A., Simone, A.-L., Walsh, S., Simmons, Z., & Felgoise, S. H. (2004). Factors supporting quality of life over time for individuals with amyotrophic lateral sclerosis: The role of positive self-perception and religiosity. *Annals of Behavioral Medicine, 28*, 119-125.

Brody, H. (2003). *Stories of sickness* (2nd ed.). New York: Oxford University Press.

Brumfitt, S. (1993). Losing your sense of self: What aphasia can do. *Aphasiology, 7*, 569-591.

Brumfitt, S. (1999). *The social psychology of communication impairments.* London: Whurr.

Bruner, J. (1987). Life as narrative. *Social Research, 54*, 11-32.

Bruner, J. (1990). *Acts of meaning.* Cambridge, MA: Harvard University Press.

Bruner, J. (1999). Narratives of aging. *Journal of Aging Studies, 13*, 7-10.

Bruner, J. (2002). Narratives of human plight: A conversation with Jerome Bruner. In R. Charon & M. Montello (Eds.), *Stories matter: The role of narrative in medical ethics* (pp. 3-9). New York: Routledge.

Bruner, J. (2003). *Self-making narrative.* In R. Fivush & C. A. Haden (Eds.), *Autobiographical memory and the construction of a narrative self: Developmental and cultural perspectives* (pp. 209-226). Mahwah, NJ: Lawrence Erlbaum.

Bruner, J. (2004, Fall). Life as narrative. *Social Research, 71*(3), 691-710. Retrieved June 6, 2007, from http://www.plataforma.uchile.cl/fb/cursos_area/cognit/unidad2/tema2/doc/bruner_2004_lifeasnarrative.pdf

Buck, M. (1963). The language disorders: A personal and professional account of aphasia. *Journal of Rehabilitation, 29*, 37-38.

Buck, M. (1964). Adjustments during recovery from stroke. *The American Journal of Nursing, 64*, 92-95.

Burle, A., & Caan, W. (2004). Social exclusion and embracement: A helpful concept? *Primary Health Care Research and Development, 5*, 191-192.

Bury, M. (1982). Chronic illness as biographical disruption. *Social Health & Illness, 4*, 67-82.

Byrne, D. (1998). *Complexity theory and the social sciences: An introduction.* New York: Routledge.

Caap-Ahlgren, M., Lannerheim, L., & Dehlin, O. (2002). Older Swedish women's experience living with symptoms related to Parkinson's disease. *Journal of Advanced Nursing, 39*, 87-95.

Calder, S. A., Ebmeier, K. P., Stewart, L., Crawford, J. R., & Besson, J. A. O. (1991). The prediction of stress in carers: The role of behavior, reported self-care and dementia in patients with idiopathic Parkinson's disease. *International Journal of Geriatric Psychiatry, 6*, 737-742.

Caplan, S. E., Haslett, B. J., & Burleson, B. R. (2005). Telling it like it is: The adaptive function of narratives in coping with loss in later life. *Health Communication, 17*, 233-251.

Caregivers are Really Essential (CARE). (n.d.). Welcome to CARE: For caregivers of people with Parkinson's. Retrieved October 15, 2007, from http://www.pdcaregiver.org/index.html

Carey, J. (1975). A cultural approach to communication. *Communication, 2*, 1-22.

Carson, R. A. (2002). The hyphenated space: Liminality in the doctor-patient relationship. In R. Charon & M. Montello (Eds.), *Stories matter: The role of narrative in medical ethics* (pp. 171-182). New York: Routledge.

Chambers, T., & Montgomery, K. (2002). Plot: Framing contingency and choice in bioethics. In R. Charon & M. Montello (Eds.), *Stories matter: The role of narrative in medical ethics* (pp. 77-84). New York: Routledge.

Charlton, G. S., & Barrow, C. J. (2002). Coping and self-help group membership in Parkinson's disease: An exploratory qualitative study. *Health & Social Care in the Community, 10*, 472-478.

Charmaz, K. (1983). Loss of self: A fundamental form of suffering in the chronically ill. *Sociology of Health and Illness, 5*(2), 168–195.

Charmaz, K. (1993). *Good days, bad days: The self in chronic illness and time.* New Brunswick, NJ: Rutgers University Press.

Charon, R. (2001). Narrative medicine: A model for empathy, reflection, profession and trust. *Journal of the American Medical Association, 286*, 187–190.

Charon, R. (2002). Time and ethics. In R. Charon & M. Montello (Eds.), *Stories matter: The role of narrative in medical ethics* (pp. 59–68). New York: Routledge.

Charon, R. (2006). The self-telling body. *Narrative Inquiry, 16*(1), 191–200.

Charon, R., & Montello, M. (Eds.). (2002). *Stories matter: The role of narrative in medical ethics.* New York: Routledge.

Chia, A., Gauthier, A., Montuschi, A., Calvo, A., Di Vito, N., Ghiglione, P., et al. (2004). A cross sectional study on determinants of quality of life in ALS. *Journal of Neurology, Neurosurgery & Psychiatry, 75*, 1597–1601.

Cifu, D. X., Carne, W., Brown, R., Pegg, P., Ong, J., Qutubuddin, A., et al. (2006). Caregiver distress in Parkinsonism. *Journal of Rehabilitation Research & Development, 43*, 499–507.

Clarke, P. (2003). Towards a greater understanding of the experience of stroke: Integrating quantitative and qualitative methods. *Journal of Aging Studies, 17*, 171–187.

Cohen-Schneider, R. (2007, September). *The clinician's role in enabling successful living with aphasia: An underexamined factor.* Poster presented at the Living Successfully with Aphasia: Intervention, Evaluation and Evidence Conference, Toronto, Canada.

Cole, M. (1985). The zone of proximal development: Where culture and cognition create each other. In J. V. Wertsch (Ed.), *Culture, communication, and cognition: Vygotskian perspectives* (pp. 146–161). New York: Cambridge University Press.

Connelly, J. E. (2002). In the absence of narrative. In R. Charon & M. Montello (Eds.), *Sto-*

ries matter: The role of narrative in medical ethics (pp. 138–146). New York: Routledge.

Cooley, C. M. (1902). *Human nature and the social order.* New York: Charles Scribner's & Sons.

Corbin, J. M., & Strauss, A. (1991). A nursing model for chronic illness management based upon the Trajectory Framework. *Scholarly Inquiry for Nursing Practice, 5*, 155–174.

Cruice, M., Worrall, L., & Hickson, L. (2006). Quantifying aphasic people's social lives in the context of non-aphasic peers. *Aphasiology, 20*, 1210–1225.

Cruice, M., Worrall, L., Hickson, L., & Murison, R. (2003). Finding a focus for quality of life with aphasia: Social and emotional health, and psychological well being. *Aphasiology, 17*, 333–353.

Cruice, M., Worrall, L., Hickson, L., & Murison, R. (2005). Measuring quality of life: Comparing family members' and friends' ratings with those of their aphasic partners. *Aphasiology, 19*, 111–129.

Csikszentmihalyi, M. (1990). *Flow: The psychology of optimal experiences.* New York: Harper, Collins and Row.

Damasio, A. (1999). *The feeling of what happens: Body and emotion in the making of consciousness.* New York: Harcourt.

Damiano, A. M., Snyder, C., Strausser, B., & William, M. K. (1999). A review of health-related quality-of-life concepts and measures for Parkinson's disease. *Quality of Life Research, 8*, 235–243.

D'Andrade, R. (1987). A folk model of the mind. In D. Holland & N. Quinn, *Cultural models in language and thought* (pp. 112–148). Cambridge, UK: Cambridge University Press.

Darling, R. B. (2003). Toward a model of changing disability identities: A proposed typology and research agenda. *Disability and Society, 18*, 881–895.

Davison, K. P., Pennebaker, J. W., & Dickerson, S. S. (2000). Who talks? The social psychology of illness support groups. *American Psychologist, 55*, 205–217.

Douglas, K. (2003). *My stroke of luck.* New York: Harper Collins.

Dowd, J. J. (1980). *Stratification among the aged.* Monterey, CA: Brooks/Cole.

Dowd, J. J. (2004). Social identities across the life course: A review. *Contemporary Sociology, 33,* 300-301.

Elman, R. (Ed.) (2006). *Group treatment of neurogenic communication disorders: The expert clinician's approach* (2nd ed.). San Diego, CA: Plural.

Erikson, E. H. (1963). *Childhood and society* (2nd ed.). New York: Norton.

Erikson, E. H. (1968). *Identity: Youth and crisis.* New York: Norton.

Faircloth, C. A., Boylstein, C., Rittman, M., & Gubrium, J. F. (2005). Constructing the stroke: Sudden-onset narratives of stroke survivors. *Qualitative Health Research, 15,* 928-941.

Faircloth, C. A., Rittman, M., Boylstein, C., Young, M. E., & Van Puymbroeck, M. (2004). Energizing the ordinary: Biographical work and the future in stroke recovery narratives. *Journal of Aging Studies, 18,* 399-413.

Feldman, S. (1999). Please don't call me "dear:" Older women's narratives of health care. *Nursing Inquiry, 6,* 269-276.

Fischer, W. (1987). *Human communication as narrative.* Columbia, SC: University of South Carolina Press.

Fivush, R. (1991). The social construction of personal narratives. *Merrill-Palmer Quarterly, 37,* 59-82.

Fivush, R., & Haden, C. A. (Eds.). (2003). *Autobiographical memory and the construction of a narrative self: Developmental and cultural perspectives.* Mahwah, NJ: Lawrence Erlbaum.

Frank, A. W. (1995). *The wounded storyteller: Body, illness, and ethics.* Chicago: University of Chicago Press.

Frank, A. W. (2002). *At the will of the body: Reflections on illness.* New York: Houghton Mifflin.

Frank, A. W. (2005). Foreword—Stories by and about us. In L. M. Harter, P. M. Japp, & C. S. Beck (Eds.), *Narratives, health, and healing: Communication theory, research, and practice* (pp. xi-xvii). Mahwah, NJ: Lawrence Erlbaum.

Ganzer, C. (2007). The use of self from a relational perspective. *Clinical Social Work Journal, 35,* 117-123.

Ganzer, C., & England, S. E. (1994). Alzheimer's care and service utilization: Generating practice concepts from empirical findings and narratives. *Health & Social Work, 19,* 174-181.

Gardner, H. (1975). *The shattered mind: The person after brain damage.* New York: Knopf.

Garfinkel, H. (1956). Conditions of successful degradation ceremonies. *The American Journal of Sociology, 61,* 410-424.

Geertz, C. (1973). *The interpretation of cultures.* New York: Basic Books.

Gibson, F. (2004). *The past in the present: Using reminiscence in health and social care.* Baltimore: Health Professions Press.

Giddens, A. (1976). *New rules of sociological method: A positive critique of interpretive sociologies.* London: Hutchinson.

Giddens, A. (1991). *Modernity and self-identity: Self and society in the late modern age.* Cambridge, UK: Polity Press.

Giles, H., & Reid, S. A. (2005). Ageism across the lifespan: Towards a self-categorization model of aging. *The Journal of Social Issues, 61,* 389-404.

Gladwell, M. (2005). *Blink.* New York: Little, Brown and Company.

Glass, T. A., & Maddox, G. L. (1992). The quality and quantity of social support: Stroke recovery as psycho-social transition. *Social Sciences & Medicine, 24,* 1249-1261.

Goffman, E. (1959). *The presentation of self in everyday life.* Garden City, NY: Doubleday (Anchor Books).

Goffman, E. (1963). *Stigma: Notes on the management of spoiled identity.* New York: Simon & Schuster.

Goldstein, L., Atkins, L., & Leigh, P. (2002). Correlates of quality of life in people with motor neuron disease (MND). *Amyotrophic Lateral Sclerosis & Other Motor Neuron Disorders, 3,* 123-129.

Gooberman-Hill, R., Ayis, S., & Ebrahim, S. (2003). Understanding long-standing illness among older people. *Social Science & Medicine, 56,* 2555-2565.

Gover, M. R., & Gavelek, J. (1996). *Persons and selves: The dialectics of identity.* Michigan State University. Retrieved August 4, 2005, from http://www.msu.edu/user/govermar/ident.htm

Grady, D. (2006, October 24). Self-portraits chronicle a descent into Alzheimer's. *The New York Times*, retrieved October 7, 2007, from http://www.nytimes.com/2006/10/24/health/24alzh.html

Gregg, G. S. (2006). The raw and the bland: A structural model of narrative identity. In D. P. McAdams, R. Josselson, & A. Lieblich (Eds.), *Identity and story: Creating self in narrative* (pp. 63–87). Washington, DC: American Psychological Association.

Grenier, A. (2006). The distinction between being and feeling frail: Exploring emotional experiences in health and social care. *Journal of Social Work Practice, 20,* 299–313.

Grenier, A., & Hanley, J. (2007). Older women and frailty: Aged, gendered and embodied resistance. *Current Sociology, 55,* 211–228.

Gubrium, J. F. (1986). The social preservation of the mind: The Alzheimer's disease experience. *Symbolic Interaction, 9,* 37–51.

Gubrium, J. F. (2003). What is a good story? *Generations, 27,* 21–24.

Gubrium, J. F., & Holstein, J. A. (1997). *The new language of qualitative method.* New York: Oxford University Press.

Gubrium, J. F., & Holstein, J. A. (2001). *Institutional selves: Troubled identities in a postmodern world.* New York: Oxford University Press.

Guendouzi, J., & Müller, N. (2006). *Approaches to discourse in dementia.* Mahwah, NJ: Lawrence Erlbaum.

Hagstrom, F. (2001). Using and building theory for clinical action. *Journal of Communication Disorders, 34,* 371–384.

Hagstrom, F. (2004). Including identity in clinical practices. *Topics in Language Disorders, 24,* 225–238.

Hagstrom, F., & Wertsch, J. V. (2004). Grounding social identity for professional practice. *Topics in Language Disorders, 24,* 162–173.

Haidet, P., Kroll, T. L., & Sharf, B. F. (2006). The complexity of patient participation: Lessons learned from patients' illness narratives. *Patient Education and Counseling, 62,* 323–329.

Haight, B. K., Bachman, D. L., Hendrix, S., Wagner, M. T., Meeks, A., & Johnson, J. (2003). Life review: Treating the dyadic family unit with dementia. *Clinical Psychology and Psychotherapy, 10,* 165–174

Harman, G., & Clare, L. (2006). Illness representations and lived experience in early-stage dementia. *Qualitative Health Research, 16,* 484–502.

Harré, R. (1991). The discursive production of selves. *Theory and Psychology, 1,* 51–63.

Harrison, T., & Kahn, D. L. (2004). Perceived age, social integration, and disability: A case study of aging women. *Journal of Loss and Trauma, 9,* 113–129.

Harter, L. M., Japp, P. M., & Beck, C. S. (Eds.). (2005). *Narratives, health, and healing: Communication theory, research, and practice.* Mahwah, NJ: Lawrence Erlbaum.

Harter, L. M., Japp, P. M., & Beck, C. S. (2005). Vital problematics of narrative theorizing about health and healing. In L. M. Harter, P. M. Japp, & C. S. Beck (Eds.), *Narratives, health, and healing: Communication theory, research, and practice* (pp. 7–29). Mahwah, NJ: Lawrence Erlbaum.

Hatakeyama, T., Okamoto, A., Kamata, K., & Kasuga, M. (2000). Assistive technology for people with amyotrophic lateral sclerosis in Japan: Present status, analysis of problem and proposal for the future. *Technology & Disability, 13,* 9–15.

Heidrich, S. M. (1999). Self-discrepancy across the life span. *Journal of Adult Development, 6,* 119–130.

Heidrich, S. M., & Ryff, C. D. (1993). Physical and mental health in later life: The self-system as mediator. *Psychology and Aging, 8,* 327–338.

Heidrich, S. M., & Ryff, C. D. (1993). The role of social comparison processes in the psychological adaptation of the elderly. *Journal of Gerontology: Psychological Sciences, 48,* P127–P136.

Hepburn, K. W., Caron, W., Luptak, M., Ostwald, S., Grant, L., & Keenan, J. M. (1997). The Family Stories Workshop: Stories for those who cannot remember. *The Gerontologist, 37,* 827–832.

Herman, D. (2000). Narratology as a cognitive science. *Image and Narrative, 1,* 1–21.

Hevern, V. W. (2004, November). Neuropsychology and Cognitive Psychology. *Narrative psychology: Internet and resource guide.* Retrieved January 3, 2008 from the Le Moyne College Web site: http://web.lemoyne.edu/~hevern/nr-neuro.html

Hevern, V. W. (2007). Theorists and key figures: Index. *Narrative Psychology Internet and Resource Guide.* Retrieved October 7, 2007, from http://web.lemoyne.edu/~hevern/nr-theorists.html#gergen_k

Hewitt, J. P. (1989). *Dilemmas of the American self.* Philadelphia: Temple University Press.

Hinckley, J. J. (2007*). Narrative-based practice in speech-language pathology: Stories of a clinical life.* San Diego, CA: Plural.

Hinton, W. L., & Levkoff, S. (1999). Constructing Alzheimer's: Narratives of lost identities, confusion and loneliness in old age. *Medicine & Psychiatry, 23,* 453–475.

Hodgson, J. H., Garcia, K., & Tyndall, L. (2004). Parkinson's disease and the couple relationship: A qualitative analysis. *Families, Systems & Health, 22,* 101–118.

Hofvander, C. (n.d.) My aphasia. Retrieved October, 15, 2007, from http://www.aphasiahope.org/experience

Holland, A. L. (2007). *Counseling in communication disorders: A wellness perspective.* San Diego, CA: Plural.

Holland, A., & Sarno, M. T. (2007, September). *Stepping back and looking forward: A conversation.* Keynote address presented at the Living Successfully with Aphasia: Intervention, Evaluation and Evidence Conference, Toronto, Canada.

Holstein, J. A., & Gubrium, J. F. (2000). *The self we live by: Narrative identity in a postmodern world.* New York: Oxford University Press.

Holstein, J. A., & Gubrium, J. F. (2001). *Institutional selves: Troubled identities in organizational context.* New York: Oxford University Press.

Hopper, J. (2001). Contested selves in divorce proceedings. In J. F. Gubrium & J. A. Holstein (Eds.), *Institutional troubled identities in selves: A postmodern view* (pp.127–141). New York: Oxford University Press.

Horton, S. (2007). Topic generation in aphasia language therapy sessions: Issues of identity. *Aphasiology, 21,* 283–298.

Huberman, B. A., Loch, C. H., & Onculer, A. (2004). Status as a valued resource. *Social Psychology Quarterly, 67,* 103–114.

Hurwitz, B. (2000). Narrative and the practice of medicine. *The Lancet, 356,* 9247.

Hux, K., Manasse, N., Weiss, A., & Beukelman, D. (2001). Augmentative and alternative communication for persons with aphasia. In R. Chapey (Ed.), *Language intervention strategies in aphasia and related neurogenic disorders* (4th ed., pp. 675–687). Philadelphia: Lippincott, Wolcott, and Wilkins.

Institute of Medicine. (2007, April). *Report brief: The future of disability of America.* Available at http://www.nap.edu

James, W. (1950). *Principles of psychology* (Vols. 1 & 2, Authorized ed.). New York: Dover. (original work published 1890)

James, W. (1963). *Psychology.* Greenwich, CT: Fawcett. (Original work published 1892)

Jenkinson, C., Fitzpatrick, R., Brennan, C., & Swash, M. (1999). Evidence for the validity and reliability of the ALS assessment questionnaire: The ALSAQ-40. *Amyotrophic Lateral Sclerosis & Other Motor Neuron Disorders, 1,* 33–40.

Jenkinson, C., Peto, V., Fitzpatrick, R., Greenhall, R., & Hyman, N. (1995). Self-reported functioning and well-being in patients with Parkinson's disease: Comparison of the short-form health survey (SF-36) and the Parkinson's Disease Questionnaire (PDQ-39). *Age & Ageing, 24,* 505–509.

Kagan, A. (2005, November). *Living with aphasia: Framework for outcome measurement (A-FROM).* Paper presented at the Annual Convention of the American Speech-Language-Hearing Association, San Diego, CA.

Kagan, A. (2007, September). *Assessment of living with aphasia: An application of A-FROM.* Poster presented at the Living Successfully with Aphasia: Intervention, Evaluation and Evidence Conference, Toronto, Canada.

Kagan, A., Simmons-Mackie, N., Rowland, A., Huijbregts, M., Shumway, E., McEwen, S., et al. (2007). Counting what counts: A framework for capturing real-life outcomes of aphasia intervention. *Aphasiology, 21,* 39-66.

Kalkhoff, W., & Thye, S. R. (2006). Expectation states theory and research: New observations from meta-analysis. *Sociological Methods Research, 35,* 219-249.

Kent, R. (1990). Fragmentation of clinical service and clinical science in communicative disorders. *National Student Speech-Language Association Journal, 17,* 4-16.

Kenyon, G. M. (2003). Telling and listening to stories: Creating a wisdom environment for older people. *Generations, 27,* 30-43.

Kenyon, G. M., & Randall, W. L. (1997). *Restorying our lives: Personal growth through autobiographical reflection.* Westport, CT: Praeger.

Kerby, A. (1993). *Narrative and the self.* Bloomington: Indiana University Press.

Kimbarow, M. (in press). Foreword. *Topics in Language Disorders.*

Kitwood, T. (1993). Person and process in dementia. *International Journal of Geriatric Psychiatry, 8,* 541-545.

Kitwood, T. (1993). Toward a theory of dementia care: The interpersonal process. *Ageing & Society, 13,* 51-67.

Kitwood, T. (1997). *Dementia reconsidered: The person comes first.* New York: Open University Press.

Kleinman, A. (1988). *The illness narratives: Suffering, healing and the human condition.* New York: Basic Books.

Konstam, V., Holmes, W., Wilczenski, F., Baliga, S., Lester, J., & Priest, R. (2003). Meaning in the lives of caregivers of individuals with Parkinson's Disease. *Journal of Clinical Psychology in Medical Settings, 10,* 17-25.

Kovarsky, D. (2007). Foreword: Explorations in clinical discourse. *Topics in Language Disorders, 27,* 3-4.

Kovarsky, D., & Curran, M. (2007). A missing voice in the discourse of evidence-based practice. *Topics in Language Disorders, 27,* 50-61.

Kovarsky, D., Duchan, J., Mastergeorge, A., & Nichols, L. (2003, November). *Construction of identity in clinical discourse.* Paper presented at the meeting of American Speech-Language-Hearing Association, Chicago.

Krasner, J. (2005). Accumulated lives: Metaphor, materiality, and the homes of the elderly. *Literature and Medicine, 24,* 209-230.

Kubler-Ross, E. (1997). *On death and dying.* New York: Scribner.

Langdon, S. A., Eagle, A., & Warner, J. (2007). Making sense of dementia in the social world: A qualitative study. *Social Science & Medicine, 64,* 989-1000.

LaPointe, L. L. (1999). Quality of life with aphasia. *Seminars in Speech and Language, 20,* 5-17.

Lawton, M. P., Kleban, M. H., Moss, M., Ravine, M., & Glicksman, A. (1989). Measuring caregiving appraisal. *Journal of Gerontology, 44,* P61-P71.

Lazarus, R., & Folkman, S. (1984). *Stress, appraisal, and coping.* New York: Springer.

Leeds-Hurwitz, W. (1993). *Semiotics and communication: Signs, codes, cultures.* Hillsdale, NJ: Lawrence Erlbaum.

Levin, T., Scott, B. M., Borders, B., Hart, K., Lee, J., & Decanini, A. (2007). Aphasia talks: Photography as means of communication, self-expression, and empowerment in persons with aphasia. *Topics in Stroke Rehabilitation, 14,* 72-84.

Lieberman, M. A., Winzelberg, A., Golant, M., Wakahiro, M., DiMinno, M., Aminoff, M. S., et al. (2005). Online support groups for Parkinson's patients: A pilot study of effectiveness. *Social Work in Healthcare, 42,* 23-38.

Liechty, J. A. (2006). On the tip of my tongue: Living with aphasia. *Journal of Christian Nursing, 23,* 32-33.

Lindbergh, R. (2001). *No more words: A journal of my mother, Anne Morrow Lindbergh.* New York: Touchstone.

Linell, P. (1992). The embeddedness of decontextualization in the contexts of social practices. In A. H. Wold (Ed.), *The dialogical alternative: Towards a theory of language and mind* (pp. 253-271). Oslo, Norway: Scandinavian University Press.

Livneh, H., & Antonek, R. F. (Eds.). (1997). *Psychosocial adaptations to chronic illness and disability.* Gaithersburg, MD: Aspen.

LPAA Project Group. (2001). Life participation approach to aphasia: A statement of values for the future. In R. Chapey (Ed.), *Language intervention strategies in adults with aphasia* (4th ed., pp. 235-245). New York: Williams and Wilkins.

Lubinski, R. (2001). Environmental systems approach to adult aphasia. In R. Chapey (Ed.), *Language intervention strategies in aphasia and related neurogenic disorders* (4th ed., pp. 269-296). Philadelphia: Lippincott Williams & Wilkins.

Luria, A. R. (1981). *Language and cognition.* New York: John Wiley and Sons.

Luterman, D., & Luterman, D. M. (2001). *Counseling persons with communication disorders and their families* (4th ed.). Austin, TX: Pro-Ed.

Lyon, J. G. (1998). *Coping with aphasia.* San Diego, CA: Singular.

Lyotard, J. F. (1979). The postmodern conditiion: A report on knowledge. Manchester, England: Manchester University Press.

Ma, E. P.-M., Worrall, L., & Threats, T. T. (Eds.). (2007). Introduction: The International Classification of Functioning, Disability and Health (ICF) in clinical practice. *Seminars in Speech and Language, 28,* 241-243.

MacGill, V. (n.d.). Chaos and complexity tutorial. Retrieved October 15, 2007, from http://complexity.orcon.net.nz/intro.html

MacIntyre, A. (1981). *After virtue* (2nd ed.). London: Duckworth.

Mackay, R. (2003). "Tell them who I was": The social construction of aphasia. *Disability & Society, 18,* 811-826.

Malinowski, B. (1923). The problem of meaning in primitive languages. Supplement to C. K. Ogden & I. A. Richards (Eds.), *The meaning of meaning: A study of the influence of language upon thought and the science of symbolism* (pp. 451-510). London: Routledge & Kegan Paul.

Manor, Y., Posen, J., Amir, O., Dori, N., & Giladi, N. (2005). A group intervention model for speech and communication skills in patients with Parkinson's disease: Initial observations. *Communication Disorders Quarterly, 26,* 94-101.

Markova, I. (2003). Constitution of the self and intersubjectivity and dialogicality. *Culture & Psychology, 9,* 249-259.

McAdams, D. P. (1988). *Power, intimacy, and the life story: Personological inquiries into identity.* New York: The Guilford Press.

McAdams, D. P. (1993). *Stories we live by: Personal myths and the making of the self.* New York: William Morrow.

McAdams, D. P., Josselson, R., & Lieblich, A. (Eds.). (2005). *Turns in the road: Narrative studies of lives in transition.* Washington, DC: American Psychological Association.

McAdams, D. P., Josselson, R., & Lieblich, A. (Eds.). (2006). *Identity and story: Creating self in narrative.* Washington, DC: American Psychological Association.

McAdams, D. P., Josselson, R., & Lieblich, A. (2006). Introduction. In D. P. McAdams, R. Josselson, & A. Lieblich (Eds.), *Identity and story: Creating self in narrative* (pp. 3-11). Washington, DC: American Psychological Association.

McFadden, S. H. (2005). Creating and sustaining selfhood: Autobiographical memories from early childhood through old age. Review essay. *The Gerontologist, 45,* 414-418.

McKevitt, C. (2000). Short stories about stroke: Interviews and narrative production. *Anthropology & Medicine, 7,* 79-96.

McNamara, P., & Durso, R. (2003). Pragmatic communication skills in patients with Parkinson's disease. *Brain & Language, 84,* 414-424.

Melton, A. K., & Shadden, B. B. (2006). Linguistic accommodations to older adults in the community: The role of communication disorders and partner motivation. *Advances in Speech Language Pathology, 7,* 233-244.

Menninger, K. (n.d.). Listening. Retrieved October 15, 2007, from http://www.menninger-clinic.com/about/early-history.htm

Miller, N., Noble, E., Jones, D., & Burn, D. (2006). Life with communication changes in Parkinson's disease. *Age & Ageing, 35,* 235–239.

Mills, H. (2004). *A mind of my own: Memoir of recovery from aphasia.* Bloomington, IN: AuthorHouse.

Miner-Rubino, K., Winter, D., & Stewart, A. (2004). Gender, social class, and the subjective experience of aging: Self-perceived personality change from early adulthood to late midlife. *Personality and Social Psychology Bulletin, 30,* 1599–1610.

Mockford, C., Jenkinson, C., & Fitzpatrick, R. (2006). A review: Carers, MND and service provision. *Amyotrophic Lateral Sclerosis, 7,* 132–141.

Mold, F., McKevitt, C., & Wolfe, C. (2003). A review and commentary of the social factors which influence stroke care: Issues of inequality in qualitative literature. *Health & Social Care in the Community, 11,* 405–414.

Monks, J. A. (2000). Talk as social suffering: Narratives of talk in medical settings. *Anthropology & Medicine, 7,* 15–38.

Montbriand, M. J. (2004). Seniors' life histories and perceptions of illness. *Western Journal of Nursing Research, 26,* 242–261.

Moore, O., Kreitler, S., Ehrenfeld, M., & Giladi, N. (2005). Quality of life and gender identity in Parkinson's disease. *Journal of Neural Transmission, 112,* 1511–1522.

Moran, W. R. (2006, May/June). Kate's journey. *Stroke Smart Magazine,* 34–37. Retrieved October 15, 2007, from http://www.kates journey.com/KatePDFjune2006.pdf

Moreira, T., & Palladino, P. (2005). Between truth and hope: on Parkinson's disease, neurotransplantation and the production of the "self." *History of the Human Sciences, 18,* 55–82.

Morganroth-Gullette, M. (2003). From life storytelling to age autobiography. *Journal of Aging Studies, 17,* 101–112.

Moss, B., Parr, S., Byng, S., & Petheram, B. (2004). "Pick me up and not a down down, up up": How are the identities of people with aphasia represented in aphasia, stroke and disability websites? *Disability & Society, 19,* 753–768.

Murphy, J. (2004). "I prefer contact this close": Perceptions of AAC by people with motor neuron disease and their communication partners. *AAC: Augmentative & Alternative Communication, 20,* 259–271.

Muscular Dystrophy Association. (n.d.). Amyotrophic Lateral Sclerosis. Retrieved October 15, 2007, from http://www.als-mda.org

Nakano, E. V., Hinckley, J. J., & Paul, C. (2007, September). *Changes in the perception of self in individuals with aphasia.* Poster presented at the Living Successfully with Aphasia: Intervention, Evaluation and Evidence Conference, Toronto, Canada.

National Alliance for Caregiving & AARP. (2004). *Caregiving in the U.S.* Retrieved October 15, 2007, from http://www.caregiving.org/pubs/data.htm

National Institute on Deafness and Other Communicative Disorders. (n.d.) Aphasia. Retrieved October 15, 2007, from http://www.nidcd.nih.gov/health/voice/aphasia.asp

National Parkinson's Foundation. (n.d.). Parkinson's disease. Retrieved October 15, 2007, from http://www.parkinson.org

National Stroke Association. (n.d.) What is stroke? Retrieved October 15, 2007, from http//www.stroke.org/

Nelson G. K. (2002). Context: Backward, sideways, and forward. In R. Charon & M. Montello (Eds.), *Stories matter: The role of narrative in medical ethics* (pp. 39–47). New York: Routledge.

Nelson, K. (Ed.). (1986). *Event knowledge: Structure and function in development.* Hillsdale, NJ: Erlbaum.

Nelson, N. W., & Butler, K. G. (2007). From the editors: Explorations in clinical discourse. *Topics in Language Disorders, 21,* 1–2.

Newborn, B. (1997). *Return to Ithaca: A woman's triumph over the disabilities of a severe stroke.* Newport, MA: Element Books.

Norlin, P. F. (1986). Familiar faces, sudden strangers: Helping families cope with the crisis of aphasia. In R. Chapey (Ed.), *Language intervention strategies in adult aphasia* (2nd ed., pp. 174–186): Baltimore: Williams & Wilkins.

Nuland, S. B. (1994). *How we die*. New York: Alfred A. Knopf.

Nygren, I., & Askmark, H. (2006). Self-reported quality of life in amyotrophic lateral sclerosis. *Journal of Palliative Medicine, 9*, 304-308. Retrieved May 20, 2007, from http://www. liebertonline.com/doi/abs/10.1089/jpm. 2006.9.304

Obler, L. K. (1980). Narrative discourse style in the elderly. In L. K. Obler & M. L. Albert (Eds.), *Language and communication in the elderly: Clinical, therapeutic, and experimental issues* (pp. 75-90). Lexington, MA: D. C. Heath and Co.

O'Rourke, N., & Tuoko, H. (2000). The psychological and physical costs of caregiving: The Canadian study of health and aging. *Journal of Applied Gerontology, 19*, 389-404.

Parkinson's Disease Foundation. (n.d.). Parkinson's disease: An overview. Retrieved October 15, 2007, from http://www.pdf.org/ AboutPD

Parkinson's Living. (n.d.). About Parkinson's disease. Retrieved October 15, 2007, from http://parkinsonsliving.com

Parr, S. (2001, August). *Psychosocial aspects of aphasia*. Keynote presentation at the 25th World Congress of the International Association of Logopedics and Phoniatrics, Montreal, Canada.

Parr, S., Byng, S., Gilpin, S., & Ireland, S. (1997). *Talking about aphasia: Living with loss of language after stroke*. Buckingham, UK: Open University Press.

Parr, S., Pound, C., Byng, S., & Bridget, L. (2000). *The stroke and aphasia handbook*. London: Connect Ltd.

Pasupathi, M. (2006). Silk from sows' ears: Collaborative construction of everyday selves in everyday stories. In D. P. McAdams., R. Josselson, & A. Lieblich (Eds.), *Identity and story: Creating self in narrative* (pp. 151-172). Washington, DC: American Psychological Association.

Pearlin, L. I., Mullan, J. T., Semple, S. J., & Skaff, M. M. (1990). Caregiving and the stress process: An overview of concepts and their measures. *The Gerontologist, 30*, 583-594.

Pell, M., & Leonard, C. L. (2005). Facial expression decoding in early Parkinson's disease. *Cognitive Brain Research, 23*, 327-340.

Platt, M. M. (2004). Identity and Parkinson's disease: Am I more than the sum of my parts? *Journal of Loss & Trauma, 9*, 315-326.

Powell, W. E. (1988). The "ties that bind": Relationships in life transitions. *Social Casework, 6*(9), 556-562.

Prather, H. (1970). *Notes to myself: My struggle to become a person*. Lafayette, CA: Real People Press.

Queensland University Aphasia Group. (n.d.). Stories from Queensland University aphasia groups/stories. Retrieved October 15, 2007, from http://www.shrs.uq.edu.au/cdaru/aphasia groups/Stories/Stories.html

Quittenbaum, B. H., & Grahn, B. (2004). Quality of life and pain in Parkinson's disease: A controlled cross-sectional study. *Parkinsonism & Related Disorders, 10*, 129-137.

Randall, W. L. (1995). The stories we are: An essay on self-creation. Toronto: University of Toronto Press.

Randall, W. L. (1999). Narrative intelligence and the novelty of our lives. *Journal of Aging Studies, 13*, 11-28.

Randall, W. L., & Kenyon, G. M. (2000). *Ordinary wisdom: Biographical aging and the journey of life*. Westport, CT: Praeger.

Randall, W. L., Prior, S. M., & Sarborn, M. (2006). How listeners shape what tellers tell: Patterns of interaction in lifestory interviews and their impact on reminiscence by elderly interviewees. *Journal of Aging Studies, 20*, 381-396.

Rappaport, J. (1993). Narrative studies, personal stories, and identity transformation in the mutual help context. *The Journal of Applied Behavioral Science, 29*, 239-256.

Rappaport, J. (2004). On becoming a community psychologist: The intersection of autobiography and history. In J. B. Kelly & A. Song (Eds.), *Six community psychologists tell their stories: History, contexts, and narrative* (pp. 271-294). New York: Haworth.

Raskin, A. H. (1992). The words I lost. Retrieved October 15, 2007, from http://www.aphasia.

org/aphasia_community/the_words_i_lost. html (Originally published in *New York Times* Op-Ed, Saturday, September 19, 1992)

Redmond, S. (2003, June 18). Abstract from *The Cripples Palace*. Retrieved October 15, 2007, from http://www.alsindependence.com/ The_Cripples_Palace.htm

Richter, M., Ball, L., Beukelman, D., Lasker, J., & Ullman, C. (2003). Attitudes toward communication modes and message formulation techniques used for storytelling by people with amyotrophic lateral sclerosis. *AAC: Augmentative and Alternative Communication, 19*, 170-186.

Ricoeur, P. (1980). Narrative time. In W. T. Mitchell (Ed.), *On narrative* (pp. 165-186). Chicago: University of Chicago Press.

Ricoeur, P. (1992). *Oneself as another* (Trans.). Chicago: University of Chicago Press.

Ritchie, C. (n.d.). Living in a silent world: Husband with aphasia. Retrieved October 15, 2007, from http://www.aphasiahope.org

Rittman, M., Faircloth, C., Boylstein, C., & Gubrium, J. F. (2004). The experience of time in the transition from hospital to home following stroke. *Journal of Rehabilitation Research and Development, 41*, 259-268.

Roberts, L. J., Salem, D., Rappaport, J., Toro, P. A., Luke, D. A., & Seidman, E. (1999). Giving and receiving help: Interpersonal transactions in mutual-help meetings and psychosocial adjustment of members. *American Journal of Community Psychology, 27*, 841-868.

Rosel, N. (2003). Aging in place: Knowing where you are. *International Journal of Aging & Human Development, 57*, 77-90.

Ross, A., Winslow, I., Marchant, P., & Brumfitt, S. (2006). Evaluation of communication, life participation and psychological well-being in chronic aphasia: The influence of group intervention. *Aphasiology, 20*, 427-448.

Rusesabagina, P. (with Zoellner, T.). (2006). *An ordinary man: An autobiography*. New York: Penguin Books.

Sabat, S. R. (1991). Turn-taking, turn-giving and Alzheimer's disease: A case study of conversation. *The Georgetown Journal of Languages & Linguistics, 2*, 161-175.

Sabat, S. R. (2001). *The experience of Alzheimer's disease: Life through a tangled veil*. Oxford, UK: Blackwell.

Sabat, S. R. (2003). Malignant positioning and the predicament of the person with Alzheimer's disease. In F. M. Moghaddam & R. Harré (Eds.), *The self and others: Positioning individuals and groups in personal, political, and cultural contexts* (pp. 85-98). Westport, CT: Greenwood.

Sabat, S. R. (March, 2007). *Selfhood and the subjective experience of people with Alzheimer's disease: Implications for treatment strategies*. Paper presented at a conference on Untangling Selfhood: The History and Experience of Alzheimer's Disease, marking the 100th anniversary of Alzheimer's disease as a diagnostic category, College Station, Pennsylvania State University.

Sabat, S. R., & Harré, R. (1992). The construction and deconstruction of self in Alzheimer's disease. *Ageing and Society, 12*, 443-461.

Sacks, O. (2005, October 31). A neurologist's notebook: Recalled to life. *The New Yorker*. Retrieved October 15, 2007, from, http:// www.aphasia.org/naa_materials/sacks_recall edtolife.pdf

Sakalys, J. A. (2003). Restoring the patient's voice: The therapeutics of illness narratives. *Journal of Holistic Nursing, 21*, 228-241.

Sarbin, T. R. (1986). *Narrative psychology: The storied nature of human conduct*. New York: Praeger.

Sarbin, T. R. (1986). The narrative as a root metaphor for psychology. In T. Sarbin (Ed.), *Narrative psychology: The storied nature of human conduct* (pp. 3-21). New York: Praeger.

Sarbin, T. R. (2005). If these walls could talk: Places as stages for human drama. *Journal of Constructivist Psychology, 18*, 203-214.

Sarno, M. T. (1997). Quality of life in aphasia in the first post-stroke year. *Aphasiology, 17*, 665-678.

Sarno, M. T., & Peters, J. F. (Eds.). (2004). *The aphasia handbook: A guide for stroke and brain-injury survivors and their families*. New York: National Aphasia Association.

Schulz, R., Newsom, J. T., Mittlemark, M., Burton, L. C., Hirsch, C. H., & Jackson, S. (1997). Health effects of caregiving. The Caregiver Health Effects Study. *Annals of Behavioral Medicine, 19*, 110-116.

Shadden, B. B. (Ed.). (1988). *Communication behavior and aging: A sourcebook for clinicians.* Baltimore: Williams & Wilkins.

Shadden, B. B. (1988). Interpersonal communication patterns and strategies in the elderly. In B. B. Shadden (Ed.), *Communication behavior and aging: A sourcebook for clinicians* (pp. 24-41). Baltimore: Williams & Wilkins.

Shadden, B. B. (1994, November). *Stroke support groups revisited: Facilitating communication recovery in aphasia.* Part of a miniseminar presented at the Annual Convention of the American Speech-Language-Hearing Association, New Orleans.

Shadden, B. B. (1997). Language and communication changes with aging. In B. B. Shadden & M. A. Toner (Eds.), *Aging and communication* (pp. 135-170). Austin, TX: Pro-Ed.

Shadden, B. B. (1999, November). *Fatigue and stress: Impact on spouse interactions with an aphasic adult.* Poster session presented at the Annual Convention of the American Speech-Language-Hearing Association, San Francisco.

Shadden, B. B. (2001, August). *Psychosocial aspects of aphasia: Whose perspectives?* Discussant presentation as response to keynote address at the 25th World Congress of the International Association of Logopedics and Phoniatrics, Montreal, Canada.

Shadden, B. B. (2005). Aphasia as identity theft: Theory and practice. *Aphasiology, 19,* 211-223.

Shadden, B. B. (2006). Rebuilding identity through stroke support groups: Embracing the person with aphasia and significant others. In R. Elman (Ed.), *Group treatment of neurogenic communication disorders: The expert clinician's approach* (2nd ed., pp. 113-128). San Diego, CA: Plural.

Shadden, B. B., & Agan, J. P. (2004). Renegotiation of identity: The social context of aphasia support groups. *Topics in Language Disorders, 24,* 174-186.

Shadden, B. B., & Hagstrom, F. (2007). The role of narrative in the life participation approach to aphasia. *Topics in Language Disorders, 27,* 319-333.

Shadden, B. B., & Koski, P. R. (2007). Social construction of self for persons with aphasia: When language as a cultural tool is impaired. *Journal of Medical Speech Pathology, 15,* 99-105.

Shadden, B. B., Raiford, C. A., & Shadden, H. S. (1983). *Coping with communication disorders in aging.* Portland, OR: C. C. Publications.

Shadden, B. B., & Toner, M. A. (Eds.). (1997). *Aging and communication.* Austin, TX: Pro-Ed.

Shotter, J. (2003). "Real presences." Meaning living movement in a participatory world. *Theory and Psychology, 13,* 435-468.

Shotter, J. (2005). Acknowledging unique others: Ethics, "expressive realism," and social constructionism. *Journal of Constructivist Psychology, 18,* 103-130.

Simmons-Mackie, N. (2000). Social approaches to management of aphasia. In L. Worrall & C. Frattali, (Eds.), *Neurogenic communication disorders: A functional approach* (pp. 162-188). New York: Thieme.

Simmons-Mackie, N. (2004). Using the ICF framework to define outcomes. *Perspectives on Neurophysiology and Neurogenic Speech and Language Disorders, 14,* 9-11.

Simmons-Mackie, N., & Damico, J. (1999). Social role negotiation in aphasia therapy: Competence, incompetence, and conflict. In D. Kovarsky, J. Duchan, & M. Maxwell (Eds.), *Constructing (in)competence: Disabling evaluations in clinical and social interaction* (pp. 313-341). Hillsdale, NJ: Lawrence Erlbaum.

Simmons-Mackie, N., & Damico, J. S. (2007). Access and social inclusion in aphasia: Interactional principles and applications. *Aphasiology, 21,* 81-97.

Simmons-Mackie, H., Elman, R. J., Holland, A. L., & Damico, J. S. (2007). Management of discourse in group therapy for aphasia. *Topics in Language Disorders, 27,* 5-23.

Simmons-Mackie, N., & Kagan, A. (2007). Application of the ICF in aphasia. *Seminars in Speech and Language, 28,* 244-253.

Singer, J. (2004). Narrative identity and meaning making across the adult lifespan: An introduction. *Journal of Personality, 72,* 437-460.

Skultety, K. M., & Whitbourne, S. K. (2004). Gender differences in identity processes and self-esteem in middle and later adulthood. *Journal of Women & Aging, 16,* 175-188.

Smith, M. (2007, September). *My aphasia and me.* Poem read at the Living Successfully with Aphasia: Intervention, Evaluation and Evidence Conference, Toronto, Canada.

Smith, P., Crossley, B., Greenberg, J., Wilder, C., & Carroll, B. (2000). Agreement among three quality of life measures in patients with ALS. *Amyotrophic Lateral Sclerosis & Other Motor Neuron Disorders, 1,* 269-275.

Snaevarr, S. (2007, March/April). Don Quixote and the narrative self. *Philosophy Now, 60.* Retrieved January 8, 2008, from http://www.philosophynow.org/issue60/60snaevarr.htm

Sneed, J., & Whitbourne, S. I. (2001). Identity processing styles and the need for self-esteem in older adults. *International Journal of Aging and Human Development, 52,* 323-333.

Sneed, J. R., & Whitbourne, S. K. (2003). Identity processing and self-consciousness in middle and later adulthood. *The Journals of Gerontology: Series B. Psychological sciences and social sciences, 58B,* P313-P319.

Sneed, J. R., & Whitbourne, S. K. (2005). Models of the aging self. *The Journal of Social Issues, 61,* 375-388.

Sorin-Peters, R. (2003). Viewing couples living with aphasia as adult learners: Implications for promoting quality of life. *Aphasiology, 17,* 405-416.

Stanley, P. (2004). The patient's voice: A cry in solitude or a call for community. *Literature and Medicine, 23,* 346-363.

Stier, A., & Hinshaw, S. P. (2007). Explicit and implicit stigma against individuals with mental illness. *Australian Psychologist, 42,* 106-117.

Sullivan, H. S. (1953). *The interpersonal theory of psychiatry.* New York: Norton.

Sundin, K., Norberg, A., & Jansson, L. (2001). The meaning of skilled care providers' relationships with stroke and aphasia patients. *Qualitative Health Research, 11,* 308-321.

Swidler, A. (1986). Culture in action. *American Sociological Review, 51,* 273-286.

Swidler, A. (2001). *Talk of love: How culture matters.* Chicago: University of Chicago Press.

Tanner, D. C. (1999). *The family guide to surviving stroke and communication disorders.* Boston: Allyn & Bacon.

Tanner, D., & Gerstenberger, D. (1988). The grief response in neuropathologies of speech and language. *Aphasiology, 2,* 79-84.

Tappen, R., & Williams, C. (1998). Attribution of emotion in advanced Alzheimer's disease: Family and caregiver perspectives. *American Journal of Alzheimer's Disease, 13*(5), 256-264.

Taylor, R. (2007). *Alzheimer's from the inside out.* Baltimore: Health Professions Press.

Threats, T. (2004). The use of the ICF in intervention for persons with neurogenic communication disorders. *Perspectives on Neurophysiology and Neurogenic Speech and Language Disorders, 14,* 4-8.

Threats, T. T., Shadden, B. B., & Vickers, C. P. (2003, November). *Assessment and intervention with older adults using the ICF framework.* Workshop presented at the annual conference of the American Speech-Language-Hearing Association, Chicago.

Tobin, S. S. (1988). Preservation of the self in old age. *Social Casework, 69*(9), 550-555.

Trethewey, A. (2001). Reproducing and resisting the master narrative of decline. *Management Communication Quarterly McQ, 15,* 183-226.

Tucker, K. (2006, June). *Adler Aphasia Center.* Presentation at the National Aphasia Association Speaking Out Conference, Boston, MA. Retrieved March 6, 2008, from http://wingoglobal.com/transcripts/0606-Adler-Aphasia-Center.doc

Usita, P. M., Hyman, I. E., & Herman, K. C. (1998). Narrative intentions: Listening to life stories in Alzheimer's disease. *Journal of Aging Studies, 12,* 185-198.

Vollmer, F. (2005). The narrative self. *Journal for the Theory of Social Behaviour, 35*(2), 189-205.

Vygotsky, L. V. (1971). *The psychology of art* (Scripta Technica, Trans.). Cambridge, MA: MIT Press.

Vygotsky, L. S. (1987). *Thinking and speech* (N. Minick, Trans.). New York: Plenum.

Walsh, I. P. (2007). Small talk is "Big Talk" in clinical discourse: Appreciating the value of conversation in SLP clinical interactions. *Topics in Language Disorders, 27,* 24-36.

Wertsch, J. V. (1985). *Vygotsky and the social formation of mind.* Cambridge, MA: Harvard University Press.

Wertsch, J. V. (1991). *Voices of the mind: A sociocultural approach to mediated action.* Cambridge, MA: Harvard University Press.

Wertsch, J. V. (1998). *Mind as action.* New York: Oxford University Press.

Wertsch, J. V. (2002). *Voices of collective remembering.* New York: Oxford University Press.

Wertsch, J., Tulviste, J., & Hagstrom, F. (1993). A sociocultural approach to agency. In E. Forman, N. Minick, & C. Stone (Eds.), *Contexts for learning* (pp. 336-356). New York: Oxford.

Whitbourne, S., Sneed, J., & Skultety, K. (2002). Identity processes in adulthood: Theoretical and methodological challenges. *Identity: An International Journal of Theory and Research, 2,* 29-45.

Willis, P. (1977). *Learning to labour: How working class kids get working-class jobs.* New York: Columbia University Press.

Woodruff, R. (Prod.). (2007, August 28). Senator's road to recovery. Feature story on *Nightline* [Television broadcast]. New York: American Broadcasting Company. Retrieved November 7, 2007, from http://abcnews .g o.com/Nightline/Story?id=3532159&page=4

World Health Organization. (2001). *International Classification of Functioning, Disability and Health.* Geneva: World Health Organization.

Worrall, L. (2006). Professionalism and functional outcomes. *Journal of Communication Disorders, 39,* 320-327.

Worrall, L. (2007, September). *What people with aphasia want: Towards person-centered goal-setting in aphasia rehabilitation.* Poster presented at the Living Successfully with Aphasia: Intervention, Evaluation and Evidence Conference, Toronto, Canada.

Worrall, L. E., & Hickson, L. M. (2003). *Communication disability in aging: From prevention to intervention.* San Diego: CA: Singular.

Worrall, L., Ma, E. P.-M., & Threats, T. (Eds.). (in press). ICF and speech-language pathology: Framing and expanding the scope of practice [Special issue]. *International Journal of Speech-Language Pathology, 10*(1-2).

Wrigley, M. (2001, March). Real stories or storied realism? [Review of the article Introducing narrative psychology: Self, trauma and the construction of meaning, by M. L. Crossley, 2000]. *Forum Qualitative Sozialforschung/ Forum: Qualitative Social Research* [On-line journal], *2*(2). Retrieved December 7, 2007, from http://qualitative-research.net/fqs/fqs-eng.htm

Wulf, H. (1986). *Aphasia, my world alone.* Detroit, MI: Wayne State University Press.

Index